D1560257

Discharge Planning Guide for Nurses

Judith Waring Rorden, RN, BEd, MSN
K.O.A.L.A. Associates
Los Altos, California

Elizabeth Taft, RN, MSN, MA
Discharge Planning Coordinator
Stanford University Hospital
Palo Alto, California

1990
W.B. SAUNDERS COMPANY
Harcourt Brace Jovanovich, Inc.
Philadelphia   London   Toronto   Montreal   Sydney   Tokyo

W. B. SAUNDERS COMPANY
Harcourt Brace Jovanovich, Inc.

The Curtis Center
Independence Square West
Philadelphia, PA 19106

Library of Congress Cataloging-in-Publication Data

Rorden, Judith Waring.

   Discharge planning guide for nurses / by Judith Waring Rorden
and Elizabeth D. Taft.

   p.   cm.

Includes bibliographical references (p.

ISBN 0–7216–2845–1

1. Hospitals–Admission and discharge.   2. Nurse and
   patient.   I. Taft, Elizabeth D.   II. Title.

RA971.8.R568   1990

362.1′1–dc20   89–70132
                                                          CIP

Editor: Thomas Eoyang
Designer: Terri Siegel
Production Manager: Linda R. Turner
Manuscript Editor: Kendall Sterling
Illustration Coordinator: Lisa Lambert
Cover Designer: Joan Wendt

Discharge Planning Guide for Nurses   ISBN   0–7216–2845–1

Printed in the United States of America.

Last digit is the print number: 9   8   7   6   5   4   3   2   1

Preface

Throughout the history of nursing, nurses have been concerned with the whole person who becomes a patient. They have recognized the psychological and social implications of medical care. They have been alert to family interaction and cultural values as they influence the patient. In spite of the demands that technology has placed on their skills and the limits that shorter hospital stays have placed on their ability to communicate fully with patients and their families, nurses continue to be concerned about the people who are their patients. Within this context, discharge planning is a process that is part of nursing care, not an activity separate from it. The skills needed for effective discharge planning are the assessment, communication, and teaching skills that the nurse uses throughout the nursing process. In this *Guide for Nurses,* we seek to show nurses how to use those skills and focus their concerns so that discharge planning is both effective and efficient. The first part of this book examines various aspects of discharge planning as a process and how they fit together. Case examples have been used to demonstrate the practical application of the principles discussed. The second part of the book guides the nurse through the construction and documentation of discharge plans. It is designed to act as a reference for the practicing nurse as well as a learning tool for the student.

Rapid changes in the health care delivery system in the United States have placed increasing emphasis on discharge planning as a process that expedites the progress of patients through acute care to community care. This book reflects that emphasis in that discharge planning is discussed as a process that begins with admission to acute care. The authors, both of whom have a community health background, hasten to add that discharge planning in this sense is only one part of the care planning that extends throughout the well-ness-illness continuum of an individual. Nurses in many settings other than hospitals use their professional skills to help people plan for their future health and well-being. The principles that are discussed in this book apply to them in their nursing practice as well as to the hospital nurse.

A great many people contributed to the preparation of this book, including staff members of discharge planning units and nurses in a number of hospitals in the San Francisco Bay area. We would particularly like to acknowledge the contributions of Mimi Martucci of Petaluma Valley Hospital, Linda Dupre of El Camino Hospital in Mountain View, Mary Alice Thornton of Mills Hospital in San Mateo, and Rhoda Paulo of Stanford University Medical Center. Other staff members of the Department of Nursing and the Department of Social Services and Discharge Planning of Stanford University Medical Center also contributed generously of their time and interest in this project. Our thanks to them and to the family members and friends who gave us their support and encouragement.

JUDITH WARING RORDEN
ELIZABETH D. TAFT

Contents

PART ONE

How the Discharge Planning Process Works

The process of discharge planning often resembles the construction of a jigsaw puzzle: available pieces are placed carefully in relationship to other pieces so that together they contribute to the wholeness of the picture. The challenge of discharge planning, like that of completing a puzzle, is to find missing pieces that are just the right size and shape and then place them securely in the right position. A clear idea of the finished picture or goal improves the effectiveness of this process. The first portion of this book seeks to help nurses develop a clear view of the "picture" of discharge planning. In it we explore the factors that influence discharge planning and give practical guidance for working toward realistic goals for patients' continuing care.

Throughout these pages, we have used the phrase "discharge planning" to refer to the process that occurs within a patient care setting and that anticipates changes in patient care needs. "Continuing care" is the goal and planned outcome of this process. Effective planning results in smooth transitions in care and "continuity," another term often associated with the discharge planning process.

In the first part of this book, each of the major "pieces" of the discharge planning puzzle are examined. Special attention is given to the role of the nurse as communicator and coordinator.

Chapter 1 presents an overview of the discharge

1

planning "picture." It begins with a discussion of factors that have led to the development of discharge planning as practiced today. There follows a description of the economic, political, and medical care influences that are currently shaping that practice. A model is then presented that helps the reader understand the process as a whole and analyze the importance of each of the component parts of the "puzzle." Finally, the specific role of the nurse in helping patients deal with transitions in their care and plan for continuing care is discussed.

Chapter 2 takes an in-depth look at the assessment, communication, and teaching skills that the nurse brings to the discharge planning process. Practical guidance is given for the application of each of these skills to specific patient care situations. The quality of interpersonal communication with patient and family are emphasized. The nurse's ability to determine patient needs, assess strengths in the patient and in the patient's support system, help patient and family learn how to plan realistically, and work effectively with other health professionals are key factors in the success of continuing care.

Chapter 3 is devoted to helping the nurse more clearly understand what the patient brings to the discharge planning process. We begin with a discussion of how stress affects a person's health balance and then look at personality and the influence of beliefs on a patient's responses. We then explore the dynamics of influence by other people within the socio-cultural context. Finally, financial concerns are discussed in realistic terms.

Chapter 4 focuses on the knowledge, skills, and abilities that other health professionals are able to contribute to the discharge planning process and how these can be coordinated through a team approach. The role of the nurse in working with a discharge planning team is discussed and guidance given for promoting good team communication. Ways in which the patient and family can be helped to participate in planning and decision-making conclude the chapter.

Chapter 5 helps the nurse look beyond the walls of a medical care setting to the resources that exist in the surrounding community. We begin with guidance on how to survey community resources and follow this with notes on what kinds of sources of care and support to look for. The special kind of communication involved in making effective referrals and enlisting the help of community resources are then explored. Finally, we examine psycho-social aspects of accepting help and offer guidance for the nurse in helping patients reach "supported self-reliance": a state in which appropriate help is accepted without relinquishing independence and self-esteem.

Chapter 6 focuses on how the pieces of the discharge planning "puzzle" can be fitted together to ensure continuing care. We start with a discussion of the kinds of information the nurse uses in assessing patient needs and how discharge planning goals are reached. We then look at motivation as it affects each step of the planning process and enables patients and families to implement continuing care. Specific guidance is offered to the nurse in encouraging positive motivation. Proceeding on to the final phase of discharge planning, we examine the steps that can be taken by the nurse to confirm all aspects of the plan and ease the patient's transition to community care. The chapter ends with a discussion of the important steps of follow-up and evaluation.

Chapter 7 steps back from the discharge planning process to look briefly at some of the ethical considerations that surround it. Using case examples as the basis for our discussion, we ask who should make decisions about discharges and how quality- versus quantity-of-care issues can be resolved. We end with some ideas about how involvement in discharge planning benefits nurses. Our goal in this chapter is to stimulate nurses to explore their own attitudes, values, and roles in an area in which ethical, economic, and legal dilemmas abound.

This book is called a "Guide" because it offers nurses practical guidance for actually *doing* discharge planning; it endeavors to teach skills as well as promote knowledge and understanding. For this reason, many examples and case studies are used to illustrate ideas, concepts, and suggestions. Important points are highlighted in the text for easy reference, and an annotated bibliography at the end of each chapter in Part I will guide the reader to further reading to enhance his or her knowledge and skills. Study questions and exercises based on these seven chapters follow Chapter 7. They are appropriate either for classroom use or independent study.

1

Overview of the Discharge Planning Process

The goal of this chapter is to present a very broad view of the discharge planning "puzzle." In it many of the factors that influence the planning of continuing care and the issues surrounding them are discussed. In the first section, the historical context is explored, and in the second, we analyze the impact that recent social and economic changes have had. In Section 1.3 a model of the discharge planning process is presented and the factors influencing it are defined. The final section looks at the role of the nurse in planning continuing care, particularly the nurse's responsibilities and involvement in quality-of-care issues.

Although one usually thinks of "discharge" planning as a set of activities related to the patient's transition away from acute care, the process of planning also is appropriate to other kinds of transitions in care, for example, from an Intensive Care Unit to a medical or surgical unit; from a skilled nursing facility to acute care; and from home care to a hospice unit. In each case, the objective of discharge planning is continuing care organized to meet patient needs. This broad definition of discharge planning will be used throughout these pages.

1.1 DISCHARGE PLANNING:
EVOLUTION OF AN IDEA

A great many things about the provision of medical and health care have changed radically during the course of medical history and continue to change at an ever increasing rate. The basic *goals* of that care, however, have been remarkably stable. Since ancient times, caregivers have sought to help the ill and injured to recover their health and regain their ability to function at optimum levels within their society. For the terminally ill, caregivers have sought to help patients meet death with peace and dignity. As time has passed and care has become more institutionally based and more technologically sophisticated, the transitions between hospital and home, and between acute care and rehabilitation, have become more dramatic. With these changes has come an increased awareness that planned and supported transitions in care contribute significantly to a person's future health and well-being. In this section, we will look at how planning for continuing care has evolved.

Early Development of Health Care Organizations

Concern for the ill and injured is reflected in the writings of virtually every culture and civilization. This concern took basically two forms in the early history of health care: (1) restrictions on certain foods and activities, and (2) the offering of care to supplement the family. An example of the former is the Biblical injunction against eating shellfish and pork. An example of offered help was recorded by St. Paul who described the visits of Phebe to the homes of the sick around 60 A.D. (Leahy *et al.*, 1977, p. 350).

> *Visits to the sick and injured by designated helpers to supplement care by the family are recorded throughout history. These were early examples of "extended" or continuing care.*

The modern development of visiting nurse services, public health nursing services, and home care agencies all have their roots in a health care tradition that is thousands of years old.

During the Crusades, pilgrims were subject to disease and injury but were often far removed from caring family members and the resources of home. The monasteries that opened their doors to such travelers became the first hospitals. Wars, likewise, encouraged the development of special centers for the care of the injured and led to improved understanding of physiology and insight into treatment methods.

By the mid–1700s, major changes were occurring in the largely rural populations of Europe and Britain leading up to the Industrial Revolution (Hobson, 1975, Ch 1). Large numbers of people congregated in cities where filth, poverty, and waves of epidemic disease were common. Although hospitals had become an integral part of urban society, their purpose was to provide a facility for care rather than cure.

One of the consequences of the population shift to cities was an increasing sense of social responsibility for the welfare of others. This humanitarian attitude was reflected in the development of nursing services by religious orders in both hospitals and communities. The work of St. Vincent de Paul, whose visits to the sick and poor had begun in the early 1600s, was a model for other such services. One of the first nonreligious community health organizations was begun by William Rathbone of Liverpool, England in 1859. He saw the nurses as not only representing the "new" perception of social justice and humanity, but also offering patients "knowledge of modern medical science" (Leahy *et al.,* p. 352). Florence Nightingale was a vocal proponent of skill-based nursing services in the community as well as in hospitals.

Hospital and Community Services Expand in the United States

In the United States, care of the sick in their homes began in New York City in 1877 (Roberts, 1954, pp. 14–15). Nine years later, district nursing associations were started in Boston and Philadelphia. These were followed by similar organizations in other cities, numbering approximately 20 by 1900. The first formal continuing care agreement of record in the United States was that of 1886 in which the Boston Visiting Nurse Association agreed to follow up discharged patients of Children's Hospital (Dempsey, 1974, p. 13).

The establishment in 1909 of the famous Henry Street Settlement Program led by Lillian Wald, both a nurse and a social worker, was an important milestone in continuing care. Sponsored by the Metropolitan Life Insurance Company, it provided home nursing care to its policy holders. When the program was shown to have decreased hospital stays and neonatal deaths, it was emulated by other insurance companies and public health agencies across the nation (Roberts, 1954, Ch 9). This development acted to dispel the idea that continuing care services were only for the poor. Meanwhile, the number of hospitals continued to increase as anesthesia, surgery, and pharmacology improved.

The next two decades were punctuated by the crises of World War I and the Depression. Within a few years of the end of the war, the number of community health nursing services increased from 100 to 1200 and were distributed throughout rural as well as urban areas (Roberts, 1954, p. 193). Most of these were sponsored by the American Red Cross and employed nurses returning from the war. These nurses not only provided care in the home but also took an active role in identifying problems that needed medical attention and referring people for care. Once home care became available, referrals from hospitals to community agencies were increasingly common. Discharge planning was further stimulated by increased access to social work services in hospitals and a growing awareness of the social and economic factors surrounding illness.

The market crash of 1929 initially threw many nurses out of work but also prompted cooperation between nursing organizations for the first time. They became more vocal in promoting health and social welfare programs and more powerful in bettering work conditions for nurses.

In 1935 the Social Security Act was passed by Congress. Its provisions benefited dependent and crippled children, the blind and the aged, as well as programs devoted to maternal and child welfare and public health (Public Law No. 271, 74th Congress, H. R. 7260). Good communication between health and welfare professionals became more important as more people were affected by government-sponsored programs.

The next few years were ones of consolidation. The quality of nursing education received much attention. By the time World War II broke out, better educated nurses were able to take their place as contributors to advances in medical science. In the 1940s and 1950s, the surge of interest in the social sciences and the growing body of nursing theory led to the definition of principles that continue to guide nursing practice:

1. *Nursing care should be based on clearly identified patient NEEDS, and*
2. *TOTAL PATIENT CARE is an appropriate goal of nursing care.*

These principles had particular importance in the development of discharge planning and the implementation of continuing care.

The Hill-Burton Act of 1946 was enacted as a response to an increasing demand for acute care services. It resulted in the widespread establishment of hospitals even in small communities.

Discharge Planning Gains Momentum

By the early 1960s a number of factors converged to increase concern about access to medical care, particularly for the aged, the poor, and the disabled. Acute care hospitals were available in virtually all communities. Private insurance agencies such as Blue Cross and Blue Shield had grown rapidly, and medical insurance was now a common employee benefit, making care financially accessible to the employed and their families. The Kerr-Mills legislation of 1961 was the first major entry by the federal government into sponsorship of direct medical services to individuals by authorizing payment of care for the "medically needy." In most instances, medical care was defined as physician and hospital services. Home care was seen as "nursing" care and not similarly supported (Hall, 1985, p. 12).

Many nursing leaders did, however, recognize that medical and health care goals could not be met without community-based programs that would provide a wide range of continuing care services. In the early 1960s public health nursing services were widespread, but home care of the sick was not. One study showed that 30% of cities with populations of more than 25,000 were without such services (Freeman, 1963, pp. 21–24). Even where services were available, they were not necessarily adequate to meet the needs.

Foreseeing the importance of such programs, a landmark publication on the topic of home care was given to all participants in the 1963 convention of the National League for Nursing. Entitled *Nursing Service Without Walls* by Edith Wensley (1963), it gave step-by-step guidance for organizing a multidisciplinary home care program that would provide specialized therapists, social work, and homemaker services as well as nursing services to the ill and disabled. This work was based on a research study conducted by Louise C. Smith and reported as "Factors Influencing Continuity of Nursing Service" (1962).

In 1965, Medicare was enacted by Congress as an amendment to the Social Security Act. It provided for reimbursement for much of the medical care expense for the nation's aged as part of the Social Security benefit.

The accompanying Medicaid legislation provided federal support to states for reimbursement of medical costs for welfare recipients. The federal goal of assisting U.S. citizens to secure medical care was now backed by legislation that made the government financially responsible for meeting that goal. Even more importantly, the federal government was now in the position of setting the standards and expectations for health care delivery. Although Medicare and Medicaid applied to only a minority of citizens, their care represented a large portion of health care dollars spent. The health care industry could not afford to ignore the regulations, with the result that the provision of care to all citizens was effected.

At the same time, aspects of the *quality* of medical and health care were being examined, in particular the more effective linkage of hospital and community services. This concern was reflected in a gathering of nursing leaders in 1965 sponsored by The Catholic University in Washington, D.C. The conference was devoted to the role nurses could and should play in meeting new demands for continuity of patient care. The result was a broadened definition of continuing care that included coordination of care within a hospital setting as well as referral to post-discharge community care (Straub and Parker, 1966).

Meanwhile, a number of hospitals established discharge programs to facilitate referrals to community agencies. These usually consisted of a public health nurse or social worker acting as a coordinator of information collected from nurses, physicians, the patient, and the patient's family.

Example 1.1 Centralized Discharge Planning Begins

In September of 1967, Elizabeth Taft, P.H.N., M.S.N., was appointed to the new position of "Post-Hospital Nursing Care Coordinator" at Stanford University Medical Center. Her background as a public health nurse in an adjoining community and therefore her knowledge of community resources made her especially well-suited for her principal role as liaison between hospital and community services. Some of her recollections of those early years as a discharge planner are as follows:

"Since hospital stays were longer, there was no particular pressure to start discharge planning activities early. Patients were further along on the road to recovery when they were discharged so that home care was much less complex than it is today. I used to say that it took me five days to put a good plan together; I don't have that luxury now, although it is often necessary to plan for 'high tech' care to continue in the home.

"The main focus of my job then was planning for the elderly—defined as 65 and over. High risk is now defined here as 75 and over, and I see many patients over 90.

"Twenty years ago referrals for home care went to visiting

nurse associations and newly formed home health care agencies. Many of the latter have ceased to exist.

"Because my position was a new one, I did a lot of case-finding myself. Nurses and physicians had to be taught how to use the kind of service I was offering. Today nurses are very much aware of the need for discharge planning to begin early. They take a much larger role in assessing a patient's future needs and getting the discharge planning team involved."

It quickly became apparent that Medicare and Medicaid were going to be very much more expensive than anticipated. Within the next five years there were a number of legislative attempts to stem the flow of reimbursements. One approach was to re-define who was eligible for Medicaid (Leahy *et al.*, 1977, p. 192). Another was to tighten utilization review procedures with the intention of limiting overuse of institutional care. Pressure increased to discharge patients promptly from the hospital to less expensive community care. As part of the movement toward "de-institutionalization" large numbers of chronically mentally ill and developmentally disabled patients were discharged from institutions, often without adequate supportive services awaiting them in the community.

Recognizing the importance of better communication between institutional and community services, another amendment to the Social Security Act in 1972 made discharge planning services a specific requirement:

"Skilled nursing facilities (and hospitals) must maintain centralized, coordinated programs to ensure that each patient has a planned program of continuing care which meets his post-discharge needs . . . ." (Public Law 92–603)

Having such a discharge planning program was a condition for an organization's participation in Medicare and Medicaid.

Use of the word "centralized" in the legislation is especially important to the direction discharge planning has taken since that time. Growing awareness of the psycho-social aspects of illness and the increasing complexity of eligibility requirements for financial assistance had led to the establishment of social work departments in most larger hospitals and access to at least part-time social work consultation at most nursing homes. Although as noted previously, there were instances of a hospital nurse or a public health nurse becoming the leader of a discharge planning program, this responsibility was most frequently incorporated into the social work function. At about the same time, the Joint Commission on Accreditation of Hospitals saw discharge planning as a nursing responsibility:

"The nursing care plan should be initiated upon the admission of the patient and, as part of the long-term goal, should include discharge plans." (1973)

In 1976 the National League for Nursing published a guide called *Discharge Planning for Continuity of Care*, which had been developed two years earlier by the Virginia Regional Medical Programs. It spelled out the practical details of setting up a multidisciplinary discharge planning program. It emphasized the importance of having a person (or department) specifically designated as responsible for discharge plans.

A Prospective Payment System for Medicare Is Adopted

Unlike the Medicare and Medicaid amendment of 1965, which was debated at length over several years, the 1982 legislation was quickly enacted as a reaction to staggering cost increases. A 1980 report showed that national hospital expenditures had risen from $13.9 billion in 1965 to $99.6 billion—an increase of 717 percent (Gibson and Waldo, 1980). Making reform even more urgent, it was estimated that fraud and unnecessary program costs amounted to over $10 billion per year (Halamandaris, 1985, p. 25).

The new legislation directed the Department of Health and Human Services to develop a *prospective* payment plan for Medicare-covered hospital services to replace the former reimbursement system. The resulting plan called for the use of "Diagnosis Related Groups" (DRGs) to establish the amount of payment. This system was phased in beginning in October of 1983. Some of the issues surrounding this dramatic change and their effect on continuing care are discussed in Section 1.2. Suffice it to say that prospective payment has increased both the visibility and the workload of discharge planners significantly.

In 1985, the National League for Nursing reissued its guide, *Discharge Planning for Continuity of Care* (Hartigan and Brown). The revised edition still strongly advocated a multidisciplinary team approach to discharge planning but also emphasized the importance of documentation and evaluation through quality assurance methods. Included in the guide is the report of a study by Feather and Nichols (1985) that compares discharge planning services before and after the introduction of DRGs. They found that by August of 1984 discharge planners had more work to do but had earlier access to patients and used multidisciplinary teams to a greater extent. Hospital stays were reported to have shortened by an average of three days. By the end of 1987, a nationwide shortage of nurses was complicating the health care picture, and there were increasing reports of abuse of the prospective payment system.

The nature of discharge planning will continue to change over the coming years, reflecting pressures to limit services and to justify the cost benefit of services to patients. New methods of evaluation of continuing care will evolve, and new extended care facilities will develop. In spite of all this anticipated change, the nurse's assessment, communication and coordination skills will continue to be central to effectively planned continuing care—just as they have been throughout history.

Example 1.2 Facts about Medicare Coverage*

MEDICARE is a federal program with no income or resource requirements. It provides health insurance for persons 65 or over who are eligible for Social Security or are federal employees, and for disabled workers of any age who have been eligible for Social Security disability payments for two years. Other persons 65 or over may buy into Medicare. It provides Hospital Insurance (Part A) and Supplemental Medical Insurance (Part B). Participants pay copayments, deductibles and monthly payments for Part B. Medicare does not pay for all medical expenses.

PART A—Hospital Insurance
Part A Hospital Insurance covers inpatient hospital services, nursing facility care, home health and hospice. Acute care hospital coverage is unlimited after paying a $592 annual deductible. There are no longer "lifetime reserve days" or limitations on the number of days covered in a hospital. You do have to pay for the first 3 pints of blood you need.

Skilled nursing home care is now covered up to 150 days a year. However, now a copayment of $25.50/day for the first 8 days is required. Medicare covers, on the average, about 2 weeks in a skilled nursing facility. It does not pay for what it calls "custodial care," but only for what it considers "medically necessary" skilled nursing care, usually requiring the services of a nurse. You no longer have to be hospitalized before going into a nursing facility in order to be covered under Medicare.

---

*Excerpts quoted with permission from the Medicare Fact Sheet prepared by Senior Program, CRLA Foundation, Sacramento, Calif., 1989. Note that charges and deductible amounts change annually.

Certified hospice care is unlimited for certified terminally ill persons.

Home health care is covered . . . under parts A and B when it is "medically necessary," and the person is home-bound and requires skilled care under a doctor's orders. There are no deductibles or copayments.

PART B—Supplemental Medical Insurance

Part B pays for many doctors', ambulance and outpatient hospital services, physical therapy, a second medical opinion and certain other services and tests. In addition to monthly premiums of $33.90, you pay a deductible and copayments . . . up to $75 for covered services each year.

Expenses Not Covered Under Part A or Part B

Medicare does not cover "custodial" or ongoing care in a skilled nursing facility, intermediate nursing facility care, residential care, outpatient medicines, routine check-ups, most dental care, eyeglasses, hearing aids and other items. It never covers any treatment, hospitalization or other service which it does not consider "medically necessary."

The reader will find additional information about Medicare coverage, and in particular, the provisions of the Medicare Catastrophic Act that became law in 1988 in Appendix B of this book.

1.2 THE CHANGING CONTEXT OF DISCHARGE PLANNING

Since the enactment of Medicare and Medicaid legislation in 1965, changes in American society in general, and in health care organizations in particular, have dramatically affected the planning of continuing care. As we described in the previous section, discharge planning services were initiated as an attempt to improve the quality of patient care, particularly for the aged and those with long-term health care problems. The planning process has faltered when community facilities were unavailable, communication and coordination were poor, or financial resources limited. What had been a desirable but unevenly practiced service to patients has now been transformed into a requirement of law, although many of the barriers to effective planning still exist. The legal necessity to provide discharge planning has raised questions about the degree of control governments should have over health care, the measurement of "quality" and "access," the role caregivers should have in justifying what they do for patients, and the place of cost in deciding how much care a patient needs (see Chapter 7 for a discussion of ethical considerations).

These kinds of issues concerning the quality and quantity of medical and health care are now under intense scrutiny. In order to better understand the context within which these issues are being raised, we explore three aspects of current "history."

What Is Happening in Society That Affects Health Care?

Since Medicare was originally enacted, a wide range of social and economic changes have taken place that have had a major impact on the provision of medical and health care. Some of these are summarized in the paragraphs below.

The *structure of the family,* society's basic unit, has changed dramatically. When Western societies became more urban than rural, the extended family was reduced in size, and members tended to disperse rather than stay in the same community. From a health care point of view, this meant that an individual had fewer family resources to look to in the event of illness. Then as technology improved, mobility increased. People stayed in one community for less time and often moved far away from other family members in the quest for satisfactory employment. Not only did individuals now have limited family resources, but they often stayed in one community too short a time to establish a secure social support system of friends. In recent years a high divorce rate has greatly increased the number of single-parent families. Economic necessity keeps families small and parents employed outside the home. Lack of finances, time, and suitable accommodation keep more families from providing custodial care for their elderly members.

The *"graying" of America* is now a widely reported phenomenon. In 1900, 4% of the population was over 65. It is projected that by the year 2000, the percentage will have risen to 13. The fastest growing segment of the population is the over–85 group. The "old-old" comprised only 0.2% of the U. S. population in 1900. By 1980, that had risen to 1% and is expected to be over 5% by 2050 (O'Hare and Terry, 1988, p. 27). This kind of social restructuring causes some basic changes in health care. Because of the increased incidence of chronic illness and long-term disability in the elderly, a disproportionate share of medical care resources are required by them. Because the quality of their continuing care is dependent on available nursing home beds, frail-aged facilities, and community services, these now represent "growth industries." Mental health is also of growing concern. Older people who have outlived their spouse and have only limited contact with family members suffer from loneliness, social isolation, and depression as well as physical ailments.

The *cost of medical and health care* continue to rise rapidly. In 1986, health care costs totaled 10.6% of the nation's gross national product (GNP), up from 5% in 1960. Those numbers translate into higher insurance premiums, higher deductible amounts, and increased copayments for individuals. People on relatively low or fixed incomes increasingly find that care is inaccessible due to cost. For example, Frank reports that the percentage of care *not* covered by Medicare in 1985 equaled the amount paid by the elderly in 1964 when Medicare was enacted to relieve the "burden of medical bills" (Frank, 1988, p. 23). Revisions in the tax code have recently raised the threshold for deductions of out-of-pocket medical expenses, increasing economic pressure on lower-income individuals.

The *expectations* of the American public with regard to health care have also changed. Since the advent of employer-paid medical insurance and Medicare, people have come to assume that they are entitled to comprehensive medical and health care. This expectation has led to over-use of medical resources in some instances. At the same time, there has been a public outcry when limitations are imposed, access to care reduced, or copayments increased. In recent years there has also been greater emphasis on the legal liability of both individual practitioners and institutions. More lawsuits lead to increases in liability insurance premiums, and these increases are passed along to patients. Many employers are reducing their contribution to medical coverage or eliminating this as an employee benefit altogether. Some would rather give staff members a cash grant and let them try to provide their own medical care coverage. Health Maintenance Organizations have increased in popularity because they offer less expensive premiums—but this benefit comes at the price of limited freedom of choice of medical institution or physician. The old public expectations that care was available to everyone and that caregivers were without exception trustworthy have been eroded.

Finally, the *health and fitness movement* has gained momentum in recent years. Individuals have increasingly taken responsibility for protecting their health by becoming more knowledgeable about risk factors, by placing greater value on exercise, and by modifying their diets. For example, the announcement in early 1988 that small doses of aspirin reduces the risk of heart attack had an immediate impact on the everyday routines of thousands of people (*Newsweek*, Feb. 8, 1988).

These and other social changes have altered the attitudes of individuals toward health care institutions and toward medical professionals. Indicative of this attitude change is the common use of the impersonal terms "consumer" and "provider" of medical care. Likewise, the attitudes of caregivers toward patients have altered to include awareness of patients' rights, their own legal liability, and cost consciousness. The numbers of caregivers involved in any one incident of illness has increased with technology and the complexity of care. The mobility of society has led to less continuity in the relationship between patient and caregiver.

> *Social changes have combined to make care less continuous and seem less individualized. The relationship of trust that has traditionally characterized good care is now much more fragile than in the past.*

Society will continue to change in these directions in the foreseeable future. The challenge to governments and health care providers is to develop systems that meet patient needs efficiently and cost-effectively while still maintaining a priority on high quality, personalized care.

What Is Happening in Hospitals That Affects Discharge Planning?

Historically, the health care system in the United States has been hospital oriented. This orientation contrasts with systems in other countries, especially those with tax-supported health care (see McClelland, 1985, Ch. 5). The American free enterprise, profit-based economy has encouraged the development of high technology care delivered by specialists in well-equipped institutions. Consequently, there has been considerable emphasis on getting people with medical problems TO hospitals for cure, and much less on discharging them FROM hospitals to community care. As Buckwalter (1985, p. 8) described the problem:

"The institutionally based medical model of U.S. health care (actually 'acute illness care') has rendered many health care providers unaware of other health care options and settings such as home care or adult day care services."

The passage of Medicare and Medicaid in 1965 acted to reinforce the priority on institutional care. By providing reimbursement for services already delivered, there was little incentive to discharge patients early or to limit the number of acute care procedures offered to them (Hall, 1985, p. 12).

The impact that federal legislation has had upon the delivery of health care in general is enormous. While Medicare appears to affect only a small segment of the population, the government paid 39.7% of *all* individual medical care costs in 1984 (U. S. General Accounting Office, Sept. 30, 1985). Legislation also provides a pattern often followed by private insurers in setting their guidelines for payment. Any system, human or organizational, responds to a set of rewards by altering its behavior. Retrospective reimbursement stimulated the health care system to respond by over-utilizing that which was rewarded. The tremendous cost increases that resulted, viewed in this way, are not surprising.

In 1982, the reward system was effectively reversed; with prospective payment, it is in a hospital's best economic interest to speed up discharges. Again, not surprisingly, organizations have responded to the new rewards with behaviors that limit services and encourage early discharge. As a consequence, discharge planning is an organization's best ally in moving patients out quickly. As Halamanderis points out, it is somewhat ironic that it was not until prospective payment legislation took effect that having a discharge planning program was made a requirement of institutions paid by Medicare (1985, p. 26). They almost certainly would have established such programs in response to prospective payment, even without the imposition of regulations.

If "overutilization" was an issue for health care providers in late 1960s and 1970s, "quality of care" is the issue of the 1980s and 1990s. Discharge planners find themselves at the center of this issue. Just as legislative attempts to control overutilization were enacted establishing Professional Standards Review Organizations (PSROs) and a variety of Utilization Review procedures, so legislation is now attempting to ensure quality of care. In 1986 the Medicare Quality Protection Act (also known as the Heinz-Stark Bill) required hospitals to:

- provide discharge planning,
- develop a uniform needs assessment instrument, and
- provide a written statement of discharge rights (O'Hare and Terry, 1988, pp. 15–16).

Meanwhile, private insurers have also shifted to prospective payment systems by using Diagnostic Related Groups (DRGs) as a basis of payment or by requiring authorization and medical review prior to hospitalization. Whether they are Medicare recipients or not, patients are being discharged from hospitals significantly earlier after acute care than in the past (Feather and Nichols, 1985). Discharge planning departments are generally not able to offer services to all patients, but only to those meeting specific criteria (see Section 6.1 for a discussion of such criteria). It can be argued, however, that *every* patient needs help with planning his or her discharge.

Nurses hold the key to assessing patient needs and to

helping patients and families plan appropriately for transitions in care.

This nursing contribution to the quality of patient care is even more important in the current climate of early discharges than it ever has been.

What Is Happening in the Community That Affects Continuing Care?

It is obvious that discharge planning is effective only if there are sources of care able to meet patient needs at the end of the process. In many instances, early identification of post-hospital needs, combined with teaching and counseling, allow patients to care for themselves with the aid of family members. In many other instances, especially when the patient is seriously or chronically ill or aged, the help of outside resources are essential. Early drafts of the Medicare legislation recognized the importance of a wide range of extended care services in the community. As Medicare coverage has evolved, however, extended care has a distinctly *medical* bias. Care in a skilled nursing facility or nursing home is covered only when care is certified to be "medically necessary," and then for only a short time. The services of home health agencies are also limited to skilled care under a doctor's orders (see Example 1.2 for a description of some of the regulations).

For many chronically ill or aged persons, medical care is not the most pressing issue; they need help with everyday tasks such as shopping, house cleaning, cooking, and bathing. This kind of assistance would allow many people to stay at home (a much less expensive alternative than institutionalization). It was originally proposed that the cost of "home health aides" to do such tasks would be reimbursable. Current regulations, however, do not allow this. Hall (1985) makes the point that home health aides have been seen by largely male legislators as a "maid service" whose assistance does not constitute a "health service." His conclusion is that discharge planners are forced to institutionalize people rather than send them home (p. 18). Meanwhile nurses in the community also face dilemmas such as that posed by one staff nurse: "Can you limit yourself to Medicare's definition of skilled nursing care when your patient is cold, wet, or hungry?" (J. B. Smith, 1987, pp. 305–6).

Private insurers have followed much the same pattern as Medicare in their coverage. For these reasons, Health Maintenance Organizations (HMOs), which provide a wide range of acute and extended care for a single insurance premium, have gained acceptance. Traditionally, government-supported public health nursing services and non-profit visiting nurses associations have been the primary sources of home care even to those not covered by Medicare or other insurance. Public health services are now being drastically reduced due to budget cuts (Suther and Ricciardelli, 1985, p. 129). Taking their place are proprietary home health care agencies operated for profit and not always certified to provide care under Medicare and Medicaid.

Economic issues are at the heart of some developing approaches to medical care that reduce hospital use and therefore cost. Many larger hospitals now have "In-and-Out" surgical facilities in which patients come for relatively minor procedures on the day of surgery and are discharged the same day. "Free-standing" surgical centers not associated with a hospital have developed in some parts of the country. In recent years more and more procedures have been added to the list of operations done without hospitalization. While certainly limiting costs, these facilities pose another kind of problem in discharge planning. There is no time to adequately teach patients how to care for themselves post-operatively or to plan individualized follow-up. Written instructions sometimes do not suffice to reassure anxious patients or help them diagnose a possibly dangerous complication.

Another development, notably in California, has been free-standing "Emergency" or "Urgent Care Centers." The names can be somewhat misleading as they are not generally equipped to treat serious medical emergencies such as heart attacks. These readily accessible facilities do, however, offer basic diagnosis and treatment of routine medical complaints. They have a licensed physician in attendance and often provide some short-term teaching or counseling services. They do not require an appointment to be made ahead, and there is a minimum of paperwork. While they are sometimes called "Docs-in-a-Box" in reference to their similarities to fast food operations, they do seem to fulfill a need for basic medical help in a very accessible form at relatively low cost.

Increasing medical care costs will continue to inspire development of new approaches to meeting patient needs. One such response has been renewed public interest in maintaining health. Exercise and fitness programs, as well as health education programs, now have large numbers of enthusiastic participants. Nurses can contribute a great deal to such programs because of their assessment and teaching skills.

The success of community-based medical and health care programs is dependent upon client education in self-care, self-assessment, and appropriate use of resources.

In summary, this section has explored some of the changes and issues currently affecting discharge planning. We have sought to help readers better understand the social and economic context within which continuing care is planned so that they are prepared to approach patient care challenges realistically.

1.3 UNDERSTANDING THE DISCHARGE PLANNING PROCESS

Having explored some of the history of discharge planning and the current context of issues surrounding it, we will now focus intensively on the process itself, its component parts, and how it leads to continuing patient care. We begin by defining some of the words that are used in connection with this process. A model is then presented that outlines the scope of discharge planning. Finally, the dynamics of the process are discussed, with an emphasis on the importance of communication and coordination.

What Discharge Planning Is—And Is Not

Since first identified as a discrete activity with specific goals and outcomes, discharge planning has been defined in a variety of ways. Early in the use of the term, it meant those activities leading to referral of a patient to a community service or facility after discharge from acute care. Some of the first discharge planning coordinators were called "Referral Nurses." Within this context, discharge planning was focused on a single event: the moment when the patient physically departed from the hospital. Because of this very limited definition in its past, some authors have argued that the phrase "discharge planning" is now out of date and should be replaced (McClelland *et al.*, 1985, p. vii). Unfortunately, most of the terminology suggested as replacement, such as "planning for continuity of care" or "patient planning," are either cumbersome or so general as to be confusing.

> *The phrase "discharge planning" will be used in this text to refer to a process made up of several steps or phases whose immediate goal is to anticipate changes in patient care needs and whose long-term goal is to insure continuity of health care.*

By including the idea of "process" within the definition, we emphasize the dynamic, interactive, patient-centered aspects of discharge planning.

Most modern definitions of discharge planning include the notion of helping patients through transitions from one level of care to another.

No more is the focus only on moving patients out of the hospital, but rather on helping them progress through a number of levels of care intensity. The discharge planning process may therefore have as its immediate goal the successful transition of a patient from intensive care to intermediate care, from a surgical unit to a rehabilitation program, or from home care to a hospice unit.

Discharge planning is NOT:

- limited to concern about the physical transfer of the patient;
- focused only on the physical care needs of the patient;
- an activity that is done *to* or *for* the patient without his active involvement; or
- the responsibility of a discharge planning specialist alone.

One of the more intriguing definitions that we came across described discharge planning as the "vehicle which moves the patient to the proper level of care" (Bristow *et al.*, 1976, p. 5). In the current climate of early discharges, patients may well sometimes perceive the vehicle as a bulldozer!

Discharge planning, however, IS a process that:

- begins with early assessment of anticipated patient care needs;
- includes concern for the patient's total well-being;
- involves patient, family and caregivers in dynamic, interactive communication as planning progresses;
- places a priority on collaboration and coordination among all health care professionals involved;
- results in mutually agreed upon decisions about the most economic and appropriate options for continuing care; and
- is based on thorough, up-to-date knowledge of available continuing care resources.

Although the process is complex, the basic concept is straightforward: discharge planning helps the patient progress toward a return to health. A diagrammatic representation of this concept is shown in Figure 1–1. In it the discharge planning process is shown to parallel and remain supportive to the person's progress through a continuum of care.

Figure 1–1. *Discharge planning and the continuum of care.*

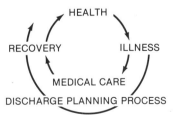

As a dynamic process, discharge planning begins with an assessment phase, continues to planning, is then implemented, and finally evaluated. The effectiveness of each phase depends upon the thoroughness and care with which the previous phase was completed. Like other dynamic processes such as the nursing process and the problem-solving process, feedback in the form of added information, clarified communication, or modified goals continues to sharpen the focus of the discharge planning process throughout its phases.

Every patient who receives medical treatment will make at least one transition during care (from acute care to the community, for example) and perhaps several (between various levels of care). In preparation for these changes, the patient may have the help of a multi-professional discharge planning team or the help of a nurse or physician, or may be offered no help at all related to the transition. Typically, transitions in care involve changes in caregiving personnel and different roles for the patient, the family, and the physician. Whenever such changes in roles or participants occur, the patient is likely to experience some unevenness of care. Like shifting gears in a car, there may be a momentary discontinuity in its otherwise smooth performance. The greater the adjustment in level of care, the more possibility there is of discontinuity and the more anxiety-producing the transitional period is for the patient. It can be terribly frightening to be unsure of what is expected of you and uncertain whether new caregivers will do their part to help you.

> *Discharge planning reduces uncertainty and stress in patients by helping them understand what to expect and reduces the possibility of discontinuous care by coordinating services. Every patient needs this kind of help whenever he makes a transition to a new level of care.*

Nurses are key figures in providing transitional care. Because they have more continuing contact with patients and their families than do other members of the health care team, they are in the best position to begin an early assessment of the patients' anticipated needs. They are the professionals who are most likely to have relationships of trust with patients within which reassurance and support can be given effectively and efficiently. (The nurse's role in discharge planning is discussed in detail in Section 1.4.)

A Model of Phases of Care and the Discharge Planning Process

In order to help the reader better understand the scope and complexities of the discharge planning process, a diagram representing some of its important aspects is shown in Figure 1–2. In it, the patient is depicted as a three-dimensional figure. That figure contains all of the strengths, needs, resources, and concerns that patients bring with them to the medical care situation. Each surface of the figure represents the patient's needs and resources for a particular level of health care. In the following paragraphs, we will describe the various elements of this model.

Patients entering the *acute phase* present needs for care that cannot be met without additional resources. In cases of physical distress, the needs for medical attention may well dominate all other concerns and needs. Even awareness of patients' personal strengths and ongoing psycho-social needs are pushed to the side in the face of a medical emergency, although they continue to influence responses to treatment. The diagram shows that factors such as financial resources and the psychological support of family and social system are present but temporarily overshadowed by patients' intense concern about acute care.

Underlying immediate medical and health care requirements are patients' previous experiences and beliefs. Their interpretation of how "good" or "poor" their health has been, optimism about recovery, and former experiences with health professionals and institutions all influence their perceptions of what is happening to them during acute care. (See Chapter 3 for a discussion of how experiences and beliefs affect patient needs.)

As patients begin to enter the *transitional phase*, new needs emerge. Although the need for acute care is still present, its urgency is reduced, and patients begin to turn their attention toward the future. The wide array of exposed needs make them especially vulnerable to the effects of stress and anxiety. To begin to plan positively for continuing care is both reassuring and stress provoking. An examination of patients' personal strengths, available resources, and the quality of family and social support systems will naturally raise concerns about whether their needs will be met in another setting. It is during this time that the trust relationships patients have formed with caregivers during acute care are most important. They allow patients the freedom to plan honestly and realistically for their continuing care.

> *A defensive or fearful patient will not be able to participate fully in planning and is much less likely to take responsibility for self-care later.*

As in the acute phase, patients' background experiences and beliefs about health continue to influence their decision-making.

The physical transfer of patients to a new care setting marks the final part of the transitional phase. After a brief period of adjustment,

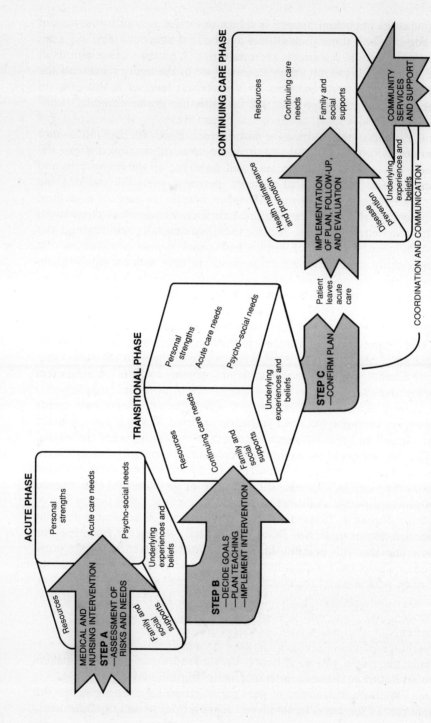

Figure 1–2. *Phases of care and the discharge planning process.*

ACUTE PHASE

Resources

Personal strengths

Acute care needs

Psycho-social needs

Underlying experiences and beliefs

Family and social supports

STEP A —ASSESSMENT OF RISKS AND NEEDS

MEDICAL AND NURSING INTERVENTION

STEP B —DECIDE GOALS —PLAN TEACHING —IMPLEMENT INTERVENTION

TRANSITIONAL PHASE

Resources

Personal strengths

Acute care needs

Psycho–social needs

Continuing care needs

Family and social supports

Underlying experiences and beliefs

STEP C —CONFIRM PLAN

Patient leaves acute care

CONTINUING CARE PHASE

Resources

Continuing care needs

Family and social supports

Health maintenance and promotion

IMPLEMENTATION OF PLAN, FOLLOW-UP, AND EVALUATION

Disease prevention

Underlying experiences and beliefs

COMMUNITY SERVICES AND SUPPORT

COORDINATION AND COMMUNICATION

they enter the *continuing care phase*. Now the plans that had been made in anticipation of needs begin to be implemented. If the patient's discharge was to home and community care, psycho-social needs can be met more directly by the support of family and friends. In the diagram, community services are shown as reinforcing and supplementing patients' other available strengths and resources.

If the patient now progresses toward recovery, *health care needs* will soon begin to emerge. They include health promotion, health maintenance, disease prevention, and access to acute care should the need arise. Self-responsibility is the most important single factor in whether the patient is able to "turn the corner" from continuing care to health care.

As patients' needs change, the medical care team uses the steps of the discharge planning process to prepare them to leave acute care.

A simple diagram cannot adequately depict a complex process appropriate to every patient. The objective here is to present a way of identifying important elements that influence the continuum of care so that they can be further discussed and analyzed.

The Dynamics of the Discharge Planning Process

Discharge planning is a service to patients and their families that helps them make appropriate use of their own and supplemental resources to meet continuing care needs. Helping patients learn of the existence of possibly useful resources, helping to anticipate probable needs and to identify ones that are certain, participating in realistic planning and decision-making, and coordinating caregivers so that their goals of care are mutually shared are all important parts of the discharge planning process. As discussed earlier in this section, the process advances through a number of steps.

In Figure 1–2, the first step toward effective discharge planning occurs early in the acute phase of care. At, or even before, admission to acute care, it is possible to begin the assessment of probable future needs. The patient paralyzed with a stroke will need rehabilitation, the elderly person with a broken hip will need help with meal preparation, safety, and possibly personal care, and the heart attack victim may benefit from diet and exercise counseling. Most institutions screen patients at admission, at least in general terms, so that the need for discharge planning services can be anticipated. For Medicare patients and others who will need extensive services or nursing home care, a referral is often made immediately to the centralized discharge planning unit. We will discuss the criteria most frequently used to make such referrals in Section 6.1.

The first step toward discharge planning is, however, more than just filling out an admission questionnaire.

It is the responsibility of every caregiver involved with a patient to remain alert to possible discharge needs throughout his or her acute care.

This continuing assessment includes not only awareness of ongoing physical needs but also *strengths* that will help them later, *psycho-social needs* that influence their relationships with others, the *experiences and beliefs* that influence their attitudes, and the framework of *resources and support* that are available to them. Much of this information is acquired from the nursing assessment completed early in the patient's care supplemented in informal ways: by conversing with the patient, by observing responses to treatment, and by watching for clues in interactions with friends and family members. More formal interview procedures are also used in many situations. These are helpful in giving detailed, quantitative information. They also let the patient and family know that caregivers are concerned about what happens upon discharge from acute care and give the message that the patient can expect help with making continuing care decisions.

As the patient enters the transitional phase and acute care needs lessen, it is time to begin building a plan for continuing care in earnest. This step includes patient and family teaching, discussion of continuing care options, and support for decisions concerning them, and the active coordination of services and resources that will be involved in the process. It is important that planning for discharge starts early in the patient's care and not wait until assessment data seem to be complete. The nature of a dynamic process such as discharge planning dictates that feedback will continue throughout. Important items of information always are added as planning begins, no matter how carefully an assessment was made, because people faced with decision-making are stimulated to think about things not previously considered. This is why it is so critical that patients and their family members participate in all steps of the process from the beginning.

Planning cannot begin too early; planning can certainly begin too late. Planning that is not flexible or modifiable as new information comes to light is as bad as no planning at all.

It is a distressing experience for all concerned when a plan fails to meet patient needs due to lack of information that should have been added as planning progressed.

Example 1.3 Missing Information Complicates Discharge

Mr. Adams was an elderly man, but a very independent one, who lived alone. He was hospitalized after breaking his left leg in a fall. Because he was somewhat frail, he could not manage crutches very well, but he was taught to use a walker for getting around his apartment. A number of older women friends had agreed to help him fix meals and do his washing.

The day of discharge from the hospital arrived and Mr. Adams was taken to the front door, where a taxi awaited him. Studying the taxi driver, Mr. Adams said to the volunteer accompanying him: "I don't think that fellow will be able to carry me up the stairs, do you?" The information that the patient lived on the second floor of a building without an elevator had somehow been overlooked during planning.

Planning that is to avoid such complications takes place in an environment of good *communication*—both formal and informal— and of good *cooperation* between professionals. In the case example above, the primary care nurse knew that the patient lived on the second floor but had forgotten to record it or to mention the fact to the discharge planning coordinator.

The quality of communication and cooperation between professionals is determined by the amount of trust and mutual respect they are able to establish with one another. In hospitals where there is frequent staff turnover, where nurses are "floated" between units too often to get to know patients, or where some animosity exists between discharge planning specialists and unit staff, communication and cooperation is reduced and so is the effectiveness of discharge planning. Administrative support for team development work is an approach that is useful when the problem is a "turf battle" or uncertainty about roles and responsibilities. In the case of staff inconsistencies, a general attitude of goodwill toward one's colleagues as demonstrated by staff leaders can go a long way toward overcoming communication barriers. Well constructed and consistently used discharge planning documents also are critical to success. Other ideas for improving communication and cooperation in discharge planning will be discussed in Chapter 4.

There is an old saying that "the proof of the pudding is in the tasting." So it is with discharge planning; the proof is in whether the plan, when implemented, meets the patient's continuing care needs. The end of the transitional phase marks the point at which the plan becomes reality.

Plans are seldom implemented without a period of ad-

justment in which the pieces of the puzzle come together and begin functioning. The wise planner prepares the patient, family, and caregivers for this final part of the transitional phase.

Coordination of efforts and continuing communication with all concerned are essential if the plan is to actually work; we have called this step "confirming the plan" (see Section 6.3). Again, flexibility is crucial for success. This is a time of very high stress for both patient and family. Immediate responses to new caregivers, new routines, and new expectations may well reflect this stress level. Participation by patient and family in the planning process and endorsement of continuing care goals serve to lessen negative reactions during this period and smooth the transition.

One of the problems confronting discharge planners is that the ability of the planning team to follow through is limited. Not only does this situation sometimes seem like abandonment to the patient, but it also prevents planners from improving their skills based on evaluation of success. Most often, follow-up of a discharge plan involves an interview or a brief telephone conversation. If it is possible for the person who coordinated the discharge plan to clearly "pass the baton" on to a person who will coordinate continuing care, much of the potential confusion about responsibilities will be eliminated. A family member, the patient, or a health professional who will be immediately involved in care may be designated for this role and encouraged to give feedback to the planning team. (See Section 6.4 for further discussion of the evaluation of discharge planning success.)

In summary, discharge planning is a dynamic process in which communication and feedback are essential at every step. It is important that the process begin early in the patient's acute care so that future needs can be anticipated as fully as possible before planning, teaching, and the coordination of resources begin. The patient and family are the most important members of the discharge planning team, since they hold the keys to the patient's real needs and to the motivation that will mean success or failure.

1.4 NURSING ROLES AND THE PLANNING OF CONTINUING CARE

In this section, we will examine some of the forces that move nurses toward an active role in discharge planning and some that discourage nurses' participation. We will also look at the range of roles available to the nurse in response to a variety of patient needs. For the sake of this discussion we will limit the use of the term "nurse" to mean the professional caregiver involved in direct patient care. A discharge planning coordinator or specialist may also be a nurse, but we will refer to these people by their job titles in order to avoid confusion.

Factors That Promote a Nursing Role in Discharge Planning

Of the forces that encourage nurses to take an active part in discharge planning, the most compelling is that the nurse is in the best possible position to see clearly what the patient will need.

When patients leave acute care, it is changes in nursing services that affect them the most. Acute care nurses constantly assess the impact their care has on the patients' well-being and can most easily anticipate what kind of care they will need in the future.

In noting daily responses to care and treatment, the nurse has a broad view of the patient's continuum of care. If the patient has progressed slowly and seems not to be motivated to do self-care, the nurse can see that continued encouragement and care will be needed at home. If a patient has supportive family members who are willing and able to give continued care, the nurse will be able to anticipate that nursing home placement need not be the only option.

The nurse is able to do this kind of assessment of continuing care needs due to *ongoing relationships* with patients, frequent communication with them, and observation of their social support systems as represented by visitors. Transitions in care always involve changes in roles and expectations; patients need to have knowledge and understanding of these changes. If care is to be taken over by the patient or by a family member, teaching is an essential part of successful discharge. Established communication with the patient allows the nurse to teach effectively. It also allows the nurse to know WHEN the patient is ready to change levels of care.

The continuing assessment of future patient care needs is also a *legal requirement* for nurses. The Accreditation Manual for Hospitals states: "The nursing care plan should be initiated upon the admission of the patient and, as part of the long-term goal, should include discharge plans" (JCAH, 1973, pp. 55–56). Being able to show that discharge planning services are provided for patients is one of the conditions of participation in the Medicare program for both acute care hospitals and skilled nursing facilities. As noted in the excerpts of the

Medicare Fact Sheet shown in Example 1.2, payment for services other than acute care are based on the "skilled nursing needs" of the patient that are documented as "medically necessary." The professional judgment of the nurse in helping to determine patient care needs is an important factor in whether Medicare and some private insurance coverage is received.

The documentation of patient care needs and goals is a regular part of nursing practice. The *nursing process* requires the nurse to assess needs and formulate a nursing diagnosis, make plans consistent with goals of care, implement those plans, and evaluate progress. One of the reasons that nurses find it easy to participate in discharge planning is that this process uses the same steps, judgments, and often the same documents as the nursing process. Attention to discharge planning is not something that is separate from what the nurse usually does; rather it is an expansion of the nurse's view to include longer-term goals.

In summary, the nurse is encouraged to participate in discharge planning because of:

- an ongoing relationship with the patient and an awareness of patient needs over a period of time,
- legal requirements which make the nurse responsible for recording long-term patient care goals, and
- the similarity of the discharge planning process with steps in the nursing process.

Factors That Discourage a Nursing Role in Discharge Planning

There are likewise a number of reasons that nurses are reluctant to participate in discharge planning. Probably the major factor is the perception that discharge planning involves a whole new set of activities that will necessarily require a time commitment. Nurses are realistically concerned about taking time away from immediate nursing care needs, but also have to give serious thought to the overall quality of patient care. If preparing patients for transitions in level of care makes the difference in whether they progress to recovery or relapse, then the expenditure of time is certainly justified. Discharge planning means becoming aware of long-term needs, of taking opportunities to teach and to help family members understand what needs to be done after discharge, and communicating effectively with other caregivers—all things that are well within the range of excellent nursing care.

Certain aspects of coordinating and implementing a discharge plan take considerable time if the nurse does not have an effective central team to refer to. Organizing nursing home placements and learning which community services are available, for example, are time consuming. In an ideal situation, the nurse who identifies a patient's continuing care needs can call upon specialists who then work together with the nurse and patient to make and implement a plan.

Yet the very existence of a specialist team leads to two reasons why nurses are sometimes reluctant to get involved in the discharge planning process. The first is that it is tempting to imagine that they are therefore responsible for all discharge planning activities. The person with this kind of attitude mentally declares: *"Let the experts do it!"* Such an attitude is the result of seeing discharge planning as a process quite apart from nursing care. It also assumes that a team of specialists is able to offer planning assistance to all patients who need this service. The coordinators of several discharge planning departments in a metropolitan area recently estimated that they are involved in less than 20% of hospital discharges and focus their attention mainly on Medicare and Medicaid recipients. None were able to offer help with transitions in care that occur within the hospital.

Wherever a group of professionals of different disciplines attempt to work together on shared goals there is a potential for *role confusion* and sometimes competition. Unfortunately, it is the patient who suffers most from this kind of struggle. All caregivers need to be alert to problems of this sort and work to resolve them. It is also important that administrators prevent "turf battles" by clarifying policies and supporting efforts at team building.

In summary, some of the factors that discourage nurses' participation in discharge planning are:

- concerns about the time it takes,
- failure to recognize the discharge planning needs of all patients,
- willingness to leave the responsibility to others, and
- intra-disciplinary struggles or role confusion.

Nursing Roles That Reflect a Range of Discharge Planning Needs

Patients' needs for discharge planning services vary as they progress on a continuum of care from illness to health. The roles that are appropriate for the nurse in meeting their changing needs vary from basic communication to intense involvement in the coordination of services. Roles may blend and overlap according to patient needs and the nurse's skills and resources. A list of some possible nursing roles is shown in Figure 1–3. They are arranged to show the least complex at the bottom and the most complex at the top of the graph. In most cases, a particular role will include and be built upon those that are below it; in order to share useful information with other professionals, for example, the nurse will have had to make a full needs assessment. The line represents the increasing amount of knowledge, time, and skills required of the nurse fulfilling roles of increasing complexity.

Starting with the first level, *exchanging information* with patients is the least complex, in that it involves activities that are part of nursing care. By developing good communication with patients, the nurse is able to gather information upon which an assessment of discharge planning needs can be based. The nurse also invites patients' participation by answering questions and helping them understand aspects of their care.

Identifying the full range of patients' discharge planning *needs* is the next role level. Note that this activity is less complex for the nurse with easy access to patients and continuing relationships with them than it would be for other professionals who do not know them as well.

The next more complex level of nursing role is the gathering of information appropriate to making a discharge plan and *communicating* it to a specialist planning team. As part of this role, the nurse collects and organizes patient data and helps to clarify the role of the planning team for patients and their families.

Coordinating a transition in care within an institution is less complex than a community discharge because of the proximity of the caregivers who will continue the patient's care. Cooperative effort, communication, and feedback on patients' progress can usually be accomplished efficiently. It is important that patients and their families understand why a transition is planned and are helped to learn what to expect. Introducing them to a nurse who will be continuing their care in the new setting will greatly reduce their anxiety.

Helping patients learn about themselves, their care, and what to expect is part of every step in the discharge planning process. When

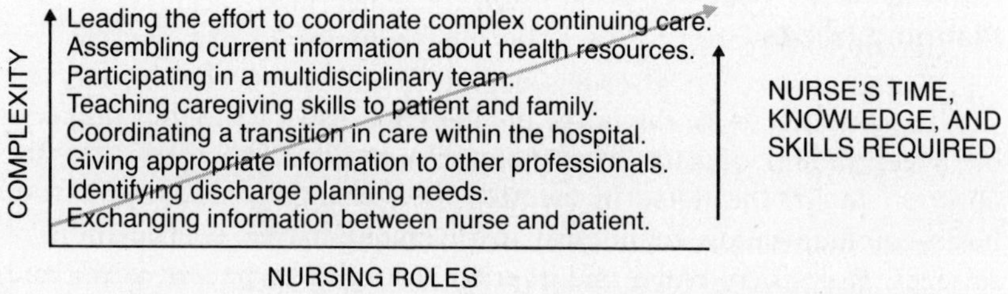

COMPLEXITY

Leading the effort to coordinate complex continuing care.
Assembling current information about health resources.
Participating in a multidisciplinary team.
Teaching caregiving skills to patient and family.
Coordinating a transition in care within the hospital.
Giving appropriate information to other professionals.
Identifying discharge planning needs.
Exchanging information between nurse and patient.

NURSE'S TIME, KNOWLEDGE, AND SKILLS REQUIRED

NURSING ROLES

Figure 1–3. *Range of nursing roles in discharge planning.*

patients or family members need to learn special knowledge or skills that will allow them to take over responsibility for continuing care, it can add a great deal of complexity to the discharge plan. *Teaching* is a role that is very well suited to the skills of nurses and is positively essential to the success of many discharges. Good teaching takes good planning, however; clear teaching goals must be selected, rapport built with patient and family, and time set aside for instruction and practice well in advance of the patient leaving the hospital.

Participation in a discharge planning team involves the nurse not only in knowing what other professionals can contribute to a patient's discharge, but also in coordinating information effectively, following through on plans to be sure they are implemented, and ensuring the participation of patient and family. In most instances the nurse will take responsibility for patient and family teaching as part of the team effort.

If a specialist discharge planning consultant or team is unavailable, the nurse will need to *assemble detailed current information* about sources of medical and health care in the community. Ideally the nurse should not wait to begin this process until discovering that a patient needs the help of community agencies or services, although information should be updated whenever a referral seems likely (see Chapter 5).

Finally, the highest level of complexity is taking the *leadership role in discharges* of patients with long-term or difficult-to-meet continuing care needs. Again, expert communication and teaching skills are necessary, as well as a thorough knowledge of sources of care and support.

In order to fully meet the continuing care needs of a particular patient, the nurse may play several of these roles. The following case examples demonstrate nursing involvement in the discharge planning process.

Example 1.4 Coordinating a Transition in Care

Mr. Barnes, age 58, had been admitted to the Coronary Care Unit after collapsing with an apparent myocardial infarction at his office. Tests revealed only minor damage due to the attack, but a serious degree of vascular occlusion. He was advised by his doctor that bypass surgery was indicated. Surgery was scheduled for the next morning.

Julie Wilson had been Mr. Barnes' primary care nurse since his admission the day before. As part of her initial care, she described cardiac function to him, explained use of the monitor, and answered his questions about medications. She had gotten to know him well enough, even in a short time, that she was immediately aware that Mr. Barnes was unusually upset by his session with the doctor. A few questions revealed that a close friend of many years had died following complications of bypass surgery. Julie first encouraged him to talk about his friend and his fears. She then arranged to spend some time with him and his wife during visiting hours later in the afternoon. Returning to the nurses' station, she called the doctor to inform him of the patient's unusual degree of anxiety, and then she reserved use of the videotape machine. She also telephoned the Intensive Care Unit to arrange for one of the nurses on duty the next day to come and meet Mr. and Mrs. Barnes.

In her session with them, Julie again encouraged both husband and wife to talk about their fears and uncertainties. When they began to ask questions about what would happen, she suggested they come with her to view a videotape made specifically to help patients understand the procedures. She had just begun to answer their questions following the video when the Intensive Care nurse arrived. She joined in the question-and-answer session and instructed Mr. Barnes on the deep breathing that she would be asking him to do following surgery.

In this example, the nurse *exchanged information* with the patient early in his hospitalization, thereby forming a relationship of trust with him and finding out about him, his priorities, and his knowledge base. This information laid the foundation for the later identification of discharge planning needs. This early assessment allowed the nurse to quickly identify Mr. Barnes' state of anxiety and fear while she still had time to intervene. Recognizing the importance of the patient's mental state, the nurse then *gave appropriate information* to the patient's doctor. By arranging and participating in a meeting with the patient's future caregiver, the nurse *coordinated the transition of care*. The performance of these three roles ensured uninterrupted, supportive continuing care for Mr. Barnes.

In the following case example, the nurse confronts a complex discharge planning need.

Example 1.5 A Crisis of Home Care

It was a cold November night when police finally brought Nellie Costa into the Emergency Room. She had been reported missing from her daughter's home that afternoon. Nellie, a 68-year-old, partly blind woman, suffered from Alzheimer's disease. She had wandered away before, but had always been found quickly by her family. This time it was decided to admit her overnight for observation.

Nellie's daughter and her husband, Nancy and Rick Yass, were clearly very upset over the incident. While waiting in the hallway for the doctor to finish his examination, the nurse overheard Rick say to his wife: "This is the last straw! We just can't continue to keep your mother at home. You're exhausted all the time, and it's not fair to the boys." A few minutes later, the nurse was able to take the time to initiate a conversation with Nancy and Rick. They readily expressed their concern over their ability to continue to care for Nellie, but had not as yet investigated any alternatives. The nurse suggested that they talk over the situation with the doctor while he was there. The doctor later put a note on the chart requesting referral to the discharge planning team. The nurse gave the family a pamphlet describing the functions and members of the team and set up a tentative appointment with the social worker for the next morning.

In this case example, the nurse was alert to the *identification* of discharge planning needs. She took the time to gather information and to be sure that the doctor was aware of the needs. Since this hospital had a multidisciplinary discharge planning team, the nurse's immediate role was to *coordinate the referral* and be sure the family knew what to expect of the service. She would later work with the team to assess Nellie's continuing care needs and help the family develop a plan. Her involvement with the plan's implementation would depend on the decisions made and the community resources available.

> *The roles of nurses in discharge planning are initially determined by their awareness of patient needs for continuing care, their ability to gather relevant information, and their skills in quickly forming trust relationships with the patient and family members.*

In the next chapter we will look at how the nurse's skills can be used to best advantage for a full range of discharge planning roles.

SUMMARY

This chapter has taken a broad view of the discharge planning "puzzle." The historical, social, and economic contexts within which discharge planning operates have been explored. Discharge planning has been described as a process that begins upon admission to acute care and proceeds through several phases. The importance of patient and family involvement in each phase has been emphasized. The roles of nurses in this process depends upon their identification of patients' needs, the resources available to them, and the complexity of the issues involved. Although a specialist team may help to plan the discharge of some patients, the nurse has a responsibility to be involved in the continuing care plans of all patients, whether they are experiencing transitions in levels of care within the hospital or preparing for discharge and community care.

In the next four chapters we take a close look at four major pieces of the discharge planning puzzle, starting with the skills that nurses bring to the process. In subsequent chapters we focus on the patient, on the contribution of other health professionals, and on resources for continuing care in the community.

FURTHER READING

Harris, Richard. *A Sacred Trust.* New York: The New American Library Inc., 1966.
Originally written as a series of essays for The New Yorker *magazine, this book presents an easy-to-read history of the events leading up to the passage of the Medicare and Medicaid legislation in 1965.*

Hartigan, Evelyn G. and D. Jean Brown (eds.). *Discharge Planning for Continuity of Care* (Publication No. 20–1977). New York: National League for Nursing, 1985. *This is an expanded and updated edition of the original 1976 publication. Every nurse should have access to this book, because it presents a brief but clear description of the discharge planning process and the issues surrounding its practice. It includes an extensive bibliography, historical statistics, a glossary, and examples of record forms. This book is available from the N.L.N. at 10 Columbus Circle, New York, NY 10019–1350.*

McClelland, E., K. Kelly, and K. Buckwalter (eds.). *Continuity of Care: Advancing the Concept of Discharge Planning.* Orlando: Grune & Stratton, Inc., 1985. *Each chapter in this work is separately authored. Part A, A Conceptual and Historical Framework for Continuity of Care, containing four chapters, is especially relevant to the material in this chapter, as are Chapters 7 and 10 on roles and DRGs, respectively.*

Wensley, Edith. *Nursing Service Without Walls.* New York: National League for Nursing, 1963.
This landmark publication is worth searching for in a medical library. The basic principles discussed in Part III are as valid today as they were when this was written.

How to Apply Nursing Skills to Discharge Planning

Nurses are key figures in the discharge planning process. Their skills allow them to fully assess patients' needs for continuing care and then to work with them and their families, other professionals, and community resources to meet those needs. In this chapter we review three specific skills and show how they can be applied to effective discharge planning. Our focus is on assessment, communication, and teaching. Other important skills that nurses bring with them to discharge planning are discussed elsewhere in this text. They include the skills of coordination, motivation, goal-setting, and recording.

2.1 HOW TO APPLY ASSESSMENT SKILLS TO DISCHARGE PLANNING

The gathering of patient data is the acknowledged first step in the nursing process. The information collected is used by nurses to identify nursing care needs and by other health professionals to determine the goals of their intervention. As medical care has become more specialized and more health professionals are involved in one patient's care, the importance of data that takes into account many aspects of the patient's functioning has been demonstrated. Nurses are in a unique position among caregivers to be able to gather and assess data concerning the *whole* patient and the full range of needs. The nursing assessment and resulting nursing diagnosis have proven their worth by facilitating more comprehensive and more consistent care. As Yura and Walsh note in their work on the Nursing Process:

The nurse's function is to assess the existence and extent of wellness or illness. . . . In contrast to goals of other members of the health profession, the nurse is involved with human needs that affect the *total* person rather than one aspect, one problem, or a limited segment of need fulfillment. (1983, p. 135)

The broad view that the nurse brings to assessment is what makes the nurse such a valuable team member in planning for continuity of care.

What Nursing Skills Are Involved in Assessment?

The nursing assessment generally proceeds through three phases, although they may not be distinctly separate: gathering data, evaluating that data, and determining the nursing diagnosis. Some of the specific skills developed by nurses in order to assess patient needs are as follows:

- *Interview* skills that include the ability to listen as well as to formulate insightful questions;
- *Interpretation* skills that allow the nurse to understand what patients say about their concerns and symptoms and transmit these in concise form and appropriate terminology to other caregivers;
- *Nonverbal communication* skills that permit the nurse to recognize even subtle responses to treatment that reflect the patient's moods, attitudes and psycho-social needs;
- *Relationship* skills that cut across potential social and cultural barriers to promote a climate of trust with patients, family members, and professional colleagues;
- *Observational* skills that allow the nurse to distinguish normal from abnormal functioning and to recognize changes in patient responses to treatment;
- *Evaluation* skills that permit the nurse to consider not only the facts about a patient's condition but also the interconnections and balance between relative strengths and deficits; and
- *Goal-setting* skills that help the nurse see beyond immediate needs to identify intermediate and long-term goals of care.

These kinds of skills, together with the nurse's *educated sensitivity* (which helps anticipate the impact that actions will have on the patient), make the nursing assessment of patient needs a crucial part of the discharge planning process.

The collection and evaluation of patient data are done in varying degrees of formality and cover varying lengths of time. Sometimes an interview, physical examination, questionnaire, or combination of these are part of the admission procedure for every patient. Sometimes nurses take a much less formal approach and simply talk with patients with the principal intent of getting to know them. In these cases, specific questions may be limited to inquiries about birthdate, address, onset of symptoms, and allergies. In either case, a nursing diagnosis is usually recorded following the admission procedures.

Patient data gathered on admission will alert the nurse to potential discharge planning needs, but additional data will be needed as the patient's treatment progresses.

As we pointed out in Section 1.1, discharge planning cannot begin too early, but it can be completed too early. Occasionally one finds a well-intentioned caregiver who uses admission data and diagnosis to decide FOR the patient what should happen on discharge. This person is usually quite dismayed when patient or family react negatively to what they may regard as unnecessarily controlling or even hostile behavior. Having not been part of the planning, they certainly cannot be expected to take responsibility for implementation.

To avoid this kind of problem, one needs to be aware not only of the *range of data* required by effective discharge planning but also the importance of the *dynamics of caregiving* and patients' responses. Items such as the degree to which patients progress in accepting their illnesses and any future limitations imposed, the sources of stress in their lives, and details of their financial situations usually come to light slowly within the context of an ongoing trust relationship with caregivers. Yet, each of these is as important to a patient's future well-being as knowing whether she or he lives on the second floor of an apartment building (see Example 1.3). The problem for the nurse is finding a way to organize the wealth of patient information collected so that it can easily be used to assess the patient's continuing care needs.

Using the Patient's Health Balance as a Guide for Assessment

An assessment tool that seems well suited to the needs of the discharge planning process is the "health balance." By using it, the nurse and other caregivers can gather important patient data over a period of time in an organized fashion. It emphasizes the dynamic relationships between positive and negative factors that influence health and well-being.

A representation of the health balance is shown in Figure 2–1 using the concept of a child's seesaw. Needs and demands are balanced by strengths and resources, just as children might balance on a seesaw. As long as there is a balance between factors (or children), there can be movement within a dynamic range; a person whose health is in balance can adjust to a range of changes and challenges. Illness or distress occurs when one or more of the factors overwhelm the adaptive powers of the balance by becoming too "heavy" or too "light." For example, a person whose resources for personal attention and emotional support are lacking may suffer decreased self-esteem and resulting depression. The person whose immune system (a strength) is overwhelmed by an infection seeks medical assistance to meet an increased level of need.

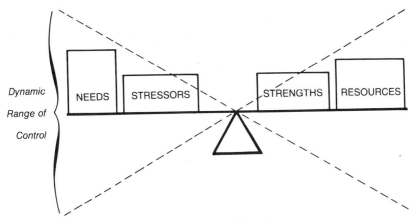

Figure 2–1. *The health balance.*

While in acute distress, only a patient's needs may be obvious. Yet if the health balance is to be restored, other factors must be investigated and their relationship to one another considered.

> *The assessment required for effective discharge planning is more extensive than that necessary for meeting immediate medical needs.*

The health balance model helps the nurse keep these factors, as well as their interaction, in perspective while beginning the planning process. The factors that influence the health balance are described in the following paragraphs.

Needs or Deficits. This factor includes basic human needs that all people share, as well as those individual and personal needs perceived by the person as deficits. They may be either acute, demanding prompt attention by caregivers, or chronic, requiring continued work over a longer time. For example, a patient may *need* immediate information and reassurance about survival and safety. The health balance may also be affected by what the patient sees as a *deficit* of close and loving relationships, or the need for a greater sense of fulfillment on the job. (See Section 6.2 for a discussion of needs as they influence motivation.)

Demands or Stressors. This factor is made up of the demands placed on a person from a variety of sources and stressors in the environment. They may be physical, emotional, or social. (See Section 3.1 for a discussion of increased stress as a result of transitions in care, and Section 3.3 for a description of social and cultural factors in planning care.) For example, a patient who has been injured in a traffic accident away from home may experience *stress* owing to physical impairment, emotional distress owing to inability to contact and receive support from family members, and concern about being absent from work. Other *demands* on time and energy that could affect the patient's ability to regain a health balance may include financial responsibility for a young family, less-than-adequate housing, or marital discord.

Strengths. A person's strengths include physical, intellectual, motor, and affective or emotional abilities. The knowledge, attitudes, and skills gained through previous experience make a major contribution to a person's present strengths. If, for example, the accident victim is in good physical condition as a result of regular exercise, has previously had experience walking with crutches, has good problem-solving ability, and is even-tempered and emotionally stable, the accident will have less negative impact than it would if these internal strengths were not present.

Resources. Another factor whose presence positively influences health is the external resources to which a person has access. These may include material resources, access to health care, and the emotional support of other people. A hospitalized patient, for example, who has good medical insurance coverage and sick leave benefits and whose church membership provides strong personal support and emotional care may well regain his or her health balance after an illness more quickly than someone without these resources. The improvement of health resources and community services such as paramedic teams, trauma centers, home care programs, and public health screening programs positively affects the health balance of all community members.

Each of the component parts of these four factors contributes positively or negatively to a person's present health balance. In determining what is needed to restore balance, the *interaction* between factors becomes important. For example, a patient's needs may be balanced by improved strengths and resources if meeting them directly is not possible. Reducing the intensity of demands may also be feasible.

Realistic planning for continuing care begins with careful assessment of the factors contributing to the patient's health imbalance and extends to an appreciation of the interaction of factors necessary to restore balance.

The following case example shows how the nurse's skills are used to assess a patient's health balance as part of the discharge planning process.

Example 2.1 Assessment of Health Balance Factors

Sylvia Donner was a 34-year-old, unmarried executive in the fashion industry. She had recently noticed a lump in her left breast. Mammography revealed an irregular growth the size of a large marble. A simple mastectomy was performed following confirmation of malignancy by biopsy. The following items were among those recorded by Sylvia's primary care nurse as having relevance for her continuing care. They are summarized on a chart, which also shows the effect of each on health balance factors and the skills used by the nurse in making this assessment.

ITEM	BALANCE FACTOR	NURSING SKILL
* Reduced mobility, left arm	Increased need Decreased strength	Observation
* Good sick leave and medical benefits	Good resource	Interview
* Concern over recurrence of cancer; positive family history	Increased stress	Relationship Interpretation Interview
* Prides self on high achievement; enjoys demanding work	Good resources High stress normal	Relationship Nonverbal comm. Interpretation
* Physical attractiveness very important; expresses concern about impact of surgery	High self demands Increased stress Decreased strength	Interview Evaluation Goal-setting

In this case example, the nurse used a range of skills to identify some of the changes in this patient's health balance as a result of surgery. She also identified some pre-existing factors that could contribute to recovery, such as the resource of paid sick leave, the resource of job satisfaction and sense of achievement, and some self-imposed stresses and demands. These assessment items together with other patient data allowed the nurse and her professional colleagues to work with the patient in planning her continuing care. The use of the health balance as a basis for assessment helped the nurse see connections between physical and psycho-social aspects of care.

In summary, all of a nurse's interactional skills as well as skills of observation are necessary if the assessment of nursing care needs is to be extended to provide data upon which discharge planning can be based. Because of ongoing relationships with patients and their family members, the nurse is in a unique position to quickly and effectively assemble such information. The skills of interpretation, evaluation, and goal-setting make the nurse's assessment accessible to colleagues. The health balance model has been described as one way of organizing data and giving appropriate attention to the interconnections between positive and negative factors.

2.2 HOW TO APPLY COMMUNICATION SKILLS TO DISCHARGE PLANNING

If a broad-based assessment is the first step toward effective discharge planning, communication is the means by which this and subsequent steps are accomplished. Communication provides the energy that sorts out the puzzle pieces and connects them together.

The first goal of nurse-patient communication is to establish a relationship of trust. The effectiveness of discharge planning depends on meeting that goal. In this section we will look first at how the nurse encourages trust and then examine the specific skills of nonverbal and verbal communication. Use of communication skills to facilitate coordination and cooperation with colleagues will be discussed in detail in Chapter 4.

How to Encourage Trust

Any student of human nature knows that few people have simple, straightforward life situations. When problems arise, the concerns they have and the conditions they experience are, as Gerard Egan (1975) expressed it, "messy." They are messy partly because feelings are such an important part of a person's functioning. Emotions such as anxiety, sadness, fear, and resentment interfere with rational thinking and problem solving. Few experiences of acute or chronic medical difficulties are *not* "messy."

For the nurse attempting to communicate effectively with patients, the presence of strong emotions offers a complex challenge. On the one hand, the nurse must recognize that people do not readily share their feelings with others. They may tell the *facts* as they see them, but unless they have active reason to trust the nurse, worries, concerns, and emotional responses will not be shared. On the other hand, without access to the subjective as well as objective experiences of patients, the nurse will be unable to assess their needs or help them plan for the future.

> *It is important that both the facts of patients' situations and their emotional responses be taken into account when planning continuing care. Failure to do so risks failure of the plan.*

How then does the nurse quickly break down the natural barriers to revealing feelings and encourage trust in patients and their family members? Clinical and counseling psychologists have found that it is not so much what the nurse does, but the attitudes that are demonstrated. (For example, see Rogers, 1961; Egan, 1975; Muldary, 1983.) Most patients assume that their caregivers are "trustworthy" in the sense that they will do nothing injurious to them and will treat information confidentially. On the basis of this assumption, patients generally put up with invasions of their personal privacy and try to answer direct questions. The first thing that nurses must do then is to show themselves worthy of at least this basic level of trust. This is done by treating the patient with respect as an individual and by demonstrating a caring and concerned attitude. The nurse attempts to make the person physically comfortable; offers information about what is happening; explains why questions are being asked or procedures done.

If a deeper level of communication is to be reached that includes feelings as well as facts, however, the nurse must direct energy to encouraging greater trust.

It is the nurse's responsibility to initiate a relationship in which trust can be developed.

There are four basic *qualities* that the nurse needs to do this effectively. It is from these qualities that attitudes spring. These have been variously named, but we will use the terms *warmth, respect, empathy, and genuineness.*

Warmth. This is a quality that helps others feel accepted. Nurses who communicate warmth are willing to extend themselves to other people with openness, expressing their own feelings appropriately. Rather than being cold, expert, or disapproving, they acknowledge their own and other people's humanness. Their behavior reflects the attitudes of self-respect, self-acceptance, and genuine concern for the welfare of others. People respond by feeling that they can safely be themselves in the nurse's presence.

Respect. This quality means treating another person as a worthwhile and unique individual and giving consideration to his or her personal attributes, such as personality, preferences, culture, and opinions. Respect shares with warmth the valuing of other people as equals even though their characteristics, opinions, and background are quite different from one's own. To respect does not necessarily mean to like, but to accept and value. Carl Rogers (1961) called the attitude by which respect is shown "unconditional positive regard." By this he meant that the caregiver should value others without any "strings attached," viewing their capabilities optimistically. For the nurse who is helping the patient with discharge planning, this involves believing in a person's self-responsibility for problem solving, even though decisions or actions might not be what the nurse would choose.

Respectful attitudes are reflected in a variety of ways, some of which are simple politeness. Addressing people who are older than oneself as Mr., Mrs., or Ms. until invited to use their first names denotes respect, as does ensuring physical privacy when possible and refraining from the use of jargon or abbreviations that are possibly not known to the person. Respect means avoiding "overpowering" the patient or family by insisting that things be done a certain way or at a certain time unless absolutely necessary, and then only when an adequate explanation is offered. Patients who are consulted about events in their care, or even just advised before something happens, feel that they are being respected and treated as individuals, not just as bed numbers or disease entities.

Empathy. This quality means helping people feel understood. The empathic nurse suspends judgment about patients' actions or words and instead tries to think and feel *with* them rather than *about* or *for* them. The word empathy derives from the German word *Einfühlung*, meaning "feeling into." This means actively tuning into the feelings and thoughts behind the words and gestures so that the whole picture of a person's experience can be appreciated. It also means letting go of stereotypes and prejudices that may cloud the nurse's view of the person.

Empathy is an essential ingredient in trust relationships. If patients feel that they are understood, they are much more likely to hear information presented to them and to share their deeper emotional responses. Demonstrating empathy means being willing to be involved with people and willing to exert the effort of concentration to really hear them without demanding that they feel as you imagine you would in the situation.

Genuineness. This quality, sometimes termed "congruence," helps people feel that they are interacting with a "real" person whose interest and care they can trust. Two aspects of the elusive quality of genuineness are especially important to nurse-patient trust relationships. One is that the nurse avoid "playing games" with people by attempting to manipulate the situation and their responses. Inappropriate joking, making light of a serious situation, and coldly professional and efficient "busy-ness" are examples of ways in which nurses and others sometimes avoid real, caring contact with people. Although one cannot always be intense and serious and in fact, sometimes must put procedures before people, the self-aware nurse knows when these behaviors are appropriate and when they signify avoidance.

Another aspect of genuineness has to do with being consistent. Parents know that children are good at picking up discrepancies between the verbal and nonverbal messages of adults. For example, the parent who says "no" in a pleading tone of voice or with a smile is seldom obeyed. Likewise, when concern is voiced by a nurse who fails to make eye contact with the patient, the verbal message may be disregarded or judged "put on," whereas the nonverbal message of emotional distance is considered real. Whenever there is an inconsistency between verbal and nonverbal behavior, the nonverbal will be judged the more honest.

People in stressful and threatening situations are more alert than usual to any lack of congruence in communication. Developing trust means that patients can rely on nurses to mean what they say and say what they mean.

The development of trust within the nurse-patient relationship depends on the nurse's tactful honesty and a willingness to share oneself with others.

The qualities of warmth, respect, empathy, and genuineness are reflected in the attitudes the nurse brings to all caring situations. They are detected immediately by patients, family members, and colleagues. They take no extra time apart from that necessary for good communication; indeed they hasten the development of relationships in which problem solving can be done efficiently as well as effectively.

Nonverbal Communication: Sending Behavior Messages

Nonverbal behavior often communicates more "loudly" than words. When people are troubled, anxious, or uncertain, they depend much more than usual on feedback from others. They look for clues that indicate whether caregivers are interested enough in them as individuals to pay attention to their needs and concerns. A combination of nonverbal actions and words conveys the message that the caregiver is interested and regards what the patient has to say as important. Counselors use the term *attending* to refer to the nonverbal part of this message.

The most important ingredients of attending to people and their concerns are summarized by the mnemonic C-A-R-E:

> *C-ENTERED ATTENTION*
> *A-PPROPRIATE RESPONSES*
> *R-ELAXED POSTURE*
> *E-YE CONTACT*

This mnemonic provides a kind of checklist for the nurse who is purposefully communicating attention and concern to another person.

Centered Attention. To let a person know that he or she is being attended to, the nurse stops doing other tasks and makes that person the center of attention. The nurse also mentally focuses on what the person is saying *here and now;* one does not try to anticipate what they might say or to follow one's own train of thought. This kind of concentrated listening is difficult for nurses to do for a number of reasons—many of them environmental. Distractions for the listener include a high noise level, movement of other people in the immediate vicinity, lack of privacy for confidential conversation, and a variety of interruptions.

Sometimes nurses feel defensive about "only" talking with a patient. Given other pressures on them for their skill and attention, it is easy for nurses to avoid spending time on attentive communication. Sometimes nurses are tempted to pretend that they are listening carefully, hoping that the person will not continue for too long or say anything of importance. Such a pretense is seldom convincing. It is more open and honest to say something like, "I can see that this is important to you and that you would like to talk about it. Right at the moment I cannot stop and really pay attention. I'll finish what I'm doing and come back at . . . so we can talk then." This kind of statement is generally well accepted and does not interfere with the helping relationship or the quality of the communication. The important thing is that the nurse has indicated that the patient's concern is valid and worth paying attention to.

Appropriate Responses. Full attention is usually accompanied by some sounds, even if not complete sentences, by facial expressions, and by gestures. These responses are not intended to interrupt the flow of the speaker's words or thoughts but merely to let the person know that what is said is being heard. This kind of feedback is powerful encouragement to continue. Counselors have come to call these responses "minimal encouragements to talk" (Ivey, 1971). They include verbalizations such as "um-hmmm," repetition of a significant word, and one-word questions, as well as nonverbal actions such as nods of the head, reflection of the general feeling tone in the listener's facial expressions, and various gestures. These, in combination, give the message "I'm hearing you; it's all right to continue."

Relaxed Posture. Stiff, tense, or rigid postures, collapsed or withdrawn postures, turning away from the other person, nervous squirmings, and agitated movements all communicate that the would-be listener is uncomfortable, would rather not be there, and may disappear from the scene at any moment. Good attending behavior requires a relaxed, balanced, open posture. Most people feel at least a little anxious or tense when discussing emotional events or their feelings with someone. The listener must not contribute to this tension by also showing discomfort and anxiety. Some nurses are in the habit of placing their hands on their hips when standing still; this posture is seen by others as tense and impatient and can be construed as disapproving as well.

The best listening position is one in which patient and nurse are physically at the same level. For nurses working in clinical settings, this usually means sitting down so that they do not tower over the person lying in bed. In most Western countries the appropriate distance between people who are communicating is approximately arm's length. At this distance the listener can lean forward a little without invading the other person's "personal space." Comfortable distances do, however, vary with culture (see Section 3.3).

Associated with the concept of social distance is the relative comfort with which a person accepts the touch of another. In clinical situations nurses and patients generally disregard conventions about touch in order to give and receive physical care. When discussing an emotional topic, however, touch takes on a different meaning. The nurse may pat a shoulder, stroke an arm, or hold a hand, intending to comfort the person; however, there is at least a possibility that these gestures may be considered intrusive or condescending. Nurses must use their own sensitivity and what "seems right" at the moment as a general guide to their behavior, while making no assumptions about the other person's comfort with touching.

Eye Contact. When you attend to someone, that person occupies the middle of your field of vision and you establish eye contact with him or her. Some people feel less comfortable than others about being looked at. As with social distance, eye contact is subject to cultural variation. The appropriate amount of eye contact is enough for the nurse to communicate a sincere effort to understand people and hear their concerns, but not so much as to seem intrusive. Looking at the floor or gazing past a person's shoulder indicates lack of involvement. For patients not to meet the nurse's eyes may indicate that they are uncomfortable or embarrassed about the topic of conversation and need extra assurance of the nurse's acceptance.

Nurses are educated observers of people and their surroundings. It is tempting, when talking with someone, to visually survey the room, mentally noting the availability and status of equipment. During verbal communication this behavior is the equivalent of glancing frequently at one's watch or at the door and indicates a definite lack of attention.

Although it is desirable for caregivers to fully attend to all communication, this is simply not possible. There are certain times, however, when the messages given by attending are especially important. These include:

- the *beginning* of the nurse-patient relationship. The early encouragement of trusting communication is the basis for problem solving later.

- when the person is experiencing a *crisis*. The support offered by good listening behavior helps the person get started on a resolution.
- when *planning* for continuing care is in progress. By being given "permission" to talk about ideas and concerns by the nurse's willingness to listen carefully, the patient is encouraged to think through the consequences of the plan.
- when a person is relating something that is of *special significance* to him or her. The nurse's warm acceptance by listening attentively confirms the strength of the nurse-patient relationship.

The attending behaviors of C-A-R-E help the nurse establish and maintain good working relationships of trust with patients, family members, and colleagues. The nurse gives people attention and acceptance, but also receives important information. By listening for both the facts and the feelings of people's experiences, the nurse is better able to appreciate their frame of reference and, consequently, to more accurately assess their present needs and anticipate future ones.

Verbal Communication:
Using Questions Effectively

Questions and answers are a major part of all communication with others. Some questions are part of social ritual, such as "How are you?" Some questions inquire, probe, or challenge, while others quiz, interrogate, and suggest advice (You are going to . . . , aren't you?). Some questions confirm the authority and knowledge of the questioner, and others establish mutuality in seeking an answer. Some questions demand one-word answers and others invite open-ended exploration of a problem or concern. Whether as part of a formal assessment interview or as ongoing communication with others, questions are a major part of a nurse's verbal communication pattern. They initiate most nurse-patient interaction.

Questions fall into two broad categories: closed and open. *Closed* questions are those directed toward obtaining specific pieces of information; they are fact-based. They can usually be answered in a few words and are very time efficient. The nurse uses them to gather data: "What medications are you taking?" "When did the pain begin?" "Have you been in the hospital before?" "When did you last have anything to eat?" Asking closed questions establishes the questioner as the one in control of the situation.

Open questions are those directed toward gaining understanding; they give the opportunity to share both facts and feelings. They are less time efficient than closed questions, but the answers are much more revealing about the person as well as the medical condition. Such questions as: "How did this all start?" "Could you tell me a bit more about . . . ?" "What are you most concerned about right now?" and "How do you think this is going to affect you?" give the person permission to express thoughts and feelings openly. These are followed by active listening and C-A-R-E on the part of the nurse. They establish a partnership in dealing with problems and concerns. They are an important part of finding out how best to help with planning continuing care.

The initial assessment of patient needs by the nurse is one of the most crucial times for using questions well. This early exchange allows the nurse to diagnose immediate nursing care needs, encourages the beginning of a trust relationship, and begins the nurse on the path to understanding the patient as a person. A carefully conducted interview can provide the information on which the discharge planning process can be initiated.

The CONE Assessment Interview. In working with nurses on improving their use of questions, we have found one specific approach especially helpful (Rorden, J., 1987, Ch. 3). This is a pattern for an initial assessment interview made up of sets of open and closed questions within pre-selected areas of concern. It is called a CONE interview because the focus of questions begins broadly and becomes increasingly narrow as the interview progresses, suggesting a conical shape. Each cone has four distinct steps, shown in Figure 2–2.

A reasonably broad-based interview usually consists of four or five CONEs. Without serious distractions or interruptions, each CONE normally takes 5 to 10 minutes. The nurse can therefore plan on such an interview taking between 30 and 45 minutes, including an explanation of just what will be done and why. The end of a CONE is a natural breaking point if an interruption makes continuing impossible.

Preparation for this kind of interview consists of identifying *broad subjects* of concern and, within each, *specific kinds of information* for

Figure 2–2. *Steps in the "CONE" interview.*

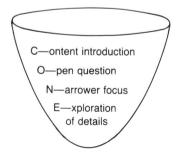

C—ontent introduction
O—pen question
N—arrower focus
E—xploration of details

which the nurse is looking. This planning may well serve, with few modifications, for all assessment interviews on a particular unit, whether they are with patients or with other people giving information about patients. For example, on a surgical unit, subjects chosen for exploration may include "previous experience and present knowledge about surgical procedures" and "the patient's experience with medications of various types." On an obstetrical unit, subjects of concern may include "preparation for parenting."

The success of the CONE interview as a method of patient data collection depends on the patient's cooperation. Those who are physically able to express themselves usually welcome the opportunity to allow the nurse to get to know them better and appreciate having their thoughts and concerns heard. It is wise and tactful to advise the patient of the confidentiality of the information he shares with the nurse. An example of a statement by the nurse to introduce the interview to the patient might be:

"Mr. Jones, I'd like to talk with you for a little while so I can get to know you better. There are some things I especially want to find out from you, so that we can give you the best possible care. Of course any information that you share with me will be used only by the professional staff immediately involved in your care."

It is important that this introductory statement be warm, genuine, and respectful, whatever words are used. It is an attempt to give the patient the message that the nurse is willing to really listen. The nurse should also be physically relaxed, unhurried, and willing to sit down. Once assured that both of them are comfortable, the nurse may proceed to the first CONE.

Step 1: Content Introduction. The purpose of a short introductory statement for each CONE of the interview is to help the patient understand *what* the subject of concern is and *why*. For example, Mr. Jones' nurse might say:

"I'm interested in the medications you have taken in the past and how they affected you so that we can better monitor the effects of those you are now taking."

Such an introduction helps to direct the patient's attention to the subject of concern.

Step 2: Open Question. This is a question that invites patients to talk freely about a subject, sharing what *they* think is important about it. What is chosen to relate gives the nurse valuable clues to a person's concerns and priorities. An open question for Mr. Jones might be:

"Can you tell me about your experience with medications before you became ill this time?"

The nurse must then listen CARE-fully to really hear the patient's response. Some parts of the response will provide material to be followed up later.

Step 3: Narrower Focus. After a full response to a broad, open question, the nurse will need to *summarize, clarify*, and ask more narrowly focused open questions. These bits of communication follow directly from what the patient has said and help the nurse more clearly understand the meaning behind the words. For example:

> "So you've been taking Lanoxin, Diuril, and Slow-K for two years now without any side effects. Is that right? (Waits for response.) Is there anything else you've taken on a regular basis? (When the patient shakes his head no, the nurse follows with a related open question.) You mentioned that you occasionally take aspirin for a headache. What's your experience been with other non-prescription medications or vitamins?"

As in the example, narrower focus questions often take the form of "You said. . . ." "Can you tell me a bit more about. . . ." This step may be repeated several times as the nurse follows up and clarifies information given in response to the initial open question.

Step 4: Exploration of Details. During this last step, the nurse seeks specific information identified during the preparation for the interview as being important but not yet discussed. Closed questions may be used to obtain this information. For example Mr. Jones' nurse might ask:

> "Did you take your morning medication before coming to the hospital?" and "Do you have your medications with you?" (If he has, she can objectively verify part of what the patient has told her.)

The CONE is brought to a conclusion by briefly summarizing the information shared by the patient during this segment and then proceeding with the introduction to the next CONE. For example:

> "You've given me a lot of useful information about your medication history. I'm also interested in finding out about. . . ."

An example of a fully planned CONE assessment interview based on the health balance model is shown in Table 2–1. Some simple modifications would make the interview useful for obtaining information about the patient from another person. By using this kind of interview format, the nurse is able to gather a wide range of subjective information pertinent to planning both immediate and continuing care. The nurse uses largely open questions that invite patients to fully express themselves but that are relatively nonthreatening to answer, because patients can choose the information they are comfortable sharing. Thus the interview is guided in specific directions without the nurse having to take an aggressively controlling or directive approach.

Table 2–1. *OUTLINE FOR HEALTH BALANCE ASSESSMENT INTERVIEW*

Purpose of Interview—to help nurse assess patient's overall health as well as present illness.

Topic for CONE A—*Strengths* of patient
  Introduction: Interest in overall health background
  Initial open question: "Can you tell me about your health before this illness/accident?"
  Looking for: Background experiences and health knowledge
                 Perception of prior physical health
                 Attitude toward present situation
                 Familiarity with hospital/clinical procedures
                 Ability to express self verbally

Topic for CONE B—*Needs* of patient
  Introduction: Interest in what is presently going on
  Initial open question: "What sorts of things most concern you right now?"
  Looking for: Unmet basic needs
                 Present anxiety level
                 Present/future orientation
                 Areas of needed information/reassurance
                 Willingness to discuss feelings
                 Motivation to learn

Topic for CONE C—*Stressors* affecting the patient
  Introduction: Interest in how patient sees his future
  Initial open question: "What kind of changes do you think will be occurring in your life now?" or alternatively, "Can you tell me about other things that are going on in your life that might affect your recovery?"
  Looking for: Socio-cultural context of illness
                 Level of awareness of consequences of illness
                 Life-style changes foreseen by patient
                 Present or impending crises
                 Attitude of patient toward changes
                 Apparent ability to cope with change
                 Motivation to participate in decisions and care
                 Areas of knowledge, attitude, or skills deficits

Topic for CONE D—*Resources* available to the patient
  Introduction: Interest in other people in patient's life
  Initial open question: "How are your family and friends affected by your illness/accident?"
  Looking for: Extent of social resources and support
                 Strength of bonds with others
                 Self-image in relation to others
                 Importance of social roles
                 Identification of people who are most significant

The overall message presented is that the nurse is genuinely attempting to hear and understand the patient as a person in order to better work *with* him or her in overcoming the present difficulty. This kind of message presented by the nurse's verbal and nonverbal behavior is a major step in encouraging the patient's trust and participation in care.

In summary, we have reviewed some basic elements of the nurse's communication skills in this section—namely, encouraging trust, using nonverbal behaviors to convey messages, and using questions as an effective part of verbal communication. Specific guidance was given in how to listen actively by using a checklist of the nurse's behavior in the form of C-A-R-E. Attention was then focused on the assessment interview as one of the most important instances of using question-asking skills. A planned format of such an interview was proposed, and its use described.

Communication skills are at the center of the nurse's contribution to discharge planning. The nurse gathers information about both facts and feelings, organizes them into an assessment of patient needs, and communicates these needs to professional colleagues. Attention to improving communication skills will allow the nurse to teach, to guide patients toward decision-making, and to coordinate patient care more effectively.

2.3 HOW TO APPLY TEACHING SKILLS TO DISCHARGE PLANNING

The one general statement that can be made about patient needs is that every patient preparing for a transition in care or discharge has a need to *learn*. In the current climate of early discharges, patients are often sent home still needing intensive care. This means that patients and their families must be coached on how to do various procedures, how to organize and coordinate ongoing care, and how to identify and respond to complications or setbacks in recovery. Patients who are discharged to another institution must learn what their options are, how their needs will be met, and how to coordinate financial aspects of the transfer. Even patients whose care is being transferred to other units within the hospital need to learn who will be caring for them and what to expect.

The nurse's ongoing relationship with patient and family members, ability to anticipate continuing care needs, and range of skills put the nurse in a unique position to help the patient with learning. In this section, we will review several aspects of patient and family teaching as they relate to discharge planning, including how learning occurs, how to plan teaching intervention, and how to teach a lesson. Our emphasis is on early identification of learning needs and on time-efficient as well as effective methods.

How Learning Occurs

The discharge planning puzzle has several very important pieces related to learning. Understanding how they fit together and contribute to the whole picture is the first step toward effective teaching. A reasonable starting point is to consider the kinds of learning that may need to take place. In general terms, these can be divided into three different categories of learning: *knowledge, attitudes,* and *skills.* The nurse's approach, choice of teaching strategy, and manner of evaluation of learning will differ for each of these. Some examples of different kinds of learning needs patients may experience are:

- Knowledge of the diagnosis and its implications for future functioning;
- Knowledge of their present treatment and what to expect of it;
- Knowledge of available resources for continuing care;
- Attitude of acceptance of present reality and any future limitations imposed by their illness;
- Attitude of trust and confidence in their caregivers;
- Attitude of self-responsibility for future health and well-being;
- Skill to carry out self-care procedures
- Skill in using and maintaining assistive devices; and/or
- Skill to communicate health care needs to caregivers appropriately.

Being able to organize potential learning needs into these three categories gets the nurse started with planning a teaching approach. Specific goals and objectives will become clear during the nursing assessment or a survey of the patient's health balance. Other learning needs will come to light as acute care develops and the nurse interacts with the patient and family. It is important that the nurse keep a perspective on what needs to be accomplished by teaching.

The goal of teaching is learning. Learning is a dynamic process consisting of three basic phases: readiness to learn; acquisition of new knowledge, attitudes, or skills; and a resulting ability to change behavior.

Once learning needs have been identified by the nurse, it is tempting to start teaching immediately. To do this, however, assumes that the patient or family member shares the nurse's view of needs and is able to concentrate on and make use of the teaching. Teachers who fall into this kind of trap find, to their annoyance, that learning has not taken place, and they must repeat the teaching again later. The problem is that the nurse has started the learning process in the middle rather than at the beginning. More effective and time-efficient teachers pause momentarily and evaluate the person's *readiness to learn* without making any assumptions. They strive to find out what pieces of the puzzle are already in place and how new learning can be made to fit into the larger picture.

There are two basic principles of learning that explain why attention to a person's readiness to learn is so important.

Principle #1: Learning progresses from simple to complex.

Learning is a building process; each new understanding rests on earlier learning, like bricks in a wall. Examples of this principle of learning are all around us. Children must learn to say words before they can structure sentences. Student nurses must have a grasp of basic arithmetic before they can accurately administer medications. Patients must understand what their options are before they can be expected to make decisions about their continued care.

For adults, life experiences provide the major sources of learning. Their attempts to solve problems lead them to develop a background of ideas, beliefs, and approaches that become their tools for solving other problems (Knowles, 1984). Before deciding how to help a person learn, the nurse needs to know something of what these experiences have been and what tools the individual brings to a new learning challenge. This knowledge will guide the nurse in planning how to begin, what kind of examples to use in explanations, and how much time to allow for reaching learning goals. For example, the person who has done the family shopping for years and the one who has seldom cooked or shopped for food represent very different starting points in learning about specific diet nutrients.

Principle #2: Learning is motivated by the perception that new knowledge, attitudes, or skills will help to meet needs or solve problems.

Without an awareness of a need to learn, a person does not pay attention to available learning opportunities or does not value them. Again, examples abound. School children often do not study a subject with intensity unless they know they will be tested on it. Nurses do not work on improving their comunication and teaching skills unless they can see that patient care will benefit. Patients are motivated to learn how to continue their treatments or medications at home only after they understand their importance to future health and well-being.

There is an old saying, often used to describe teaching, that "you can lead a horse to water but you can't make it drink." The challenge for the nurse who has limited teaching time is to make sure the horse is "thirsty"! This is done by finding out what most concerns patients and what their immediate goals are. Teaching is then tailored to these priorities, actively guiding patients' attention by helping them develop an awareness of their learning needs. The patient most concerned about whether he will be able to walk again, for example, is "thirsty" for knowledge and skills related to strengthening muscles. The nurse may have to help him understand that mobility would be better if he lost some weight and only then attempt diet teaching.

Figure 2–3 illustrates how the factors of previous experience and perception of need together with nurse-patient interaction provide the climate for learning to take place. The effective teacher helps to draw together the elements of readiness to learn and connects teaching to them.

In many patient care situations, the primary "learner" is not the patient but a family member or other significant person. Planning for continuing care often may not wait until the patient is able to actively participate. Sometimes several learners are involved. Each person will be ready to learn in his or her own way.

Effective teaching is individualized to meet the learner at his or her own point of readiness.

When one learner is ahead of another in understanding, that person might take the role of "teacher." For example, the wife of a heart disease patient might, under the guidance of the nurse, teach her husband what she has learned about cardiac function or exercise when he is able to participate. Similarly, when a number of people have the same learning needs they might be gathered together in a group and encouraged to help one another. Presenting examples and inviting discussion and questions will ensure that each person's readiness to learn is recognized.

We will examine the subject of motivation, particularly as it applies to changes in behavior, in Section 6.2.

How to Plan Teaching

Having determined what the patient must learn in order to continue care and how ready he or she is to begin learning, the nurse is ready

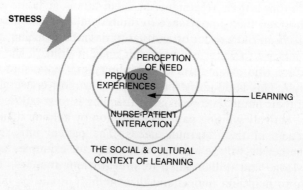

Figure 2–3. *Factors influencing readiness to learn.*

Table 2–2. *LEVELS OF LEARNING*

Knowledge	
1. Remember	To recall information
2. Understand	To grasp the meaning
3. Apply	To use the information
4. Analyze	To understand the underlying principle
5. Evaluate	To judge value and compare with other known information
Attitudes	
1. Recognize	To be aware and give attention
2. Respond	To react and give feedback
3. Verbalize	To be able to explain attitude
4. Utilize	To take action demonstrating attitude
5. Conceptualize	To make attitude part of one's larger value system
Skills	
1. Perceive	To be aware of component parts and their relationship to one another
2. Manipulate	To be able to handle parts appropriately but separately
3. Combine	To put parts together for coordinated action
4. Perform	To carry out sequenced actions and complete total task procedure
5. Adapt	To modify procedures to fit circumstances

to specifically plan a teaching approach by making a number of decisions about what should be taught, to whom, and when. These decisions will be influenced by the nurse's own knowledge base, the time and teaching resources that are available, and the learner's level of stress, ability to concentrate, and readiness to learn.

A decision about *what to teach* begins with the clear statement of the goal to be reached. Comparison of the goals with the information the nurse now has about the patient's level of learning readiness determines what the nurse starts with and how much progress needs to be made. Clearly stated learning objectives that reflect each step that needs to be taken in this process help both nurse and patient focus their attention on specific learning tasks and allows them to monitor progress as it occurs.

In his exhaustive work in identifying levels of learning, Bloom (1956) showed clearly how learning builds on previous learning. He also gave teachers a way to express exactly what they mean when they assess a person's current level of learning and state learning objectives. In Table 2–2 a simplified form of a learning hierarchy is shown. Within each domain or category of learning, five levels of complexity are named and described. Number 1 is the simplest and number 5 the most complex. The following case example shows how this learning hierarchy can be used to identify what to teach.

Example 2.2 Planning Teaching About Hypertension

Jennifer Dole was the primary care nurse for Mrs. Dorothy Ellis, a 46-year-old woman admitted for a hysterectomy.

On entry to the hospital she had been found to have hypertension serious enough to warrant treatment. In addition to post-surgical care, Jennifer's nursing care plan included helping the patient learn what *risk factors* were associated with hypertension and how *diet* and *stress* management could augment medication in lowering blood pressure.

In initiating teaching on these subjects, the nurse's first action was to assess what the patient already knew that might apply to the learning goals. By talking with Mrs. Ellis, she found out that she had had a basic biology course in college and had recently seen a television program on the link between stress and high blood pressure. Her husband had been on a low cholesterol diet, so the patient knew about dietary modifications in general, but had little specific knowledge of how to limit sodium intake.

Jennifer's assessment of Mrs. Ellis' readiness to learn was that she could "remember" some facts about the physiology of the cardiovascular system from her biology class. Reviewing this information gave her a starting point, but her goal was that she be able to "apply" this knowledge to her own situation.

From watching the television program, she could "recognize" that stress affects blood pressure, but the nurse's goal was for her ultimately to "utilize" these attitudes in her life and be able to "perform" relaxation techniques. With limited time, the nurse planned to work toward the "verbalization" level of attitude development and introduce the patient to a few simple relaxation techniques, aiming only for "perception." She would then refer her to a community education class where Mrs. Ellis could further her learning.

Mrs. Ellis indicated that she already had the skills to "adapt" her diet to meet health goals but was lacking in the knowledge of how to reduce sodium. Jennifer gave the patient some informational pamphlets on the subject and arranged for her to meet with a dietitian after she had read them to answer her specific questions.

In this case example, the nurse gave her initial attention to finding out how ready the patient was to learn and matching this with her general goals. By being very clear about what the patient already knew and what she had yet to learn, the nurse was able to teach effectively but with a minimum of time expenditure.

Utilizing previous learning as a resource on which to build means:

• taking the time to explore previous learning experiences with the patient;

- not making any assumptions about the patient's background knowledge, attitudes, or skills;
- being willing to adjust the content of teaching so that it has relevance to learners and their world of experience; and
- discovering that people learn more quickly and effectively when the nurse prepares learning experiences in this way.

The question of *when to start teaching* is answered by identification of specific learning objectives.

Generally, the length of time needed for learning increases with (a) the complexity of the new knowledge, attitude, or skill; (b) the number of people involved in a change of behavior; and (c) the degree of impact the changed behavior will have on the patient's life-style.

The nurse will want to begin teaching as soon as possible after she has determined readiness to learn. The state of mind of patient and family members needs to be considered, because learners must be able to concentrate attention and respond. Aside from obvious physical limitations owing to medical condition, disturbed concentration and response are most likely to be caused by pain or high anxiety levels. The nurse may need to give a pain medication or deal with a person's urgent concerns before attempting to teach.

Teaching related to continuing care is often left until shortly before a patient's discharge. Such teaching is uniformly ineffective for two basic reasons. One is that the patient's attention span and concentration ability will be limited because of natural anxiety about the upcoming transition in care. Another reason is that teaching done under the pressure of a deadline is seldom well presented and may sound like a tape recording played on "fast forward." The patient may be unable to make sense of a tangle of admonitions, even when they are offered with well-intentioned concern.

Decisions about *who should be included in teaching* are guided by the awareness that successful learning results in behavior changes and that those changes affect others.

Other people should be included in the teaching-learning process when (a) they will be affected by the patient's change in behavior, (b) they can lend support to a change, or (c) they share responsibility with the patient for a behavior change.

Including others in a teaching session means that the nurse must plan ahead in order to coordinate attendance and adjust teaching methods and materials. The socio-cultural aspects of decision-making and change will be discussed in more detail in Chapter 3.

How to Teach a Lesson

Exactly how the activities that make up the learning experience are planned will depend on the nurse's own knowledge in the subject area, the relationship and level of communication with the learner(s), and the available teaching materials and equipment. Added to these considerations are some factors the nurse may not be able to control, such as the environment in which teaching will take place, the amount of time available, and of course, the receptivity of the patient due to physical condition. Even though there is seldom an ideal situation in which to do patient teaching, the nurse can greatly improve learning by giving thought to the sequence of steps in each teaching-learning session or lesson. A typical pattern of steps is shown in Table 2–3.

A lesson may be only five minutes long or nearly an hour; it may be one of a series of lessons on a particular subject, or it may be a lesson planned as an isolated, individual response to a patient's question or concern. In each of these circumstances the pattern of beginning, middle, and end steps in the lesson will apply. The meshing of two gears illustrates this phenomenon: the gears are moved together and begin to engage their cogs; they are then able to run smoothly together. Finally, they disengage and move apart.

The use of several teaching strategies or methods as nurse and learner progress through a lesson sequence reinforces learning and keeps the interest of the learner.

Even short lessons may combine teaching strategies, such as explanation and discussion or demonstration and role play. They also may include different teaching materials such as pictures, written instructions, or videotapes. The following paragraphs give a brief description of each of the steps listed in Table 2–3 and explain their position in the sequence.

Step 1: Confirm Knowledge Base and Motivation. As discussed earlier in this section, the nurse needs to collect information about the learner's present knowledge, attitudes, and skills before attempting to teach. This information is used to plan relevant lessons that link new

Table 2–3. *SEQUENCE OF STEPS IN A LESSON*

BEGINNING	1. Confirm knowledge base and motivation. 2. Get learner's attention. 3. Clarify objectives.
MIDDLE	4. Present content of lesson and get feedback. 5. Provide an example.
END	6. Reinforce learning. 7. Summarize and evaluate learning.

learning with previous experience and knowledge. In this first step of a lesson, the nurse confirms that information as it applies to the subject at hand. The goal is to be sure that the learner's present levels of knowledge, attitudes, and skills have been correctly interpreted and that both learner and teacher are speaking the same "language." When complex concepts or skills are involved, the nurse will want to review material presented in previous lessons as part of this step before proceeding to new content.

Step 2: Get the Learner's Attention. It is important that the full attention of both teacher and learner be focused on the learning task at hand. This may be accomplished by telling an appropriate story or anecdote, telling the patient ahead of time to anticipate a lesson on a particular subject, having the learner perform an activity related to the subject before the lesson begins, or arranging the environment so that the learner is aware that something requiring full attention is about to begin.

Step 3: Clarify Objectives. Of major importance at the beginning of a lesson is letting the learner know what to expect. One of the best ways of doing this is to clarify what *behavior* is expected as a result of learning. This may be done verbally through explanation or discussion, nonverbally through use of a written version of the objectives and perhaps content of the lesson, or through a combination of these approaches. Learning objectives may be presented as the nurse sees them and feedback from the learner invited, or nurse and learner may decide on specific objectives together.

Sometimes an "organizer" is used to prepare the learner for the subject to be covered in the lesson; it provides a context within which to understand the new learning. A statement of objectives can serve as an organizer, as can a lesson outline. For example, the listing of detailed contents shown at the beginning of each chapter is a form of organizer, as is Table 2–3, which shows an outline of material discussed in more detail in the text. By using an organizer, the nurse can emphasize points of special importance while showing how other material relates to these points. Organizers are especially useful when the content of teaching is novel to the learner or when connections with past experiences are not immediately clear. Teaching patients about clinical procedures is often in this category.

Step 4: Present the Content and Get Feedback. This step is the lesson's "main course." The teaching strategies or methods selected may include any or several of the following.

- *Explanation.* This strategy is efficient but limited, because communication travels in only one direction, from teacher to learner. Its effectiveness is improved by using it together with other strategies. It is appropriately used for transmitting knowledge.

- *Discussion.* A two-way exchange between learner and nurse makes both equal participants in learning. This strategy takes more time initially, but can be very efficient in the long run because learning occurs at greater depth. It is appropriately used for sharing knowledge or altering attitudes.
- *Demonstration-coaching.* This multi-step strategy is ideal for teaching skills. Learners become more actively involved as their skills improve.
- *Experiential strategies (role play, behavior rehearsal, or exercises).* These strategies require careful preparation by the teacher and time to carry out, but are extremely useful in helping a learner develop connections between theory and practice.

Any of these strategies may be supported by one or more teaching materials: written materials such as instructions, outlines, or pamphlets; pictures or diagrams; audiovisual programs such as films or videotapes; or self-paced learning programs in written or computer form.

Getting feedback from learners about their comprehension, interest, and progress is a very important aspect of this step.

Step 5: Provide an Example. Most people learn specific material initially, generalizing it to concept level later. Examples and illustrations are therefore important adjuncts to teaching. Examples not only help the learner see how facts and ideas can be applied in a practical way, but also stimulate interest by helping the learner identify with the person in the case study or the problem solved in the example. This is why so many case examples and illustrations have been included in this text.

Step 6: Reinforce Learning. Just as it is important to follow through with a tennis or golf swing so that the ball gets to its destination, it is essential that the nurse follow through on teaching to ensure that the objective will be reached. Reinforcing learning is more than just repeating important points; it is helping the learner make the new knowledge, attitude, or skill his or her own. It gives the opportunity to involve the learner emotionally—and perhaps physically—as well as intellectually by applying new learning in a practical way. In most cases, the nurse will want to select a teaching strategy for reinforcement that is different from that used for Step 4. Learning is aided by involving as many of the learner's senses as possible in the learning experience: sight, hearing, touch, smell, and taste.

Step 7: Summarize and Evaluate. In this final step in the lesson sequence both teacher and learner have the chance to look back over the lesson, summarize what was learned, and decide to what extent objectives were met. In briefly reviewing the content of the lesson, the major and most important points can again be emphasized. Evaluating the lesson may be as informal as a brief discussion with the learner about progress made, or as formal as a written evaluation stating planned objectives in full and asking the learner to identify specific ways in which they were met or not met.

Both teacher and learner are, of course, evaluating the learning situation throughout the lesson. In one-to-one teaching the nurse can receive constant feedback by carefully noting the learner's nonverbal behavior as well as willingness to participate and respond verbally. This ongoing evaluation allows the nurse to alter the pace, strategy, or even content of a lesson to match the learner's needs.

In summary, several aspects of patient and family teaching have been presented in this section. We have emphasized the importance of determining the learner's readiness to learn and using this information to individualize teaching. Effective teaching takes account of the level of complexity that is needed and allows this and the person's readiness to determine what is taught and when. Planning lessons that develop through a sequence help the learner make connections between past experiences, the present learning process, and future applications for new knowledge, attitudes, and skills.

SUMMARY

In this chapter three important skills that the nurse brings to the discharge planning process have been reviewed. In each section, methods have been described for using skills in specific ways to prepare the patient for transitions in care. The health balance model has been suggested as a framework for a broad-based *assessment* of patient needs. The CONE interview format was described as a method of using a range of *communication* skills to gather important patient information. The sequence of steps in a lesson is suggested as a method of organizing learning experiences that allows the nurse to use *teaching* skills efficiently.

The effectiveness of the discharge planning process depends on the ability of the nurse to use the skills of assessment, communication, and teaching to help the patient reach beyond immediate needs to meet the long-range goals of continuing care and self-responsibility. The development and refinement of such skills is a continuous process. Nurses are encouraged to actively work on improving their skills by continuing their own education through the study of written materials such as the books described at the end of this chapter, through classes, and through honestly evaluating their use of skills to meet patient needs.

FURTHER READING

Arnold, E., and K. Boggs. *Interpersonal Relationships: Professional Communication Skills for Nurses.* Philadelphia: W. B. Saunders, 1989.
This comprehensive text covers many aspects of nurse-patient relationships including documentation, resolving conflict, and group work in addition to basic principles of communication. Exercises at frequent intervals help the reader apply concepts to practical situations and develop their skills.

Carkhuff, R. *The Art of Helping IV.* Amherst, Mass.: Human Resources Development Press, 1980.
An easy-to-read, practical guide on basic communication skills for those in helping positions by one of the leaders in counseling education.

Davis, A. Jann. *Listening and Responding.* St. Louis: The C. V. Mosby Co., 1984.
This book, written by a nurse, discusses basic communication skills for health professionals and then focuses on some specific issues concerning communication in health care settings. The chapters on Space and Communication (Ch. 3), Growing Old (Ch. 6), and The Pain Experience (Ch. 8) are especially helpful to nurses who would like to improve their sensitivity to patient needs.

Murray, R. B., and J. P. Zentner. *Health Assessment and Health Promotion Through the Life Span* (3rd ed.). Englewood Cliffs, N. J.: Prentice-Hall Inc., 1985.
Of the many approaches to helping nurses learn assessment skills, this book represents one of the more comprehensive. It uses developmental theory to organize topics for discussion. It is easy to read and has an excellent bibliography.

Rorden, J. W. *Nurses As Health Teachers: A Practical Guide.* Philadelphia: W. B. Saunders Co., 1987.
This book takes a very practical approach to patient teaching. It includes detailed material on learning principles and process as well as discussions of the health balance model and use of the CONE interview. The nurse involved in discharge planning will find the chapters on teaching strategies (Ch. 5) and teaching materials (Ch. 6) especially helpful.

3

How Patient Experience Affects Continuing Care

Sensitive understanding of the patient as a person is an important quality for health care professionals to develop in order to help patients and their families with continuing care decisions. In this chapter we explore what patients bring to the discharge planning process that affect their needs, their judgments, their medical progress, and their willingness to carry out a discharge plan. We begin with a discussion of the influence of stress on a person's health balance and why transitions in care cause an increase in stress levels. Next we explore some aspects of people's experience of themselves and how their personalities, their view of themselves as individuals, and their beliefs influence health behaviors. Moving outward to the social world that surrounds the individual, we investigate some of the social and cultural factors that influence continuing care. Finally, the realities about the financing of care and the impact of economic issues on the whole "world" of the patient are discussed.

3.1 STRESS: A MAJOR DETERMINANT OF THE HEALTH BALANCE

In the past decade "stress" has become a popular and somewhat overused term. It has been named as the cause of behaviors ranging from hysterical joy to homicide and as an explanation for athletic achievement, artistic creativity, divorce, sexual deviance, and mental illness. Stress is, indeed, common to all of us. It is a natural response to the changes that surround us. Its effects may be positive or negative, motivating or disabling, stimulating or overwhelming.

Patients are especially vulnerable to the negative consequences of stress as a result of their experience with unusual environments, unfamiliar procedures, physiological changes, and the uncertainties that accompany transitions in care. In this section we will define stress and look at how stress responses vary before focusing on stress as a factor in discharge planning.

How Stress Affects the Individual

A first step in understanding stress as an important influence on a person's health balance is to define the term. As Sorensen and Luckmann (1986) point out, usage of the word "stress" has changed over the years and still tends to have quite different definitions, depending on the author's orientation.

Hans Selye (1974), a physician and pioneer in stress research, defined stress as the "non-specific response of the body to any demand made upon it." This response involves stimulation of the hypothalamus, resulting in release of adrenocorticotropic hormone by the pituitary. By "non-specific" Selye meant that any demand, or "stressor," results in hormone-induced changes in the cardiovascular, respiratory, and gastrointestinal systems, thereby affecting the entire body. This response represents the body's normal attempt to adjust to the demand and preserve its balance, or homeostasis. Selye particularly emphasized that both pleasant and unpleasant events cause a stress response and that the body's physiological reaction is the same. Tears of joy and of sorrow are, physically, very much alike.

A principally physiological definition of stress is useful because it focuses on the individual experience of stress rather than on the many variables that might contribute to it. For our purposes here, then, we shall differentiate between a stress response and a stressor, using the following definitions:

> *Stress is the physiologic response that an individual has to a change in his or her internal or external environment. A stressor is any change that requires energy for adaptation or readjustment.*

By itself, stress is neither good nor bad; it is simply a mechanism used by the body to cope with its environment. As such, it is a normal and universally experienced response. Without some stress reflecting changes in our lives, we would be bored, static, and unmotivated to achieve or create. On the other hand, too much stress that overwhelms a person's ability to adapt is incapacitating. Selye calls this latter experience "distress." An individual's tolerance for stressful events depends upon his relative strengths, needs, and resources. (See Section 2.1 for a description of the factors affecting the health balance.)

People are often unaware of the physical effect that environmental stressors are having on them. The stress response may intensify so gradually that it is not until the person feels tired or irritable at the end of a day that a now high stress level becomes apparent.

Stress can accumulate over a period of time with both major and minor stressors, good and bad events contributing to one's current stress response level.

Holmes and Rahe (1967) showed that a major stressor may adversely affect an individual for two or more years, long after the actual stress event occurred. Chronically high levels have been implicated in cardiovascular disease, vulnerability to infection, and psychological disturbances.

A further factor in understanding the effect of stress is that a single stressor might cause responses of different intensity in different people, or even in the same person at different times. For example, a heavy rainstorm might cause annoyance in one person and near-panic in someone else. The variation in response depends on previous experience with similar events, the importance and meaning of the stressor to the person, and the already-present stress level. This makes it difficult for a nurse to assess a patient's stress response level accurately without more information than just identification of current stressors.

Knowledge of a stressor does not allow one to predict the intensity of an individual's stress response level.

In Chapter 2 (Table 2–1), an approach was suggested for obtaining basic information about a person's stress response level using an interview technique based on the health balance model. In the following case example, the patient's behavior suggested to the nurse that stress response levels needed to be investigated further.

Example 3.1 Anger Indicates High Stress Level

Frank Foster had been admitted with a diagnosis of bleeding duodenal ulcer. In the two days since admission, Mark James, his nurse, had found Mr. Foster to be very quiet but cooperative with his medical management regimen. Mark noticed that the patient had eaten very little of his breakfast and mentioned this during morning care. Mr. Foster immediately launched into an angry tirade about the tasteless food he was served, the noisy environment that kept him from sleeping, and how nothing was being done for him. The degree of anger and its vocal expression took Mark by surprise. He had been planning to discuss continuing care needs with Mr. Foster that morning, but clearly the source of his present distress needed to be investigated first.

In this case example, the sudden expression of anger seemed to indicate that the patient's stress level was extraordinarily high. The nurse needed to listen carefully to learn to what degree Mr. Foster really was upset by his hospital experiences and whether other kinds of stressors were also contributing to his discomfort. Steps to effectively reduce his stress would have to precede continuing care planning.

How Stress Response Varies

Diagrams or models are often helpful in understanding multifaceted concepts. A continuum model seems particularly useful for depicting some of the major principles of stress theory and their implications for patient care (Rorden, 1987, Section 2.5). The continuous scale of the stress gauge, shown in Figure 3–1, suggests that the buildup of stress can be gradual and that there are no clear divisions between levels. Although people's stress response level cannot be quantified like their blood pressure, the symptoms of stress that are exhibited and knowledge of stressors that may be affecting them provide clues for the nurse. Each of the four levels of stress shown on the stress gauge represents a grouping of commonly experienced responses to stressors of increasing intensity.

The stressors that produce an *alert* response are relatively minor, commonly occurring events. Their presence has enough impact to

Figure 3–1. *Stress gauge.*

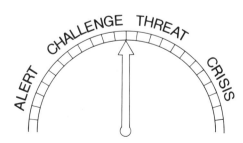

stimulate people's awareness and make them feel temporarily anxious, unsettled, or pressured, but accommodation to such events requires only straightforward problem-solving efforts. Stressors that might produce an alert response include changes in the weather requiring an alteration in clothing, inability to meet a previously planned time schedule, a temporary change in eating or sleeping pattern, or a minor physical complaint, such as a headache or mild dysmenorrhea. Each of these events would cause a normal physiological stress response, alerting the person to a higher-than-normal state of tension. As a result, the person would be stimulated to take action to minimize the disruption caused by the stressor: put on a sweater, make a telephone call, have a nap, or take an aspirin. If all of these stressors occurred in a single day, however, the person's accumulated stress response level would be high enough to make him or her much more aware of the rising stress level and somewhat uncomfortable. Consequently, the actions taken might be less effective, and the person might begin to show the effect of stress by nervous gestures or inability to concentrate.

Advertisers are aware of the usefulness of everyday, minor problems in focusing attention and stimulating interest in a better solution. Many commercial dramatizations portray just such a stressor being dealt with effectively by use of a certain product. As long as concerns experienced by their patients are not overwhelming them, as was the case with Mr. Foster, nurses can often use these concerns as a starting point for teaching or a discussion of continuing care needs. Even a complaint about hospital food indicates alertness to dietary issues and could lead to a discussion of food preparation after discharge.

The next level on the continuum model is *challenge*. A stress response at this level may include excitement, apprehension, and some temporary doubts about one's capabilities. Stressors that are likely to produce a challenge response are marriage, the birth of a child, a new job, or a move to a new community. Typically, these stressors challenge one's former roles in relation to other people or some aspects of lifestyle. They may present an opportunity for new accomplishments or creativity and a sense of personal achievement. Because a great deal of energy is required to meet the demands of these stressors, a challenging problem takes a central place in the person's life. Their full concentration is focused on it and they may not only ignore other issues but become annoyed and further stressed if forced to redirect their attention. A common response to a challenge is an attempt to learn.

Helping people meet challenges means helping them acquire information and learn new skills.

Alert and challenge stress response levels are confronted optimistically. There is no serious fear that one will be unable to meet the demands involved, although one may need to work unusually hard to accomplish the task of adjustment. This is what Selye calls good stress, or "eustress."

At a point approximately midway on the stress gauge, the optimistic viewpoint gives way to a very real fear that one may not be able to maintain control over one's life and circumstances. The upper end of the continuum is divided into two areas: threat and crisis. Others, such as Gerald Caplan (1964), use the term "crisis" to include a number of different stress levels, and some popular writers refer to stress only as a negative and destructive entity.

A *threat* response occurs when the demands placed on the individual by events or stressors are so great that they upset normal functioning. Stressors that may, by themselves, stimulate such a response are a serious illness, surgery, loss of a job, or family discord. Unlike the stressors that cause challenge, those that are threatening come on one uninvited, and often unexpectedly. They threaten some of the more basic human needs, such as safety and social belonging (Maslow, 1970). The responses they evoke may lead to loss of appetite, depression, inability to concentrate, and anger, guilt, or general anxiety. The person experiencing threat feels under attack. When a medical problem is involved, help may be sought and treatment willingly complied with, or in an effort to flee from the problem, the person may inappropriately avoid care.

People entering a hospital for care are certainly experiencing threat, if not crisis. Their personal resources are mobilized to fight off the "attack" of the stressor. Whatever caregivers can do to relieve the impact of additional psychological or socio-cultural stressors will free the person to use more of his or her energy to deal with the physical problem.

> *Information about what is happening and what to expect, recognition of individual needs, reassurance about the quality of care, and encouraging family members to show their concern and support all serve to reduce stress levels and allow the patient to focus energy on the medical problem at hand.*

Helping patients understand their diagnosis and treatment makes it possible for them to participate in care earlier and avoid being overwhelmed by a sense of powerlessness. For some people even a short period of lack of control is extremely upsetting and raises stress response to high levels (Houston, 1972; Janis and Rodin, 1979).

Many studies have shown that efforts to reduce patient stress to or below the threat level are important to the patient's acceptance of treatment, confidence in caregivers, and compliance with medical advice (Elms and Leonard, 1966; Johnson and Leventhal, 1974; Ridgeway and Mathews, 1982). Sime (1976) and others have identified some of the benefits of stress reduction as decreased need for anesthetic and pain medication and apparently improved healing.

Finally, *crisis* is a response to distress that overwhelms a person's present capacity to adapt and adjust. Stressors that cause a crisis response usually represent a sudden, traumatic loss, such as loss of personal possessions through fire or flood, loss of self-esteem through failure, loss of the relationship with a beloved person through death or separation, or loss of bodily functioning through mutilating surgery or stroke. The feelings that accompany such losses include helplessness, disbelief, shock and panic, or intense anger and guilt.

Any situation involving loss may mark the onset of a crisis response.

A great deal has been written about crisis responses, especially those prompted by death and dying. Consequently, we understand a good deal about the response mechanisms and stages of coping with this stress level. Elisabeth Kübler-Ross (1970, 1975) has been a major contributor to this understanding through her work with dying patients. A number of general principles that have evolved from this work are summarized below:

- Early identification, or anticipation, of a crisis allows help to be *immediate*. Once a person develops a maladaptive way of coping with a crisis, healthier responses are undermined. Such a coping method is difficult to change and can lead to permanent emotional dysfunction.
- A person in crisis needs support *through* the situation rather than assistance in avoiding it. Renewed strength and growth can occur only if a person confronts and fully experiences the reality of the crisis situation.
- A person in crisis should be encouraged to *express* the very strong emotions that accompany the experience. Such expressions, which might include heart-rending grief, explosive anger, or wild fantasies, help the person begin to come to terms with painful reality rather than deny it.
- A person in crisis is especially *susceptible* to influence by others. Although caregivers should avoid giving offhand advice or offering personal opinions in place of information, they do have an opportunity to encourage the person in crisis to accept appropriate help.

The early identification of a crisis response and actions based on these principles will give the patient the best chance of emerging from the crisis with coping mechanisms intact, or even strengthened.

How to Apply Stress Theory to Discharge Planning

There are two basic ways in which nurses can make use of stress theory in planning continuing care. One of these is as a basis of understanding patients' responses to treatment and to the physical and emotional demands placed on them by medical care. The second is as a guide for the nurse's own behavior in helping patients and families with discharge planning.

Early discharges do not allow patients much time to cope with their feelings of threat due to hospitalization, much less their feelings of crisis due to their medical condition. Their health balance is further disrupted if patients expect an extended period of rehabilitation or residual damage to their physical abilities. In the following case example the nurse was able to use her knowledge of stress theory to anticipate patient needs.

Example 3.2 A Distressing Diagnosis

Barry Nelson, age 30, had been a patient on Deborah Graham's unit for several days while undergoing various neurologic test procedures. As Nurse Graham passed by his room, she noticed that he was sitting on the edge of his bed in a slumped posture, apparently deep in thought. This was quite a departure from his usual display of nervous energy.

As soon as she had a few minutes that were unlikely to be interrupted, Ms. Graham went to his room, closing the door behind her, and sat down next to the bed. There was a minute or so before Barry even seemed to notice that she was there. When he looked up she could see that his eyes were red. She waited another moment and then asked gently, "Tell me about it?" The patient responded, "Yeh," and then told her that the doctor had just confirmed a diagnosis of multiple sclerosis. Barry continued to talk for some time about the likely effects of the disease on his life and his concern about his wife and young children. Nurse Graham recognized that the patient was in a state of crisis and needed support and attentive listening while he talked through his concerns. She hoped that his willingness to express his feelings to her was the first step toward his being able to use the support offered by the local Multiple Sclerosis Association, which sponsored individual and group counseling. In the limited time available for planning continuing care she would focus her efforts on giving him information about the Association and encourage his participation.

In this case example, the nurse observed a change in the patient's behavior that alerted her to his state of crisis.

The reality is that continuing care must usually be planned while patients and their families are in a state of threat or crisis.

Like Deborah Graham, the nurse will provide better discharge planning help if she or he evaluates the patient's stress level and focuses clearly on realistic objectives. Knowledge of stress theory will guide an approach to continuing care issues.

Knowing that stress is *accumulative,* the nurse will attempt to reduce the impact of environmental stressors on patient and family and actively encourage a trust relationship. The nurse will also seek information about other stressors in the patient's life. An unsupportive marriage relationship may not be the most important thing on the mind of a patient undergoing surgery, but it will have enormous impact on responses to planning care.

Knowing that stressors may cause a *variety* of stress responses, the nurse will be alert to behaviors that may signal a patient's present level. For example, Mr. Foster's anger (Example 3.1) was most likely an indication of a state of threat. A very passive, emotionally uninvolved patient may be in the "denial" stage of crisis.

Knowing that people do not begin or *progress* through a stress response at the same rates, the nurse will pay attention to the patient's family members, noting their behavior. It is quite common that a spouse will seem to be coping well with a patient's illness until planning for discharge begins. Confronted with the personal impact of caring for the ill person at home, the spouse may belatedly reach crisis.

Knowing that people experiencing threat or crisis are vulnerable to others' *influence,* the nurse will avoid making plans FOR the patient and will be alert to attempts by other caregivers to do this. Sometimes patients will ask doctors or nurses to take the responsibility for making decisions in their behalf. Not only is this professionally unwise, but it may make the situation worse for patients later; should plans not meet their needs, they will face the choice of either remaining unwilling participants or having to undo plans not of their making.

Finally, knowing that people regain their health balance in *small steps,* the nurse will begin to work with the patient and family on problem solving early in the patient's care.

> *Coping with threat or crisis is a gradual process of regaining control over one's present and, finally, one's future circumstances.*

Whatever steps, however small, the nurse can help the patient take toward making decisions and taking control of the immediate situation will contribute to reducing the overall stress level.

In summary, in this section, one of the most influential of the health balance factors, stress, has been discussed. Some principles of stress response have been reviewed along with presentation of a model that describes stress levels. We then have shown how knowledge of stress theory can influence the behavior of nurses so that the planning of continuing care is more effective.

3.2 THE INDIVIDUAL: PERSONALITY, SELF-PERCEPTION, AND BELIEFS

The individual's unique combination of characteristics and attitudes determine interactions with others, responses to experiences, and approaches to decision making. In this section, we explore some aspects of the "internal environment" of the individual as it particularly relates to health behaviors. While only a brief introduction can be offered here, these subjects bear in-depth investigation by the nurse who wishes to improve the effectiveness of continuing care planning. The Further Reading list at the end of this chapter provides some starting points.

How Personality Affects Health Care Decisions

Personality is the set of characteristics that we display to others reflecting our internal mental processes. Long before psychology was recognized as a field of study, those who were interested in human nature attempted to explain why people respond to experiences with some individual consistency. Today, thousands of volumes exist on this and related subjects. No one theory of human behavior has successfully explained all events or led to a comprehensive understanding of all people. Rather, each theory, at best, makes aspects of life a bit more understandable by presenting a generalization.

One of the theories that we have found to be of practical use in understanding nurse-patient interactions in general and health care decisions in particular is that of Carl Jung, famous psychologist and philosopher. In 1923 he proposed a theory of four personality types, or dimensions, that attempts to explain how people can have so much in common and yet function so differently.

> *Each of the four dimensions described by Jung is a pair of opposite characteristics representing a continuum. A person shares the four basic dimensions with all other people but has a unique blend of relative strengths for each characteristic.*

Jung strongly believed that one's inclination toward one or the other end of each continuum is determined at birth, but that personality continues to develop throughout life. Experience, personal insight, and the complexity of value systems all help to modify the strength of each characteristic (Schultz, 1977).

The four basic personality dimensions proposed by Jung are:

EXTROVERT ⟷ INTROVERT
CLOSURE (JUDGMENTAL) ⟷ NONCLOSURE (PERCEPTIVE)
SENSATE ⟷ INTUITIVE
THINKING ⟷ FEELING

The second and third of these are particularly relevant to health care decisions and will be reviewed briefly here. The interested reader will find a detailed description of all four dimensions in Kiersey and Bates (1978) and a discussion of how they apply to patient teaching in Rorden (1987, Section 3.4).

Closure–Nonclosure. The closure-nonclosure dimension of personality has to do with how people deal with the tasks and decisions of their lives. Jung called these "judgmental" and "perceptive," but these terms have taken on different common meanings with the passage of time. Although few persons occupy the extreme ends of this continuum, the tendency toward one or the other of these characteristics is usually clear to the sensitive observer.

Some people feel better if tasks are completed as they arise, decisions are made promptly, and their world of many roles is kept tidy. These people have a personality characteristic we will call *closure*. It greatly annoys this person to have a decision unmade or a project uncompleted. The strongly closure person can feel so driven to complete tasks efficiently that he or she sometimes draws conclusions abruptly or pushes for acceptance of a plan inappropriately. Viewed negatively, the closure person can be seen by others as being inflexible, compulsive, insensitive, and unnecessarily controlling.

By contrast, the *nonclosure* person prefers to carefully gather all relevant information before making a decision, even if it means a delay in completing a task; for the nonclosure person, a decision made is a door closed. He or she is not made uncomfortable by several things going on simultaneously, none of which may be finished within a predictable time span. This person may be viewed as being lazy or unmotivated by strongly closure people but may be appreciated for the ability to be spontaneous and flexible by those with a more positive view.

The results of surveys by the author (Rorden) of more than 300 nurses show that the great majority (85%) regard themselves as having strongly closure characteristics. It is not surprising that nurses at least behave as though they were closure types because of the diverse roles and tasks of nursing and the approval given to those who are well organized and accomplish a great deal. This characteristic, which helps nurses cope well with the diversity of their jobs, is a double-edged sword when it comes to planning continuing care. While organizational abilities are invaluable to some aspects of the discharge planning process, it may be difficult for the nurse to sit by a bedside listening attentively to a patient's response to an open question or be patient with a family's indecisiveness.

Determining whether a person leans toward the closure or nonclosure characteristic is often possible just from informal conversation about life-style and preferences. The closure person is more likely to tell stories about organizing, cleaning, and deciding, while the latter will tell of spontaneous activities.

Closure people often suffer even more than nonclosure people under the indignities of reduced privacy, feelings of helplessness, and loss of control that may accompany a medical crisis.

Their relationship with the nurse will be improved if care is taken to supply current information and include the patient in decision making as much as possible. If the nurse tells a closure patient that an event is to occur at a specific time, an unexplained delay is likely to cause some distress.

Nonclosure people are easier to get along with in a time sense, except when it comes to decision making. They also need to be given current information and data that will be important for continuing care decisions as it becomes available so that they can assimilate it slowly and not feel pressured as they near discharge.

When working with the patient's spouse or a close friend on discharge plans, the nurse may well find that this other person tends toward the characteristic opposite to that of the patient. Research has shown that, with this dimension in particular, the old adage that opposites attract does apply (see Keirsey and Bates, 1978, Ch. 3).

Sensate–Intuitive. The sensate–intuitive personality dimension relates to people's priorities and mental functions determining whether they focus on short-term or longer-term goals. Research indicates that far more people are strongly sensate than are strongly intuitive (Bradway, 1964).

The term "sensate" derives from the same root word as for "sensible." Sensate people are focused on the here and now of reality. They know that life is lived one small step at a time and are content with this. Sensates are practical, often efficient people who pride themselves on solving the problems of today without worrying especially about the distant future. For this reason they may find it difficult to set priorities or long-term goals.

The word "intuitive" is somewhat misleading, because people with a strong intuitive characteristic are not necessarily more sensitive to other people (the connotive usage of the word today). They are, however, capable of intuition, meaning that they can easily grasp the overall picture, even in a complex situation. Strongly intuitive people are basically future oriented; they are interested in what can become and what is possible in a situation. Their lives are often cluttered with unfinished projects (unless they are also strongly closure), because it is the vision of what can become that is more important than actually finishing the task. Intuitives are idealists, philosophers, business leaders, and teachers, pursuits for which a broad perspective is important.

From a practical standpoint, the nurse can assume that the majority of people encountered will be sensate. Because they assimilate knowledge *starting with the specific and working toward the general,* they will be stimulated to think about discharge planning if they are made aware of specific procedures that will need to be continued. They relate well to examples, cases, and demonstrations. The sensate stroke patient, for example, can be guided by the nurse to plan continuing care for the next three-month interval. He will also need to know how to get help with planning the next interval when it arrives.

By contrast, intuitive people assimilate knowledge *from the general to the specific.* They want to know the principle or process involved before they deal with the details. The intuitive stroke patient will want to know what the chances for long-term recovery will be. Even while planning more immediate care, this person will be acutely aware of progress toward the distant goal.

Intuitive people seem especially subject to depression and demoralization when faced with helplessness and a negative view of their personal futures. They are likely to be encouraged by a conversation with someone who has overcome their particular malady, since this gives them a positive vision to grasp. Although strongly sensate people may be overwhelmed by a similar encounter, they will probably be willing to "plug along," taking one day at a time, if they are given encouragement and continuing emotional support.

The following case example shows how one nurse used knowledge of personality differences to make discharge planning more effective.

Example 3.3 Planning a Child's Rehabilitation

Robbie Gates, age 8, had been admitted following a car accident. He had suffered head injuries in the accident, resulting in some brain damage. The most noticeable damage had been to speech centers; he had difficulty enunciating words and had regressed to using "baby talk" most of the time. Robbie's mother, Sharon, visited regularly every afternoon. Ellen White had been the nurse caring for Robbie most consistently, and she was anxious to discuss discharge plans with Sharon. Knowing how slow the school district sometimes was in responding to special needs, she wanted Sharon to contact them now about testing Robbie thoroughly and arranging special classes and a speech therapist for him. After two or three attempts at interesting Sharon in this plan, apparently without success, Ellen mentioned her frustration to Mary Rosa, a nurse who had also cared for Robbie and was acquainted with Sharon. Mary immediately suspected that the problem might be one of personalities. Her offer to talk with the mother was readily accepted by Ellen.

That afternoon Sharon arrived later than usual, explaining that she had dropped everything that morning to go help a friend hang wallpaper. When she had the opportunity, Mary suggested to Robbie's mother that they go to the conference room to talk about the child's continuing care needs. Sharon immediately brought up the other nurse's "insistence that I call the school to have him tested." She said she felt that was premature. Sharon had talked with Robbie's teacher so that she was aware of the situation. There would be a month or so during which Robbie would be recuperating at home. Sharon planned to work intensively with the child and felt that his favorite game, a computerized "Speak-and-Spell," could help him regain more normal speech. She concluded by saying: "You know, I really can only think about the next month right now." Mary's suggestion that a conference with the school's speech therapist might give her ideas about how best to help Robbie in the coming weeks was accepted as "a very good idea. I'll do that!"

Several factors may have been involved in Sharon's reluctance to implement a long-term plan for her child's continuing care. Stress would certainly have played a part, but the most relevant explanation for Mary was that the mother had demonstrated nonclosure, sensate personality characteristics. Ellen had focused on long-term needs and immediate decisions, giving evidence of a more closure, intuitive personality. An approach by Mary that took the mother's concerns into account and helped her make more effective short-term plans bridged the communication barrier.

A discussion of two of Jung's personality dimensions has been presented here to help the nurse identify some common themes in human personality and provide a way to communicate about some otherwise elusive information and observations. There is an obvious danger, however, in overgeneralizing or applying stereotypes to unique individuals. Perhaps the most useful aspect of this theoretical material will be to help the nurse identify why, as in the case example above, certain interpersonal approaches sometimes are successful and sometimes not; why the nurse sometimes relates immediately to a patient or instinctively feels that there is a barrier to trusting communication.

In Table 3–1, all four of the personality dimensions of Jung's theory are summarized, along with some suggested discharge planning approaches. It is important to remember that an individual's personality is a combination of characteristics of varying strengths. Distinct traits may not be identifiable. Like a jar containing different colors of paint, one color may be visible from one angle, yet another from a different angle; some may blend together and defy description.

How Self-Perception and Beliefs Affect Health Behavior

Self-perception is the way we see ourselves as distinct from other people (Muldary, 1983, Ch. 3). A concept or perception of self is formed as a result of interactions with one's environment. These interactions include experiences of success or failure, of support or alienation, of comfort or distress (Rogers, 1961). As a self-concept develops and a set of values are adopted, experiences that give messages that are contrary to what one has received in the past are especially upsetting. One often hears patients explain that they were motivated to seek medical care because "I just wasn't feeling like myself." In other words, their experience of self was not congruent with the way they usually experience themselves in their world.

A number of terms are used for various aspects of individuals' perceptions of themselves. One of these is "self-identity": people's view of who they are and what they are capable of. Another is "self-

Table 3–1. *SUMMARY OF JUNG'S PERSONALITY DIMENSIONS*

Dimension	Some Major Characteristics	Useful Planning Approaches
Extrovert* ↕	Sociable; easy to engage in conversation; has many visitors	Include significant others in planning sessions; use group approaches and refer to support groups.
Introvert	Seems quiet and introspective; may especially seek privacy; has few visitors, but they come frequently	Start with individual approach, encourage trust by stable staff, and show personal interest; use discussion in early planning.
Closure (Judgmental) ↕	Values organization, decisiveness, punctuality; anxious to get back to work/routine	Use structured, task-oriented approach; divide planning into small steps.
Nonclosure (Perceptive)	Values spontaneity, adaptation to circumstances; willing to take some time off to recuperate	Use open, discussion approach; connect planning with present concerns and goals.
Sensate* ↕	Values experience and practical problem solving; concerned with present reality	Start with specific and practical approaches; use examples and concrete illustrations.
Intuitive	Values imagination, insight, and speculation; lives in anticipation of the future	Start with principles and long-term goals; discuss consequences of actions in terms of fitting with future goals.
Thinker ↕	Carefully analyses new information; values rules and standards; uses few "feeling" words	Start with facts; build credibility and trust before approaching emotionally charged issues.
Personalizer	Interested in people, social values; uses "feeling" words easily; considers new information in terms of personal, emotional reaction to it	Build trust by good listening and reflection of feeling; allow person to think and talk through feelings about various care options.

*According to Keirsey and Bates (1978), there are many more people with this characteristic (3:1) than with the companion characteristic.

esteem": in what ways people like themselves, feel competent and confident, and feel likable to others. A term particularly relevant to medical care is "body-image": what people think they look like and how acceptable they feel that image is to others. All of these aspects of how people view themselves have three characteristics in common:

• Self-perception has a basis in *social* interaction. People's view of themselves is arrived at through comparison with other people. The attitudes and actions of others reinforce it or influence its change.

• Self-perception is more positive and optimistic when individuals experience a sense of *control* over the most important things in their lives. Priorities vary with personality but having personal power and control is important to all.

• One's present self-perception is potentially *threatened* by the experience of hospitalization. Loss of control by being taken care of, reduction in supportive interactions with family and friends, and changes in bodily functions and abilities all bring into question a person's view of self.

The effect of social interactions on self-perception will be discussed in Section 3.3 along with cultural aspects of discharge planning. As part of our interest in individuals and their internal mental processes in this section, however, we will explore some ideas about what a sense of personal power or control contributes to our well-being, how people sometimes "learn" helplessness, and how people's beliefs about the controllability of events determine their health behavior.

Locus of Control. A fundamental aspect of self-perception is a set of beliefs about the individual's ability to control events that affect him or her and the surrounding environment. This set of perceptions or beliefs is called one's *locus of control* and has been the subject of extensive psychological research (e.g., Phares, 1976; Lau, 1982). Unlike the personality dimensions, locus of control is vulnerable to change due to relatively brief experiences. (See discussion of "learned help-lessness".)

While people are usually classified as having an *internal* or *external* locus of control, a better representation of these concepts is a continuum. At one end are those people who believe that their own behavior is the most important influence on events in their lives; they believe that one "makes one's own luck." They are said to have an "internal" locus, or center, of control. At the other end of the continuum are those who believe that their own behavior has little impact on events in their lives. Outside forces such as God, luck, or fate are seen by them as more important influences. They are said to have an "external" locus of control (Rotter, 1966).

People's perceptions about their ability to control events in their lives determine their responses to illness and hospitalization.

The more internally focused people are, the more interested they will be in participating in their own care. Because self-responsibility is

Table 3–2. *BELIEFS ABOUT CONTROL OVER HEALTH*

Persons with these kinds of beliefs have a strongly *internal* locus of control:
1. I am basically responsible for my own health.
2. Proper nutrition, exercise, and sleep keep me healthy.
3. When I become ill, I know it is because I haven't taken proper care of myself.
4. The more I learn about my body, the better prepared I am to get well and stay healthy.
5. It's important that I work hard at getting well and staying well.

Persons with these kinds of beliefs have a strongly *external* locus of control:
1. Whether or not I become ill is a matter of luck.
2. The doctor knows best how I should take care of myself; I must do exactly what he tells me to do, even if I don't understand why.
3. Some people just catch everything that comes along no matter what they do.
4. It's not important to learn about health, because if you're meant to stay healthy, you will be.
5. If I become ill, all I can do is hope I get well soon.

Based on: Wallston, B. S., K. A. Wallston, G. D. Kaplan, and S. A. Maides. "Development and Validation of the Health Locus of Control (HLC) Scale." *Journal of Consulting and Clinical Psychology* 44(4):581, 1976.

part of their self-perception, they will welcome the chance to plan their continuing care and will take seriously recommendations about behavior changes that will benefit their health. Alternatively, strongly externally focused people may adopt a more fatalistic point of view and show little interest in planning future care.

A patient's tendency toward internal or external locus of control is usually evident in conversation and in the history of events leading up to acute care. A series of statements are shown in Table 3–2 that reflects either a strongly internal or strongly external point of view about health matters.

Those who have chosen careers in the health field typically have an internal orientation toward health beliefs. As a result, they find themselves in conflict with patients who tend toward the opposite end of the belief continuum. When the nurse does not share the patient's beliefs concerning personal power and control, ignoring the conflict or attempting to argue the person out of them will not be effective. A more useful approach is to identify some immediate concerns of the patient, establish short-term goals, and help him or her experience a measure of control in reaching them.

Example 3.4 Short-Term Goals Give Patient Control

Mrs. Hayes, age 71, was recuperating well from abdominal surgery but seemed to have little motivation to get out of bed or do things for herself. She complained bitterly about nurses who insisted she get up and who "forced" her to sit in a chair. At the same time, she frequently said—rather wistfully—that she hoped she would get stronger soon.

Martha Taylor had not previously cared for Mrs. Hayes but quickly sensed the patient's external locus of control. As she gave morning care, she talked with the patient about how she felt about her inability to "get up and about." The patient seemed genuinely concerned. Within a few minutes, Martha had helped the patient define some reachable goals; this morning she would walk with help to the chair, this afternoon they would try for the bathroom. Martha wrote the goals on a large sheet of paper and posted it on the wall so that each could be checked off as it was reached.

In this case example, an approach based on planning short-term goals with the patient was more successful than "over-powering" her.

Learned Helplessness. Hospital patients are typically subjected to stressors that undermine their sense of personal power and control (Taylor, 1979). Lack of information, inability to predict what will happen next, being treated in an impersonal manner, and loss of privacy all contribute to a temporary distortion in one's self-identity and a feeling of impotence and helplessness.

Psychologists have long been aware that repeated experiences of failure to achieve goals or exert control effectively have long-term effects on beliefs and behavior. Poverty, repeated discrimination, and long-term disability all have been shown to push a person toward an "external" locus of control. Research has shown that, in these circumstances, some people "learn" to be helpless (Seligman, 1975). They come to believe that nothing they do will affect events. Once "learned," these attitudes lap over into all areas of life, not just the one that caused the learning. People who experience intense helplessness because of a stroke, for example, may stop going for physical therapy, feel they cannot succeed in a job, and fail to make an effort to preserve their marriages. Their expectation of failure becomes a self-fulfilling prophecy (Gatchel and Baum, 1983, Ch. 4). The pervasive helplessness of a medical crisis has been shown to be very destructive for some people within a very short time.

Making decisions FOR people and in other ways contributing to their sense of helplessness may seriously affect their ability to regain control over their lives.

One of the most prevalent stressors during hospitalization—the lack or deliberate withholding of information—is also the one that can be modified most effectively by caregivers. Letting patients know in advance what kinds of tests are to be performed, for example, coaching

Table 3–3. *ELEMENTS OF THE HEALTH BELIEF MODEL*

Element	Description
Perceived susceptibility	Belief that one is in danger of contracting a given disease. When illness is present, belief in accuracy of diagnosis.
Perceived severity	Belief that the disease would/will have serious consequences for one's health, well-being, and/or daily life.
Perceived effectiveness of proposed action	Belief that a given action will be beneficial in preventing the disease or controlling its negative impact.
Perceived ability to overcome barriers to action	Belief that barriers such as cost, inconvenience, and effort are realistically surmountable.
Existence of a cue	An event, interest, or active concern that helps motivate action.

them on why those tests are important to their care, and *asking their permission* to proceed could be expected to reduce patients' accumulative stress level and increase their sense of control. (See Section 3.1.) Alternatively, frequent use of medical jargon in conversation with patients, talking "over" them with other caregivers as though they cannot interact, or referring to them by DRG classification rather than name all depersonalize patients, remove their sense of control, and greatly increase avoidable stress.

For the nurse involved in discharge planning, it is important to remember that people need a sense of control before they can be expected to make decisions or take self-responsibility for continuing care.

The patient who has been kept well informed during acute care, whose stress response has been minimized by the care of concerned staff, and who is aware of his or her rights as a decision-making adult is able to begin discharge planning earlier.

For these patients, planning is a matter of re-focusing control, not struggling to regain it before planning can begin.

Health Beliefs. In addition to general perceptions about the controllability of life's events, certain specific beliefs have an impact on health behavior. Rosenstock (1966; 1974; 1980) developed the Health Belief Model to explain why people seek medical help, take preventive actions, or plan continuing care. He identified five basic perceptions that must be present before a person is motivated to act. These elements of the Health Belief Model are listed and described in Table 3–3.

Example 3.5 Beliefs About AIDS

In 1982 the first newpaper reports began to appear about a "new" disease, acquired immune deficiency syndrome, or AIDS. This disease blocks the body's natural defenses to infection, making it vulnerable to certain rare forms of skin cancer and pneumonia. There was no known treatment, and mortality rates were virtually 100%. At first AIDS was considered to be a disease of male homosexuals almost exclusively. Then it became apparent that the incidence of the disease was, in fact, spread more widely. Intravenous drug users and those who received transfusions before effective testing was developed were especially at risk.

The 1988 publication of *CRISIS: Heterosexual Behavior in the Age of AIDS* by famed sex researchers Masters, Johnson, and Kolodny focused attention on the growing concern that heterosexuals, especially those with multiple sexual partners, were also now *susceptible* to AIDS. Surveys of young, sexually active people who were aware that they could be susceptible indicated that they considered the disease to be very *serious* and likely to be fatal within a short time of diagnosis; believed that the most *effective preventive actions* available were use of condoms and limiting or screening sexual partners; and believed that *barriers* to action such as purchase and use of condoms and changes in life-style could be satisfactorily overcome (*Newsweek:* March 14, 1988). Increasing numbers of requests by heterosexuals for testing were reported in many cities, confirming an increase in perception of susceptibility.

Cues that may have motivated action range from the many newpaper and magazine articles on the subject to knowing someone who has the disease.

In this example a series of perceptions were necessary before effective action would be taken to protect the individual. Other factors that could play a part in the health decisions of any one person are the ease with which condoms could be purchased without embarrassment and the strength of social support for a changed life-style.

These same perceptions are necessary before people will decrease their cholesterol intake, have a mammogram, take up an exercise program, lose weight, or take any other of the numerous actions to improve or protect health.

An important part of discharge planning is to be sure that a patient's health beliefs support the change in behaviors recommended for continuing care.

Only if they do will the plan be implemented effectively.

In summary, several aspects of the individual's "internal environment" have been discussed, especially as they affect health behaviors. Personality characteristics, self-perception, and beliefs about the controllability of the "world" shape a person's response to events such as illness. Two potential barriers to a patient's decision-making ability, willingness to take self-responsibility, and interest in continuing care planning have been discussed. Experiences of helplessness due to acute care or prolonged disability encourage many people to "learn" that they are unable to have much impact on what happens to them; they are at risk of adopting a long-term shift toward an external locus of control. Action to improve or protect health may also be inhibited if a person lacks a complete set of beliefs about a health threat. The sensitive caregiver takes a patient's characteristics, attitudes, and beliefs into consideration when approaching discharge planning. By building on strengths and personal resources, attempts to involve the patient in planning will be more effective and time-efficient.

3.3 THE SOCIO-CULTURAL CONTEXT OF CARE PLANNING

The social relationships that surround a person form a "world" within which life is conducted and individuality expressed. It protects and insulates the person from other dissimilar or "foreign" worlds. The patient brings his or her network of relationships to the medical care environment, and it, along with its background of ethnic patterns and cultural values, must be considered in giving care and planning discharge. In this section we will look at the issues raised by the socio-cultural world of the patient and explore how caregivers can work with it to give the best possible patient care.

There are several levels of intensity in a person's social relationships. For purposes of discussion, these can be divided into three basic groups shown conceptually in Figure 3–2.

Primary interactions are with those who know the person best and on whom she or he depends for non-judgmental support. These emotionally intense relationships are surrounded by a network of *secondary* interactions with people whose approval is important and who help an individual feel connected to the larger society but who do not share the extent of personal knowledge that family members do. Social interactions of varying intensity occur on a kind of personal

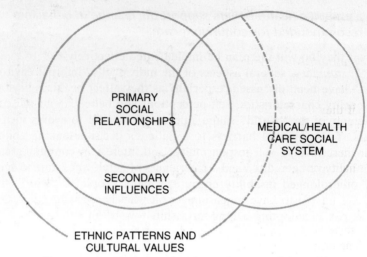

Figure 3–2. *Components of a patient's social world.*

"stage" with "scenery" made up of one's *ethnic background and cultural values.* These three levels of social interaction will be discussed in turn in the following paragraphs along with some comments about how patients are affected by the social system within medical and health care facilities.

Primary Social Relationships

For each of us, the most important or "primary" relationships within our social world are those with people who know us very well. We feel close to them and are likely to share our thoughts and feelings with them. They characteristically are familiar with many aspects of our personalities and know how we conduct ourselves within a range of life's roles. Their approval or disapproval of particular actions helps to shape our behavior, attitudes, and values (Goffman, 1971).

Those with a primary relationship to the patient are in a position to influence self-perception and the interpretation of life's events.

Although we usually think of a person's primary relationships as being largely composed of family members, this cannot be assumed. A family member may not be as close, caring, or influential in a person's life as a good friend.

The nurse generally finds it easy to identify members of the primary group of the patient because they are the ones most emotionally

involved in his or her present predicament. They either visit regularly or are referred to as wanting to be there. This small group of people represents a very significant resource for the patient. They are sought out by the nurse as having important information about the patient and as actively participating in continuing care. They are appropriately included in patient teaching and in discharge planning.

Whenever people become ill they are allowed, even encouraged, to play a special role in relation to those closest to them. This "sick" role carries with it the expectation that they will be taken care of and that their usual domestic, social, and occupational responsibilities are reduced (Gatchel and Baum, 1983). There are negative aspects to this role, however, including social awkwardness and a perception of decreased attractiveness. Individuals vary widely in the degree to which they accept and adjust to a sick role. Some people readily seek its protection while others deny their need to receive care for as long as possible. The behavior of the people in a patient's primary social group has a great deal to do with how the sick role is "played." Their acceptance, demonstrated by visiting and doing things for the patient, is generally reassuring and makes it easier for a person to make a transition to home care. Acceptance and concern become especially significant when the illness suffered has some social stigma, as in AIDS or cancer, is physically disfiguring, or is incapacitating, such as paralysis. Lack of acceptance by those close to the patient constitutes a crisis.

When those in the patient's primary social group are unable to demonstrate acceptance, they and the patient will benefit from referral to a social worker or psychologist for special help.

The nurse is in a key position to evaluate the behavior of family members and how it is experienced by the patient. Early referral for special help is a major contribution to the patient's future well-being. Some institutions have groups to which family members are invited to learn how they can best help patients with a stroke, or a burn, or a birth defect. Such groups usually deal with the issue of acceptance in addition to giving helpful information and clarifying expectations. They are a good way of involving the family in care and decision making. In the following case example, the patient's family needed special help to overcome their own fears before they could begin to help the patient.

Example 3.6 Family Resists Involvement
with Patient

Charlie Bert was admitted with a diagnosis of probable metastatic cancer of the lung. He had just recently consulted

a doctor about his increasing difficulty with breathing. A pleasant man of 62, Mr. Bert was undergoing a series of tests and biopsies to determine the extent of his disease. His history showed that he had been a heavy smoker for 40 years and that his wife had died two years before.

This was the third evening that Lisa Tanner had taken care of Mr. Bert. She was struck by the fact that he had had no visitors, although a large bouquet of flowers had appeared that day. When there was a lull in activities, she went to his room for a brief chat, hoping to find out something about him that would be of help in planning his continuing care, which was bound to become more acute. Mr. Bert had been reading but seemed happy to see Lisa. She admired his flowers and asked who they were from. He answered, rather slowly she thought, that they were from his twin brother and his wife. "Where do they live?" she inquired. "Oh, just across town," was the reply. Sensing the patient's distress, Lisa said gently, "But they haven't been in to see you." "No," he said, "I guess they just don't want to know me now." "Were you pretty close before you became ill?" the nurse asked. "Oh yes," answered Mr. Bert. "Why, I've practically lived there since my wife died."

They continued to talk for a few minutes about the events that had led the patient to seek medical care. Lisa then asked: "Do you have any idea about why your brother hasn't been here?" Mr. Bert looked away and responded slowly: "I don't know. . . . I wish I did. I guess they're scared of me now or something." Realizing that the brother and his wife represented a major personal resource for the patient, the nurse said: "You're going to need their help once you're discharged. I'd really like to see you talk with our social worker about the situation." "Well, okay," he replied, "but what can she do?" "Maybe between you, you can come up with some ideas about how to make a connection with your brother again. Seems like it might be important that this be resolved now before it goes on for too long."

In this case example, the nurse followed up on her observations and discovered information critical to the patient's future emotional, as well as physical, well-being. The crisis of his brother's sudden rejection needed to be resolved while there were resource people like the social worker available to the patient.

When people seek care from medical or health care systems, they find that those systems have social worlds all their own. Workers have

relationships of varying intensity with one another, they speak a special language of medical jargon, and a set of values and beliefs influence their priorities. Not surprisingly, most patients experience these medical "worlds" as foreign and frightening. Being cared for by "foreigners" is stress provoking, because areas of life usually reserved only for one's most trusted intimates are invaded. Having strangers see and touch their body and see their attempt to deal with pain and fear is very difficult for most people. The kind of caring and personal attention demonstrated by the nurse in the example above does two things: it reassures patients that, although largely unknown, this "foreign" world is not hostile, and it lets them know that resources not available to them before for solving problems can now be used to their advantage.

As the patient's and the medical system's worlds intersect, it is important that an attitude of equality be established by caregivers; they need to demonstrate that they will respect the patient's world and not attempt to substitute their own for it.

Doing this diminishes needless stress and anxiety for the patient and enables family members and significant others to maintain a strongly supportive position in the patient's care.

The Network of Secondary Social Relationships

If those in our primary world of social relationships know us very well in a broad sense, the people who are part of our larger social network know only one or two facets of our functioning, but may know those facets very well. This network is often role-specific: our work friends and associates form one part of it, people who share our leisure-time activities another part, and neighbors yet another. Each contributes to our sense of identity for that piece of our life. The feedback we receive from each group reassures us that we are seen by them as a "respected professional colleague," a "hard worker," a "good golfer," and a "responsible neighbor," and therefore we can see ourselves that way.

Faced with the loss of personal power that accompanies a medical crisis, our self-esteem and the security of our identity are severely threatened. (See Section 3.2 for a discussion of control and the effect of helplessness.) We acutely miss the feedback and reassurance that our secondary social network gives us. Hospital patients who are visited or sent get-well cards by members of these various groups respond with a renewed sense of belonging and wholeness. The nurse can greatly enhance the positive effect of this social feedback by showing

interest in all aspects of the patient's world. Not only is this kind of interaction interesting and stimulating for both patients and caregivers, but it also provides information relevant to discharge planning. The nurse can:

- help a patient display get-well cards on a window-sill where they can be seen easily;
- express interest in the person who visited today that the nurse did not recognize as a previous visitor;
- notice the patient's mood after visits and be willing to talk about it; or
- inquire about what the patient likes to do as leisure activities and whether group membership is part of those activities.

Pender (1982, p. 336) points out that the strength of a person's social support network affects emotional stability and the ability to cope with stress. One of the important ways this is accomplished is by reminding patients, who are likely to feel quite removed from their usual life experiences by hospitalization, of the larger reality of their lives. Concerned with one's own pain or prognosis, the patient may not be especially interested in the fact that Aunt Mathilda won a prize for her flower arrangement or that a trouble-making fellow employee has turned in his resignation, but these are items of news from the larger world that help the patient maintain a sense of perspective on reality. They also aid the preparation to re-enter that larger world upon discharge.

An important aspect of the assessment that precedes discharge planning is to determine the extent of a patient's social network.

This may be done formally or informally by a nurse, social worker, or other members of the discharge planning team. In any case, the nurse's observations are a useful adjunct to information obtained in other ways. The kinds of questions that are relevant to a social support assessment include the following (Glaser and Kirschenbaum, 1980):

- What *kind* of emotional, intellectual, and/or financial support do you receive from others?
- Who are the major *sources* of this support? Are they family members, fellow workers, or people representing other kinds of social connections?
- *How long* have they been giving this kind of support to you?
- What *groups* do you belong to and what kinds of support are offered through them? Have you received these kinds of support before?

- Do you feel that your present support network is *adequate for your present needs?* How might it be strengthened?

Whether patients are to be discharged to their own homes, to a rehabilitation program, or to other institutions, the support given by their social network will preserve their emotional health, help them remain oriented to reality, and promote their motivation to make positive changes in health behaviors.

The Influence of Ethnic Patterns and Cultural Values

America has traditionally prided itself on being a "melting pot" of diverse cultures and ethnic groups. We readily consume a range of ethnic foods from bagels to pizzas to Chinese stir-fry but often have only a very superficial knowledge of how values and social patterns are affected by cultural background. In a hospital, where all patients are expected to fit into the institutional social system, cultural differences are less obvious and can be inadvertently ignored by caregivers.

Ethnic patterns and cultural values provide the underlying structure to life; they give one a sense of historical continuity as well as personal identity with a special group. They provide general rules about behavior toward other people, define what is "right" and "proper," and determine how social roles are played. While language and religion are the most obvious differences between cultural or ethnic groups, many other attitudes and practices are influenced by ethnicity. These include rules for displaying emotion, sexual rituals and perceptions of attractiveness, and codes for nonverbal behaviors and their interpretation.

> *Because ethnic patterns and cultural values are so deeply entrenched and so pervasive in a person's life, it is important that they be identified, acknowledged, and accepted by caregivers.*

Not only do gestures of acceptance and respect give credibility to the nurse as a helper, but they make it possible to work with rather than against patients and their families in planning continuing care. For example:

- A Vietnamese patient's family brings special foods with "healing" properties to him in the hospital. Patterns of food preparation and beliefs about certain ritual foods must be taken into consideration when planning his post-hospital diet.
- A teenage patient is anxious to be discharged so that she can see all her friends. It is important to recognize the strength of the

social bond between members of this sub-cultural group and to work with the family to establish reasonable rules for visits and nutrition.

Caregivers are usually alert to the problem caused by the use of racial or socio-economic stereotypes in making assumptions about personal needs and preferences. Yet these same caregivers often fall victim to using more subtle, but just as dangerous, stereotypes in anticipating patient preferences. A nurse may erroneously assume, for example, that all Filipinos are Roman Catholic or that all Spanish-speaking South Americans have the same food patterns. In the following paragraphs a number of areas of major differences between ethnic and cultural groups are discussed briefly.

Beliefs about the Cause of Illnesses. As those who work in health care can readily attest, people have all kinds of explanations for why they became ill. Most of these represent a combination of half-understood ideas arranged to seem plausible to the person searching for a cause. Sin, scorcery, and magic are part of the explanation for illness in many parts of the world and lead people to seek the help and healing of a variety of alternative health providers (Moore *et al.*, 1980). It is not unusual, for example, for a Mexican patient to consult a *curandera* or healer and a Chinese patient an herbalist in parallel with modern medical treatment (Bauwens, 1978). The taking of vitamins and special health foods to prevent or treat illness is now very widespread in the United States. The potential interaction between these preparations and prescribed drugs should be taken into consideration for every patient.

Language. When a patient or family does not speak English, the special help of an interpreter is clearly necessary. Communication about values and beliefs is especially difficult in this circumstance. Nurses must take great care not to let stereotypes contaminate verifiable information. Not all Oriental families, for example, want to care for their elderly members at home.

There are shades of English ability that caregivers sometimes overlook. People may understand but not have the courage to try to speak English. They may be able to read English, but have difficulty writing it. A woman known to one of the authors was born in Germany but had lived in the United States for over twenty years. She seemed to speak, read, and write English flawlessly, but she was unable to phrase thank-you notes to those who had been kind to her when her husband died. The language of feeling is imbedded like an accent in one's native tongue and is the most difficult aspect of learning a second language.

Nutrition. Whatever the ethnic backgrounds of patients, it is wise

to inquire about the composition of their basic, normal diet, methods of preparation, and timing of meals before attempting to advise them on "good" nutrition. In areas where particular ethnic groups are prevalent, nutritionists will have information on how to adjust ethnic food patterns to patient needs.

Aging. Americans define the onset of old age as 65 elapsed years from birth. At this age the society expects the person to let go of various roles and "retire." This approach differs dramatically from other cultures whose definitions are based on physiologic function or newly acquired roles such as group leadership (Bauwens, 1978). There is some evidence that a person's culture influences not only when that person is regarded as old and how social roles are performed in later years, but also the physiological changes related to aging (Moore *et al.,* 1980).

Death and Dying. The way various cultures and ethnic groups handle death and dying, the rituals surrounding it, and the social significance assigned to it is a fascinating study. Nurses are encouraged to find out about the beliefs and practices of the ethnic groups in their areas. Sensitive and appropriate responses to dying patients and their family members do much to relieve the anxiety of facing death in a "foreign" place such as a hospital.

In recent years, attitudes toward approaching death have been changing in Western countries. The ethical dilemmas posed by increasing technology, gradual acceptance of patients' right to choose ahead of time whether extraordinary measures are to be used to keep them alive, the increased use of organ transplants, and the growth of hospice alternatives for the dying have all contributed to greater discussion about the issues and altered attitudes. Now that patients are more often told of their prognosis, the nurse has a greater role in giving support, helping families participate in final care, and bridging the gaps between the coldness of technology, the apparent chaos of medical crisis intervention, and human caring.

The above are just a few of the areas in which ethnic patterns and cultural values have an impact on patient care and discharge planning. In Section 2.2 we discussed aspects of communication, such as comfortable distance for conversation, touch, and eye contact, that are culturally determined. Members of other cultures often find that Americans speak too rapidly and too loudly, question too aggressively, and use first names too quickly for their comfort.

Socio-cultural barriers can complicate decision making and good communication with caregivers. The challenge for the nurse is to gather information about cultural and ethnic preferences while encouraging trust by showing respect for them.

Meeting this challenge means making no assumptions about patients' preferences and remaining alert to ethnic patterns and cultural values that affect their care.

In summary, we have briefly discussed three different levels of a person's social world: primary relationships, the network of secondary relationships, and the influence of culture and ethnic group. Patients bring all of these with them to acute care. Effective discharge planning prepares patients to return to the resources of their own social world and seeks to increase the strength of their support system by helping families learn to give support and enabling them to use community resources appropriately.

3.4 FINANCIAL REALITIES AND MEDICAL NECESSITY

Financial concerns are a pervasive part of acute medical care. They represent a major stress factor for patients and families. Financial resources determine the options available to patients in planning their continuing care. In this section we will consider some of the issues involving finances and then look at some of the realities that impose limitations on the planning of continuing care.

The Meaning of Money

In capitalist societies one is paid an amount of money for work done. This payment roughly reflects the value assigned that kind of work by the society. It is an easy and common extension of this principle to imagine that the amount of pay also reflects the value the society places on the *person* doing the work. Thus one's self-identity becomes attached to how one earns money, and one's estimate of self-worth to how much one earns. Ask most people to tell you about themselves and they will first describe their job. In American society, men are especially likely to identify personally with their job and to experience it as a crisis if they become unable to support themselves and their families.

In Section 3.2 some ideas were presented about locus of control and beliefs about personal power. Money allows us to control our world: to acquire necessities for ourselves and our families and to maintain independence from others. Abraham Maslow's hierarchy of human needs (see Figure 6–3 in Section 6.2) is reflected in how people generally use their financial resources. At the most basic level are food and shelter. If additional money is available, then the person seeks an environment that is stable and secure. Maslow described social belonging and positive regard by others as the next higher level in the hierarchy. Meeting this need can, however, involve costs for transportation and entertainment.

The length of time a person has been a part of a community and the availability of family and friends determine the amount of money that must be spent to meet social and higher-order needs.

In rural communities where extended families are common and the population stable, social needs can often be met without high cost by attending family gatherings or becoming part of community and church groups. The relationships that contribute to one's sense of belonging and experience of positive regard are relatively intense. In urban areas, higher incomes and the greater number of resources may be offset by less community stability, fewer family members and long-term friends available, and higher costs for housing, transportation, and food. Many urban elderly on limited incomes, for example, feel they cannot afford to go out or to belong to social groups and so become house-bound and lonely. They "regress" in a developmental sense to meeting only less complex needs, but this regression may well be driven by the lack of financial resources.

People who find themselves in need of medical care are especially at financial risk. Newspapers carry almost daily stories about rising medical costs and the inadequacy of federal programs and private insurance. Patients are aware that a major medical problem could jeopardize their financial as well as physical independence. They are asked when they seek care: "How is this to be paid for?" People often react to questions about financial resources in ways that signal the stress induced by the subject.

Financial Defensiveness. There are many degrees of defensiveness about financial matters, but all reflect the socially approved notion that one is personally responsible for maintaining independence. To do less represents personal failure. The defensive person regards finances as a personal and intimate subject and discusses it very reluctantly. As a result, even a spouse or children may know very little about family resources. Faced with a medical crisis, the defensive person is most likely to be willing to talk about the financial picture with someone identified as an "expert," such as a social worker, who can be depended upon to be an advocate in planning.

Financial Fantasies. This response is really one of denial, a common reaction to crisis. A person may refuse to discuss financial details, simply asserting that "everything will be all right." Similarly, a person may present a rosy, overly optimistic picture of financial resources. There is usually a large component of need for social approval as well as denial in this kind of response. The person who demonstrates a seemingly inappropriate attitude toward financial realities should be put in touch with an advisor promptly.

The above responses to potential financial crisis are complicated by the reluctance of most caregivers to discuss money matters.

> *Most nurses seem to feel that discussion of the cost of care is contrary to their altruistic ideals in providing nursing services.*

They are therefore very reluctant to broach the subject with patients or family members. They often justify this as not wanting to further increase the person's stress, but fail to realize that it is already a stress that will not be decreased by silence. Nurses also often operate on the fantasy that in order to discuss financial resources they must first be experts on the subject. While this is understandable, it is not true. Helping people begin to identify areas of financial concern, think through what they need to know, and clarify some of the financial demands of continuing care requires good communication skills but not an accountant's knowledge. Appendix B contains information on the basics of insurance coverage and financial assistance to seniors that will help nurses identify some of the problems facing patients. On this basis they can begin to formulate some of the questions that patients will need to consider while planning continuing care. In addition, nurses need to build their knowledge of sources of financial assistance so they can refer patients appropriately.

Medical Necessity and Options for Continuing Care

Discharge planning has to do with helping to determine a person's needs for continuing care and assisting him or her to select among the available options for obtaining that care. Reality is that financial considerations play a major role in availability. In the following paragraphs we will look at some of the more common sources of continuing care.

Self-care or Unassisted Care at Home. This option, in which patients care for themselves, perhaps with the temporary help of family members, is the least complex level of continuing care. Medical follow-up on an outpatient basis is usually part of this plan, and the costs are often covered by insurance. A more significant financial impact on many patients is the time they need to take off from work while they complete their recovery. Care planning that involves self-care must be supported by adequate pre-discharge teaching so that patients not only know how to take care of themselves but are also able to identify and appropriately seek help with complications (Rorden, 1987). They also may need guidance in clarifying sick leave provisions or temporary financial aid.

Family Care. When family members are available to devote the required time and energy to help with patient care, this option is usually favored. From patients' points of view, it allows them to remain in familiar surroundings with undisturbed social support. The financial burden is less severe than with institutionalization, but not absent. With early discharges, patients are often sent home with complex equipment that must be rented and which either the patient or someone else must know how to operate and "trouble-shoot." Hidden costs sometimes arise, such as needing to hire a babysitter for children while their parents provide care for the patient.

Emotional costs to family members must also be considered. A caregiver may be willing to give a patient I.V. antibiotics every four hours around the clock for a week, but the physical and emotional burden of keeping up such a schedule for a month is much greater. Cleaning up an incontinent elderly parent for a prolonged period requires enormous emotional energy as well as heavy physical labor, no matter how much that person is loved. Unfortunately, respite care allowing family members to take a break from caregiving is not readily available and/or very expensive. The cost of homemaker or companion services is seldom covered by insurance but may be available through Supplemental Security Income (SSI) or Medicaid in some states to those who qualify.

Nursing Care at Home. Intermittent skilled nursing care in the home under the direction of a physician may be available through Medicare if the patient qualifies. Otherwise, limited services may be covered by Medicaid or insurance provisions. Some policies are written broadly enough to include hospice care, adult day-care centers, or rehabilitation services. Home health agencies such as visiting nurse associations, available in most communities, sometimes offer these additional services. Hospitals are increasingly setting up home health care organizations for their own patients. The problem for medical professionals is determining what constitutes a need for "skilled" nursing care. Privately-paid-for care is expensive but may be a reasonable alternative to placement in a convalescent or skilled nursing facility.

Intermediate and Custodial Care. The frail aged and those with chronic disabilities often need help with activities of daily living. They need help getting in and out of bed, assistance with meal preparation, or help taking medications, but not "skilled" nursing care. This is a level of care that is likely to be prolonged and therefore insurance coverage for it is very expensive. Intermediate and custodial levels of care may be provided in a nursing home, in a board-and-care home, or in some retirement facilities. Costs are not covered by Medicare, but a person may be eligible for Medicaid help if his or her assets are below state limits. The financial reality is that many people must become "poor" using up much of their financial resources before they qualify for assistance. Since the cost of such care varies from $22,000 to $45,000 per year, this often does not take long; *Consumer Reports* (May 1988) estimates an average of 13 weeks. Some states, such as California, have laws that protect the spouse's resources, but the validity of these laws has been called into question by recent legislation.

Nursing Home Care. Care in an approved home is covered by Medicare but only for as long as "skilled" nursing is necessary. Prior hospitalization has now been dropped as a requirement. Many of the now proliferating nursing home insurance policies do, however, require hospitalization prior to coverage or maintain the right to disallow a claim. They are especially reluctant to provide care for patients with Alzheimer's disease or with mental disorders or alcoholism.

It is important that nurses and patients recognize that the provisions of Medicare, Medicaid, and private insurance change frequently and are interpreted differently by different people. Learning what to ask and developing a sense of assertiveness about pursuing the answers are crucial steps toward planning continuing care.

In summary, financial considerations have been discussed as having two major areas of impact on discharge planning. People's self-identity and esteem are often connected to their perception of financial "success." Because of this, it is an emotional subject that many people, including caregivers, react to with defensiveness or denial. At the same time, it is essential that economic realities be carefully evaluated as part of discharge planning since they so directly affect patients' options for continuing care. The reader is referred to Appendix B for information on insurance coverage and financial assistance to seniors.

SUMMARY

In this section we have explored some aspects of individual experience that affect the discharge planning process. Stress and stress response were the first to be examined. In most cases the planning of continuing care must take place while the patient is experiencing very high stress levels. Variations in stress response were described and some guidance was given to nurses in applying their knowledge of stress theory to more effective planning. Several aspects of a person's internal mental processes were then discussed. Personality, self-perception, and beliefs all have important implications for how planning is approached, what the patient expects, and the degree of self-responsibility that is taken for future care. A number of theories and models were presented as examples, and their application to discharge planning discussed. Next we looked at how people's values, priorities, and expectations are shaped by the social and cultural world surrounding them. We noted those aspects of the patient's social world that are especially significant in planning continuing care. Finally, financial concerns were discussed in terms of their importance as an emotional issue for many people and as a determinant of realistic options for continuing care.

FURTHER READING

Aronson, S., and M. Mascia. *The Stress Management Workbook*. New York: Appleton-Century-Crofts, 1981.
There are innumerable books on the market on stress management, but this one is recommended because it represents a unique approach to the subject. As well as presenting stress theory in a clear and readable way, it helps the reader apply the concepts of stress management to his or her own life through use of the many worksheets. Not only is this material valuable for the nurse, but it provides many good ideas about how to assess the stress levels of patients and their families.

Goffman, Erving. *Presentation of Self in Everyday Life* (1971) and *Stigma* (1968). Harmondsworth, U.K.: Penguin.
These two Penguin paperbacks are classics in the field of sociology but are easy to read and well worth the effort. In Presentation of Self, *Goffman shows how social expectations as well as self-perceptions influence how we choose a "self" to present to others. In* Stigma *he examines defensive behavior, arguing that everyone has a characteristic that they regard as a social liability. Both books lead to better understanding of others and, just as importantly, insight into one's self.*

Keirsey, D., and M. Bates. *Please Understand Me*. Del Mar, Calif.: Prometheus Nemesis Books, 1978.
This fascinating little book begins with a questionnaire that helps the reader identify his or her own Jungian personality type. It then discusses each of the personality dimensions and their combinations before describing how different personalities and temperaments complement or conflict with each other in families, marriage, work, and leadership. It is highly readable, but sometimes difficult to get from the publisher (P.O. Box 2082, Del Mar, CA, 92014).

Sampson, Chris. *The Neglected Ethic: Religious and Cultural Factors in the Care of Patients*. London: McGraw-Hill Book Co. (U.K.) Ltd., 1982.
There are many publications that are useful references for the nurse in developing understanding of different cultures, but few are as immediately helpful as this one. Written by a British nurse, it does not give information in any great depth, but it does cover facts that are essential to the nurse for giving culturally sensitive patient care. The fourth chapter, for example, lists religions alphabetically and

summarizes the special beliefs or practices of each. It includes a wide range of Eastern religions and sects.

Seligman, Marvin. *Helplessness: On Depression, Development, and Death.* San Francisco: W. H. Freeman, 1975.
Written by a major researcher in the area of learned helplessness, this book is fascinating and deeply disturbing. It is a work that needs to be read and its implications discussed and understood by all who care professionally for other people.

4

How Teamwork Contributes to Discharge Planning

Continuing care always involves a number of individuals. In previous chapters we looked at the skills brought to the discharge planning process by the nurse and the experiences, individual differences, and social network brought by the patient. In this chapter we explore how the knowledge and skills of health professionals in addition to the nurse can contribute to that process, especially its assessment and decision-making phases (see Figure 1–2). We begin by identifying professional groups that are likely to be available within an acute care setting and then discuss a variety of approaches to organizing and coordinating planning efforts. This is followed by a series of extended case examples that show how concepts of coordination and teamwork have been combined in practice. Finally, we focus on the patient and family as active participants of the discharge planning team.

Communication skills are especially important when a number of people with different backgrounds work toward a common goal. The promotion of good interdisciplinary communication is the general theme of this chapter.

4.1 IDENTIFYING HEALTH TEAM RESOURCES

While patients are receiving acute medical care, they have many more needs than usual, but they also have access to a wide variety of helping resources. As discussed in Chapter 3, the stress that patients experience as a result of medical treatment, their sudden dependency, and anxiety about their future may make them more willing than usual to reconsider their health behaviors. A person's state of crisis presents an opportunity to use the now readily available resources to acquire new knowledge, attitudes, and skills. The patient's doctor and the nurse are the key figures in beginning to assess what steps are appropriate for the person's future well-being. Even while the patient and family are struggling to cope with the acute aspects of illness, the experience of the nurse and doctor alerts them to probable and possible needs much further away in time.

> *The first step toward effective discharge planning consists of answers to the following questions: (1) Can a full assessment of the patient's health balance be made on the basis of information now available? and (2) Are the patient's strengths and resources adequate to restore the health balance after discharge?*

Other health professionals may become involved in either or both of two ways in answering these questions. One is to help gather additonal *information* about the patient's needs, stressors, strengths, and resources so that the health balance may be more fully assessed. The other is to offer *assistance* in the form of counseling, teaching, and coordination when it seems that the health balance cannot be restored without additional help.

In this section we will list those people who might be involved in discharge planning and note some areas of contribution that their professional education or experience will allow them to make. These notes are, of course, only general guidelines for nurses; in working with their colleagues they will undoubtedly discover individual talents or limitations that will modify nurses' approaches to them as sources of help.

The Core of the Team: Nurse, Doctor, and Social Worker

In addition to the nurse, the patient's physician and the social worker make up the core of the discharge planning team. They have the opportunity to work with patients and their families intensively so that transitions in care are well supported and continuing care needs met. The skills brought by the nurse to the discharge planning process have been explored in Section 1.4.

The Physician. In times past and in small communities now, the patient's doctor had/has a full picture of where the patient came from in geographical, physical, and emotional senses. Aside from providing medical care over a period of time, the doctor could be counted on to know the socio-economic context of the patient's life, if not the details of family relationships. If hospitalization was recommended, the doctor was/is involved in that hospital care and in post-hospital follow-up care. In urban America, this kind of continuity is much less common. Increasing specialization in medical practice and the mobility of the population contribute to the likelihood that a patient will see a physician for episodic care only. If a person goes directly to an emergency room for treatment, care will be directed by people unknown to him or her personally. If a person goes first to a neighborhood clinic, the physician there may not participate in hospital care. If a person belongs to the high risk group of low-income elderly, his or her medical care is commonly fragmented by inadequate communication between multiple past and present caregivers.

The doctor is often faced with the frustration of making decisions about a patient's care based on limited information.

The dilemma for physicians is that while they have legal responsibility for directing the total care of patients, they often lack information about any but the immediate pathophysiologic needs.

The problem of incomplete information becomes more complicated and communication more difficult when several medical specialists are involved in a single patient's care. If roles and responsibilities are unclear, the quality of care is quickly affected.

Sometimes physicians seem to other caregivers to have a very limited perspective of comprehensive care and be uninterested in issues beyond the pathophysiologic. There may be a number of explanations for these apparent attitudes, including time limitations and defensiveness about legal liability. A professor of internal medicine at a major teaching hospital recently noted that early discharges and higher patient acuity are responsible for an attitude shift by physicians-in-training; they see patients only in acute medical distress and often lose sight of the patient as an individual with a job, a family, a community, and a future.

Physicians have found a variety of ways to bridge the gaps between their legal responsibilities, the pressure of time, and their practical involvement in discharge planning. Some, like Master (1981), encourage nurses to assume "parallel management" responsibilities for the patient, including the initiation of the discharge planning process. Some employ physician's assistants to look after the continuing care needs of their patients. Some have developed routines for regularly referring patients to discharge planning units. Some have organized their practices so that they are able to actively participate in the full spectrum of patient care in the hospital, nursing home, and community, even though that means reducing the number of patients they serve. As legislation on medical and health care issues continues to change, so will the solutions to practical problems of patient management. In the meantime, the role of the physician in discharge planning is generally seen to include (Hartigan and Brown, 1985):

- Awareness of all those involved in a patient's care as well as potential sources of care in acute and community settings;
- Awareness of continuity of care problems and support for discharge planning activities;
- Willingness to share information about patient and family that can facilitate continuing care plans;
- Communication with patient and family to clarify available patient options and the roles of those involved in discharge planning;
- Communication of medical orders for continuing care as early in a patient's acute care as possible; and
- Approval of details of the discharge plans and referrals to other professionals or agencies.

It is the physician who is looked to by the public and his or her professional colleagues to take the lead in patient management that includes continuing as well as acute care.

The Social Worker. Historically, social workers have always been recognized as an important part of the team in planning continuing care. Their background of knowledge and skills allows them to assess the psycho-dynamic and socio-economic aspects of patient care and to help formulate a plan that meets the broad spectrum of patient needs. They have often been appointed to coordination positions in the discharge planning units of acute care institutions.

The fact that social workers are not involved in the day-to-day, minute-by-minute physical care of the patient has both advantages and disadvantages. Their willingness to form a special relationship with patient and family is greatly appreciated by those who welcome the opportunity to work through the many non-medical repercussions of a medical crisis with a competent professional. On the other hand, they may on occasion be regarded as outsiders: emotionally uninvolved authority figures who represent the institution and come to enforce painful economic realities. Social workers appropriately focus on the patient as a person with a whole spectrum of short- and long-term needs. Medically oriented caregivers may eagerly endorse this broad perspective or, faced with urgent medical needs, they may see the social worker as an unwelcome intruder.

The social worker contributes a broad perspective to acute and continuing patient care that includes psychological, social, economic, and cultural concerns.

Her or his ability to do this positively depends upon personality and communication skills as well as professional preparation, and upon the clarity of job responsibilities and degree of organizational support as well as personal competence.

Social workers have three avenues to follow in their work with patients and families: direct or case-work services, consultation, and coordination or management services (Sandman, 1981). Some of the particular contributions the social worker might make to discharge planning include:

- Detailed assessment of psycho-dynamic and socio-economic aspects of a patient's present situation and probable future needs;
- Crisis intervention with patient and family in meeting the psychological and social demands of acute care;
- Counseling and support for patient and family members;
- Consultation with other caregivers about family dynamics and the implications of ethnic patterns and cultural values; and
- Information about and coordination with sources of economic aid and community care.

The social worker is able to supply information critical to the success of discharge planning and also to function as an additional source of strength and support for patients and families. Together with the physician and the nurse, the social worker forms part of the basic discharge planning team (see Figure 4–1, page 118). It is essential that these three people work well and trustingly with one another if patient needs are to be met during transitions in care and on a continuing basis.

Clinical Consultants and Specialists

The Therapist: Physical, Occupational, Respiratory, and Speech. Each of these specialists has his or her own extremely valuable contribution to make to the discharge planning process. Any or all are appropriately involved in the assessment, treatment, and continuing care of patients who are likely to have residual impairment in functioning.

The physical therapist is concerned with restoration of physical functioning, alleviation of pain, and the prevention of disability.

The occupational therapist is concerned with regaining and maintaining the patient's ability to meet the demands of the environment including activities of daily living (ADL), use of special equipment, and a wide range of social and occupational activities.

The respiratory therapist is concerned with maintaining the integrity of the respiratory system, including analysis of requirements and energy conservation.

The speech therapist is concerned with all aspects of communication, including its development and maintenance and the treatment of disorders.

Therapists focus on the practicalities of how a patient carries out the normal functions of life. The importance of what they have to offer becomes apparent when viewed in the context of the patient's needs for a positive self-perception, independence, and sense of control. These health professionals are experts in helping patients regain or maintain physical, social, and economic functioning. Some of the particular contributions that therapists make to discharge planning include:

- Treatment during acute care to limit the long-term affects of the disease process;
- Interpretation of progress toward self-care goals;
- Assessment of continuing care needs;
- Consultation with other health professionals about patient needs and realistic plans;
- Patient and family teaching in preparation for discharge;
- Coordination with community-based therapists for continuity of care.

In some institutions the therapies are part of a department of rehabilitation. This organization often facilitates consultation with these health professionals and perhaps other allied therapists or teams such as those working especially with cardiac or stroke rehabilitation or recreation. The importance of the role therapists take in the assessment of a patient's present and future capabilities and in patient education cannot be over-emphasized.

Clinical Dietitian or Nutritionist. Like therapists, clinical dietitians and nutritionists are concerned with helping patients with the practicalities of everyday life. Food has many meanings in our society aside from pure sustenance: celebration, pleasure, stress reduction, self-control, and sharing, for example. The dietary expert takes these meanings and socio-cultural patterns into consideration as well as the patient's need for nutrients in helping construct plans for continuing care.

The clinical dietitian or nutritionist is able to assess patients' nutritional needs and make continuing care plans for dietary intake that are consistent with these needs, health care goals, and family and cultural food patterns.

The dietitian makes an extremely important contribution to continuing care through patient and family education. This may include helping them learn to plan diets, prepare foods properly, store supplies adequately, and modify food habits and behaviors appropriately. As Kearney and Gleason-Claydon (1981, p. 132) put it so graphically: "The health care facility is a learning center, and the patient participates in a 'live-in' course. The community and nutritional follow-up provided for in the discharge plan serve as the 'refresher' course."

The nutritionist or dietitian is appropriately called on by the discharge planning team to assess needs and present food patterns, observe and record nutritional intake during acute care, make dietary plans, teach patient and family, consult with other caregivers, and coordinate plans with community resources. Implementing nutritional changes to correlate with activity changes, evaluating the need for dietary supplements, and alerting the patient and medical care personnel to drug/food interactions are special contributions that are made by the dietitian to continuing care.

The Pharmacist. A sometimes overlooked member of the discharge planning team is the pharmacist; he or she may be regarded as a service rather than as a health professional able to contribute to continuing care in a variety of important ways.

The pharmacist not only supplies medications but is able to advise doctor, nurse, and patient about dosages, routes of administration, side effects, interactions, availability, and cost.

With today's complex medical treatments and early discharges that send patients home with total parenteral nutrition (TPN) and involved medication regimens, the pharmacist is an invaluable source of information and help in planning. He or she can also provide an important link with community sources of medications and medical supplies.

Other Specialists and Consultants. One of the most identifiable groups of specialists and consultants who are frequently involved in continuing care are mental health professionals. They range from nurse specialists, psychologists, and psychiatric social workers to psychiatrists. Professionals in many other specialty areas, however, may also contribute to discharge planning through assessment, patient teaching, consultation, and coordination with community services. They may include:

• Clinical nurse specialists (e.g., pediatric, ostomy, oncology);

- Counselors or psychologists (e.g., for aptitude testing, resolution of interpersonal problems, budget planning, staff support);
- Medical specialists and consultants;
- Education specialists (e.g., for teaching materials, help with teaching plans, learning evaluations);

In addition to these kinds of special resources are the representatives and consultants for community services, agencies, and groups. The contribution that these people make to the discharge planning team will be discussed fully in Chapter 5.

> *Whenever a patient has special needs or uncommon continuing care goals, the nurse is wise to look beyond the usual discharge planning team members and identify others who may give special help with problem solving.*

The nurse's creativity and resourcefulness will be well rewarded by more effective plans and better patient progress.

The Discharge Planning Coordinator. As discussed in Section 1.2, the provision of discharge planning services is one of the requirements for institutions serving Medicare patients. Although known by a variety of titles, the person who leads the discharge planning effort for Medicare and Medicaid patients is either a nurse or a social worker. In many instances, these are the *only* patients that they have time to serve.

> *While not able to be involved in the discharge of every patient, the discharge planning coordinator is a valuable resource person whose knowledge and experience contribute greatly to high quality continuing care.*

Discharge planning coordinators can point out potential problems, suggest how best to approach planning, and identify resources in both hospital and community; their willingness to share their expertise saves the nurse a great deal of time and fruitless effort.

Some hospitals have adopted a pattern of regular "rounds" with the coordinator on each patient care unit. At that time the coordinator can be consulted about the continuing care needs of any and all patients. This has proven time efficient and an effective use of coordinators' expertise in helping nurses develop discharge planning skills.

Other Sources of Discharge Planning Assistance

The Clergy. Another group often overlooked as members of the discharge planning team are the clergy. Although their contribution as a source of support and comfort in instances of terminal illness or grief is well known, their use as consultants and assessors of patient needs is not.

The clergy is a valuable resource for patients, families, and staff members about quality of life and moral/ethical issues. He or she can interpret cultural and religious priorities as well as provide special strength and support to patients.

It is often imagined by caregivers that the representative of a particular religious group has knowledge of that group only and prefers to limit his services to them. It may come as a surprise that most clergy know a great deal about other belief patterns and that they take opportunities for consultation and liaison roles as seriously as they do the direct human services and compassionate care they offer. One of the authors was once helped to a much better understanding of Jewish traditions and beliefs by a Roman Catholic nun. As discussed in Section 3.3, social and cultural considerations are enormously important to a person's self-perception and emotional health. The clergy are an important part of this aspect of continuing care.

Utilization Review Staff. In some institutions, those charged with utilization review are regarded as working against effective discharge planning; in other institutions the same person, usually a nurse called a "Patient Resources Specialist," does both review and discharge planning coordination.

If the patient's care is not to suffer, the people responsible for utilization review and discharge planning need to have a good understanding of each other's goals and effective ongoing communication, if not coordination of effort.

The antagonism that can develop between the two functions has a historical basis. Discharge planning was seen as part of quality patient care long before utilization review procedures were set up to monitor the discharge process. Confusion over legal requirements and Medicare/Medicaid qualifications has added to the problem. Generally speaking, it is the job of utilization review to see that rules for maximum reimbursement through federal and state programs are met. This means attention to timely discharges and transfer to non-acute care as soon as possible. For the nurse who has not had time to adequately prepare a patient for discharge, it may seem that the quality of care is suffering. On the other hand, a national study by Feather and Nichols (1985) shows that the majority of the hospitals surveyed (68%) report no increase in readmission rates following the introduction of DRGs. They do report that discharge planning has received more emphasis (71%) and that there is some increased use of interdisciplinary teams (39%).

It seems that it will be some years before federal and state regulations concerning reimbursements for care stabilize. In the meantime, effective communication between those giving and those monitoring care is essential. When problems arise, they must be dealt with quickly and reported carefully so that the learning by all of us can be used to benefit future patients.

The Case Manager (Insurance Company). Most of the larger insurance companies that have health insurance programs employ case managers who oversee the payment of benefits for particular clients. Although they are perhaps physically far removed from the discharge planning team, their decisions are critical to its functioning.

In the instance of a question about the patient's coverage, the case manager should be regarded as a resource person.

The forms they receive often do not adequately reflect the real human circumstances involved, and they are usually happy to have a situation clarified for them in informal conversation. The nurse should, however, take care to have all relevant information at hand before initiating this kind of contact.

Characteristics of a "STAR" Team

A "team" is more than just a collection of people who act autonomously in pursuit of a vague goal. Calling a group of people a team implies that they are working to communicate with one another and that they share a common, well-defined purpose. In the case of the effective discharge planning team, its purpose is to provide patients undergoing acute care access to professional knowledge and skills in planning for continuing care. Access is achieved when the professionals involved coordinate their efforts and cooperate with one another in *sharing tasks and responsibilities*. They must be sure, as a group, that their contributions will fit together to complete the discharge planning puzzle. Whatever their structure, groups of professionals who demonstrate this level of teamwork have a number of characteristics in common. These include:

- Willingness of all participants to communicate freely with one another;
- Clarity of focus on the unique needs of patients and their families;
- Commitment to helping patients and their families participate fully in planning;

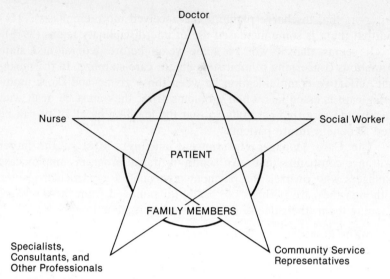

Figure 4–1. *A "STAR" team: Shared Tasks and Responsibility.*

- Cooperation with other participants in identifying tasks that need to be undertaken, in completing those tasks, and in sharing information; and
- Willingness to take mutual responsibility for planning, decision-making, and coordination.

A model of such a functioning team is shown in Figure 4–1. Communication and sharing make it "star" quality.

In summary, in this section we have identified possible members of the discharge planning team and outlined the contribution each might make. The qualities that characterize effective teamwork between professionals with diverse backgrounds have been summarized. Nurses are encouraged to develop effective communication with resource people in their organizations so that "star" quality continuing care plans are facilitated and their own skills and knowledge improved.

4.2 HOW MULTIDISCIPLINARY TEAMS WORK

As anyone who has worked with a multidisciplinary team knows, intra-professional cooperation and communication do not happen automatically; they take organization, leadership, and the building of mutual trust. The practical aspects of just how such teams come into being and how they function is the subject of this section. We will first look at how discharge planning as an activity is most commonly organized. Several different patterns of communication used in planning continuing care will then be analyzed. Finally, we will consider how communication can be improved between team members.

How Discharge Planning Teams Are Organized

The people who make up the discharge planning team are organized for the function based on an institution's size, history, and financial resources. Discharge planning may be accorded priority status and publicly lauded as an important contribution made by the institution to its patients and the community, or it may be something of an orphan, a requirement met without enthusiasm. Professional involvement in discharge planning activities may be formally organized into a unit devoted solely to that purpose or provided informally, depending on time available after other activities. The criteria for identifying patients who especially need discharge planning services may be contained in a formal document referred to routinely in patient assessment procedures, or they may exist by informal consensus in the awareness of nursing staff. Of the many organizational possibilities for discharge planning services, four general categories are described in the following paragraphs.

Separate Discharge Planning Unit. The number of professionals who staff this unit depends on the size of the institution, but it usually has either a social worker or nurse as its leader. The separate unit occupies an office of its own and a unique place in the organizational hierarchy. The unit may be responsible directly to the administration or to the nursing department. Referrals to the unit for services are made by physicians or nurses and are based on established criteria such as age, diagnosis, and the presence of certain social or financial risk factors. (See Section 6.1 for further discussion of referral criteria.)

Because the professionals appointed to a separate unit have clear discharge planning functions and an identity with the unit, cooperation and communication between them is facilitated. Difficulties may arise, however, in interpreting the unit's services and limitations to others in the institution and in gaining access to balanced information about a patient's needs. The unit's personnel may be regarded as "experts" but also as "outsiders."

Formally structured discharge planning units have, in many cases, come into existence to meet the requirements of Medicare legislation. Limited time and resources frequently mean that the services of the separate unit do not extend much further than Medicare and Medicaid patients, leaving many others with discharge planning needs to be served in less formal ways.

Decentralized Discharge Planning Unit. The decentralized unit, like the separate one, has an office and is shown separately on a diagram of the institution's organizational structure, but its personnel are deployed to specific patient care units. The person assigned to a unit acts as the initiator of discharge planning services, the conduit to broader multidisciplinary services, and the general consultant to staff about discharge planning issues. The discharge planner usually has no difficulty managing the appropriateness of referrals or having access to information because of consistency in communicating with patient care staff and proximity to patients and their families. The planner may, however, have limited identity with the discharge planning unit and therefore have less communication with coworkers there. Regular meetings and conferences between discharge planning staff help to improve communication at this level.

A Coordinated Discharge Planning Alliance. In this form of organizational structure, a coordinator or liaison officer is appointed, usually a nurse, to receive referrals and contact whatever other professionals are needed to meet a particular patient's discharge planning needs. The members of this loosely constructed team may differ for each patient. For their part, members of social work, therapy, dietary, and other potentially helpful disciplines formally agree to join the discharge planning team when needed. The coordinator, in effect, functions in a general practice role by putting nursing colleagues and patients in touch with the required specialists. The coordinator in this situation usually has responsibility for many patients or an entire institution and may therefore be limited mostly to a referral role rather than active coordination of a team.

In a small hospital or skilled nursing facility, this pattern of discharge planning services works effectively. Sometimes the director of nursing takes responsibility for this role on a part-time basis. The success of the professional alliance depends on the interpersonal and communication skills of the coordinator.

An Informal Professional Alliance. In most institutions, an informal alliance of professionals operates in parallel with the more formal discharge planning units. In some instances only 10% of patients are cared for by the formal organization, leaving a very large group with continuing care and transitional care needs that must be met in other ways. When an informal approach is used, the nurse usually functions as the coordinator, although services may be initiated by any caregiver—from physician to nursing aide—who identifies that needs exist. Unless institution-wide agreements have been reached that allow social workers, therapists, and other professionals open access to patients in need of their services, the nurse-coordinator will first need to work with the physician to obtain necessary medical orders.

There are two major problems in the effectiveness of informal discharge planning services. One is their inconsistency; the quality of services depend on the enthusiasm, sensitivity, and knowledge of the nurse who chooses to take the coordinator role. One nurse may always pay attention to the transitional and discharge planning needs of patients, while another may overlook them. The second problem is that informal systems are very vulnerable to institutional priorities; the nurse may have the support of the supervisor and hospital administration for helping patients with discharge planning, or else may be actively discouraged from taking roles other than those of direct, acute care. For example, in one hospital, access to other professionals was blocked by the administrator's demand that a very time-consuming written referral procedure be used before any consultation. This made informal discharge planning impossible until the nurses joined forces on the issue to get the policy changed.

Communication Patterns Within Teams

Whether in a formal or informal relationship, discharge planning team members develop patterns of communication with one another. These may be a result of organizational structure, habit, or the personal style of the professionals involved. The flow of communication from one person to another determines leadership responsibilities and has a profound effect on methods of problem solving. Three of the most common communication patterns are discussed in the following paragraphs, along with their implications for discharge planning teamwork.

The Open Communication Team. This is usually the kind of communication pattern meant when one speaks of teamwork. Team members regard one another as equals and see themselves as sharing team functions or tasks (see Table 4–1).

Face-to-face interaction is essential to an open communication team. They may meet several times in reference to a single case situation to set priorities, share information, and make decisions.

This kind of team is characterized by a strong sense of equality; each member is regarded as having an important contribution to make toward meeting team goals. Given this mutual regard, it is a natural pattern that they talk with each other initially to clarify their goals and decide on individual responsibilities. Each member may then proceed with his or her part of the task before meeting again to share information and assess progress. This pattern of a conference followed by individual activity may be repeated several times before the goal is reached. Rakich, Longest, and Darr (1985, Ch. 12) refer to this as an "all-channel" team or network, in recognition of the fact that no significant barriers exist to open communication. (See description of a "star" team in Section 4.1.)

Health professionals generally see the open communication team as an ideal. It is an ideal not frequently fully realized, however, due to the very high levels of coordination and excellent intradisciplinary communication required to make it work. Team members must be sufficiently autonomous that they can, as a group, independently decide on tasks and priorities without being distracted by departmental constraints. Although constructing and coordinating this kind of team seems to take an inordinate amount of time initially, that time is more than saved later due to the team's efficiency. Team members usually feel good about this kind of team effort and are satisfied with its effectiveness.

The attributes of this kind of team make it especially desirable for discharge planning teams in which patients and family members are invited to participate in team conferences as full members. The mutual *commitment* that develops within this team gives an unparalleled sense of *support* to families. They have the opportunity to share their points of view, their needs, and their strengths in team conferences. The result of involvement and communication is that plans made are much more likely to be satisfactorily *implemented* than they are with other kinds of teams. Because of their emphasis on face-to-face problem solving, open communication teams tend to be very *creative* in their approaches to problems, making them especially useful in complex situations. No one team member has to know how to make a workable plan for that patient, they just have to be willing to share their knowledge and skills within the team and to communicate openly.

Opportunities for open communication teams exist within both formal and informal organizational patterns for discharge planning so long as there is one person — usually the nurse or a discharge planning coordinator—who is willing to take the lead initially. This means contacting appropriate team members, gaining their cooperation, and setting a mutually agreeable time and venue for a first conference. This process is greatly assisted when health professionals know one another personally, have developed mutual respect and trust, and have had other experiences of working together in this way.

A diagram of the communication pattern for conferences of an open communication team is shown in Figure 4–2. This team does not necessarily have a designated leader, although it may select a coordinator. Members have equal power to initiate communication and participate in decision making. For this reason the size of the team is crucial; the ideal group consists of three to six people. Effectiveness is lost when more than six are involved. Other professionals who are

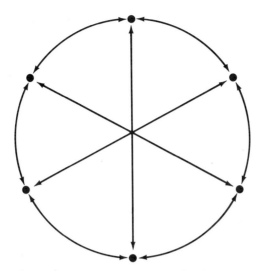

Figure 4–2. *An open communication team.*

contributing to a team task may consult with one or more team members without necessarily participating in team meetings.

The Consultation Wheel. A pattern of communication very frequently found in health care organizations, particularly large ones, is the consultation wheel. Specific people occupy positions around the periphery of the wheel. One of them initiates the discharge planning process, although this responsibility may change from time to time or from case to case. Once begun, the process proceeds from one member of this "team" to another. For example, the nurse may start the process by identifying certain discharge planning risks during the initial assessment, giving that information to the doctor with a recommendation to involve the social worker. The doctor communicates the information he or she has about the situation, along with the nurse's concern, to the social work department. The social worker may contact a home care agency or a nursing home before returning the developed plan back to the nurse. Like a snowball, the discharge plan rolls around the wheel, accumulating information as it goes. By implication, the patient is at the center of this wheel although, because participants in planning the discharge speak with the patient one at a time and may each be using a different set of information, he or she may not perceive it as a coordinated effort.

The advantages of the consultation wheel are that it is relatively efficient and makes good use of the unique knowledge and skills of each member. The professionals who are experienced with this pattern of communication develop skills in anticipating what will be required of them and organizing their "specialist" contribution to the larger picture. It works best when the positions around the wheel are firmly established so that each person knows what her or his responsibilities are and when and to whom the plan must next be passed.

The disadvantages of the wheel relate to its having no one person as the coordinator of communication. Consequently, no clear goals are established at the outset; rather, they develop out of the input of team members. If one person fails to do her or his part to pass along the plan to the next person or fails to adequately communicate with the patient, the entire process may break down.

If the patient or a family member does not take a prominent position as coordinator of the consultation wheel, useful information may bypass the patient and undermine participation in decision making.

It is especially important that a member of the team, most logically the nurse, help to coach the patient or a family member on what to expect and how to make the best possible use of the range of resources available within the wheel.

A diagram of communication flow within the consultation wheel is shown in Figure 4–3. This may be the principal communication pattern used in discharge planning or there may be a more complex pattern of other wheels, open teams, or task assignment on the periphery of the main wheel.

A Task Assignment Pattern. When time is at a premium and a number of continuing care issues must be settled quickly, a task

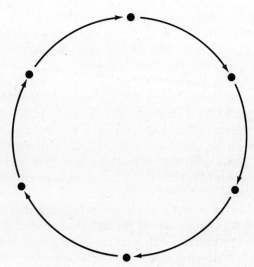

Figure 4–3. A consultation wheel.

assignment pattern may be used. This approach requires a coordinator with a clear view of the patient's multiple needs and good organizational abilities. Tasks are assigned on the basis of the discipline most involved in it; for example, the task of contacting appropriate home care agencies may be delegated to a discharge planner, and the task of investigating insurance coverage to a financial consultant. These tasks may proceed simultaneously and independently. While these two people may need to compare notes, they do so informally.

The advantage of task assignment is that it is time efficient. The major disadvantages are that the potential for fragmentation is very great and the patient and family may feel quite removed from the planning process. Because things are likely to happen quickly, they may not be able to make practical sense of information pouring in. This pattern for making discharge plans has a single leader who has power to decide what information is to be sought, how priorities are to be set, how to interpret data, and what alternatives are to be considered. For this reason flexibility and creativity in dealing with rapidly changing or highly complex situations may be limited.

While often very efficient, task assignment is a highly controlling method of planning continuing care. Efforts need to be made to involve patient and family in the process without overwhelming them with information that has no clear context.

Unlike the wheel, the structure and personnel involved in this kind of planning pattern changes with each case. Consequently, it is up to the coordinator to clarify and interpret information, putting the pieces together as imagination and ability allow.

There are some things that can be done to improve communication with the patient and family during this kind of process. For example, *consultation* during the task definition phase helps them feel part of the process, allows them to correct any misinterpretations of the patient's needs, and helps them make sense of the information they will give to and receive from other professionals. A *planning conference* that includes patient and family gives them the opportunity to ask questions, give input to decisions, and think through potential problems with implementation.

A diagram of the typical flow of communication for the task assignment pattern is shown in Figure 4–4.

The case examples in Section 4.3 demonstrate how the organization of discharge planning services and the flow of communication during the discharge planning process can be practically combined to meet continuing care needs.

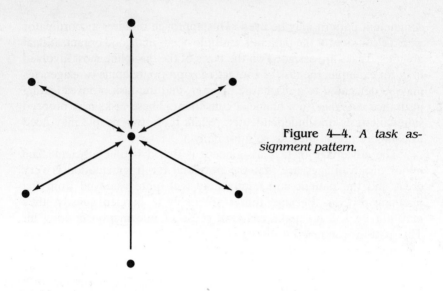

Figure 4–4. *A task assignment pattern.*

How to Improve Interdisciplinary Communication

Communications between professionals is one of those areas in which practice does not always follow theory. Each of the professions devotes a great deal of educational time and effort to teaching communication skills. It ought to be easy for nurses to apply those skills to communication with social workers and doctors to nurses. Yet people often find themselves trapped in ineffective communication patterns by feelings of competition or intimidation. Such "turf" battles are a very common experience that especially affects nurses and social workers (Terry, 1988). The literature universally decries the existence of such battles but offers little practical guidance for avoiding such problems or treating them once they arise.

Our work with multidisciplinary teams in both hospital and community settings has led to a belief that a sense of competition develops not only between nurses and social workers in particular, but also between members of other health professions, because they in fact carry out very similar functions. Their services to patients DO overlap. Each of the professions has specialties—nursing emphasizes direct care and teaching, social work emphasizes social assessment and counseling— but nurses also counsel and social workers also teach.

"Turf" battles are minimized when professionals come to see their overlapping functions as supplementary rather than competitive.

One approach to doing this is to help members of a team clarify for themselves and other team members just how they see their contributions to patient care and what functions each feels most competent performing. This is a first step toward finding ways to help each other. The list of functions for one such discharge planning team is shown in Table 4–1.

In addition to this kind of team-building exercise, there are some specific ways in which interdisciplinary coordination, cooperation, and communication can be improved.

Coordination. Good team coordination occurs when members are secure enough in their own roles and confident enough about what their colleagues have to offer that they can interpret these to patients accurately. These team members refer patients to each other easily and with continuity.

One way to encourage coordination is a follow-up exercise to the one that is described in Table 4–1. Working with a partner, one person role-plays a patient and the other (in his or her own role) describes the partner's professional strengths and abilities. For example, with the social worker playing the role of patient, the nurse partner would describe what a social worker does. This "game" allows each member a chance to correct the perceptions of colleagues and to help each learn what they would like patients to be told.

Whatever methods help team members reach consensus about *team* goals for specific patients will improve coordination.

> *Clear goals for team involvement in discharge planning and realistic expectations of fellow team members lead to improved coordination of services.*

Admonitions to "keep better records" are not enough if a group of

Table 4–1. *FUNCTIONS OF TEAM MEMBERS IN A DISCHARGE PLANNING TEAM**

Function	Nurse	Social Worker	Physical Therapist	Doctor
Assessment	+ +	+ + +	+ +	+ + +
Teaching	+ + +	+	+	+
Treatment/personal care	+ +	+	+ + +	+ +
Counseling	+	+ +	+	+
Decision-making support	+ +	+ + +	+	+ +
Coordination of resources	+ + +	+ + +	+ +	+
Referral	+	+ +	+	+ + +

*The weighting of these functions reflects the perceptions and personalities as well as the professional preparation of each of these team members. They were first asked to complete this table for themselves and the way they saw their fellow team members functioning. They then compared notes and reached consensus on the above table. In the process they worked to clarify their roles for each other.

professionals who frequently work with the same patients are failing to work together.

Cooperation. This attribute of well-functioning teams is a near relative of coordination.

> *Cooperation is the expression of a positive attitude toward teammates and the valuing of what they contribute.*

Cooperation often takes the form of negotiating functions related to a particular patient: "If you do that, I will do this." Implicit in this kind of negotiation is that the team members agree on what needs to be done.

Because it is a function of attitude, cooperation cannot be taught, but it can be encouraged and strengthened. The goal of team-building exercises is to encourage trust, helping people demonstrate the qualities of warmth, respect, empathy, and genuineness that are described in Section 2.2. (See also Muldary, 1983, Ch. 8.)

Communication. The quality of verbal communication is particularly important to good team functioning. It is in verbal interaction that attitudes are expressed and accuracy of perceptions tested. Because communication is a skill, all instances of talking with team colleagues, formally or informally, are opportunities to improve those skills and build mutual respect. Team meetings, patient conferences, and consultations provide that opportunity as long as they are conducted in an atmosphere of equality and have a goal orientation. Multidisciplinary courses and workshops sponsored by institutions for staff development also are helpful in clarifying roles and reviewing general goals.

In summary, practical aspects of how multidisciplinary teams are organized and how communication flows within them have been explored in this section. Some ideas for improving team coordination, cooperation, and communication have been presented. Teamwork is not something that occurs automatically because the people involved have a stake in the decisions made. Rather, teamwork requires the intentional development of strong interpersonal relationships over a period of time.

> *Professionals make their best contribution to families attempting to decide on continuing care issues when they are able to trust, respect, and listen to one another.*

4.3 EXAMPLES OF TEAM APPROACHES

Two extended case examples are presented in this section as demonstrations of multidisciplinary approaches to discharge planning.

Each example is analyzed in terms of the organization of services and the flow of communication between the people involved.

Example 4.1 Planning Complex Home Care

Acute Phase: Assessment of Continuing Care Needs

Shirley Stewart was a 64-year-old widow who had been living by herself until this hospital admission. She had no children of her own, but two stepsons, Russell and Brian, were in regular contact with her. Russell, who lived nearby, had been helping with shopping and transportation.

On admission it was found that Mrs. Stewart had a bowel obstruction, the result of a metastatic tumor secondary to ovarian cancer that had had surgical intervention several years previously. She was in considerable pain and was quite weak. It was clear to her primary care nurse that Mrs. Stewart would need help at home, particularly if a course of chemotherapy increased her fatigue and weakness. The patient's internist and a consulting surgeon decided that further surgery was not advisable. Plans were made to start her on total parenteral nutrition (TPN) and a self-administered subcutaneous pump for morphine. The internist and nurse consulted together and decided that the doctor would talk with the patient and her stepson about the prognosis and planned treatment. The nurse would initiate referral to the discharge planning coordinator for that unit (from a decentralized discharge planning department).

The nurse completed the formal referral form and also consulted verbally with the coordinator to arrange an introduction to the patient and an initial discharge planning meeting with her and Russell. The goals of this meeting were to clarify the roles of the coordinator and nurse in helping to plan for Mrs. Stewart's continuing care, to assess her psychological state following discussion with the doctor, and to evaluate the support offered by her stepsons (see Figure 4–5).

This meeting was proposed to the patient as a "team" meeting and was conducted in an open style, although the nurse remained the informal leader. During this meeting Mrs. Stewart was able to say that although she felt depressed, the prognosis came as no surprise to her. She expressed a great deal of uncertainty about how she would be able to cope at

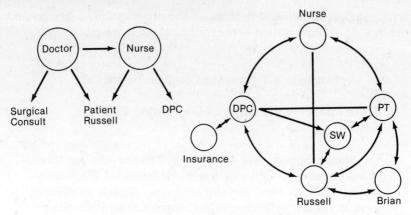

Figure 4–5. *Communication patterns during assessment. Left, Initiation of services using a consultation wheel. Right, Formation of the team. DPC = discharge planning coordinator; PT = physical therapist; SW = social worker.*

home. Russell was obviously quite devoted to his stepmother but unable to take her into his home. He had recently married, his wife was working, and he was going to school part-time. The possibility of being able to stay with the other stepson, Brian, was discussed briefly. It was suggested that the social worker who was part of the discharge planning department be consulted. All agreed to this plan, and the coordinator took responsibility for contacting the social worker about the case (see Figure 4–5).

The social worker met with Mrs. Stewart and Russell separately the next day. She later saw the coordinator in the hallway and reported that the patient had seemed eager to talk about her feelings and about not wanting to be a burden on her stepsons during her terminal care. Russell had already talked with his brother, Brian, who lived in a metropolitan area 200 miles away. Brian had a large house and only one teenager still at home. He and his wife agreed to discuss the possibility of having his stepmother come to stay with them. The social worker suggested she telephone them that evening. Meanwhile, the coordinator had found out that the patient's insurance would cover 100% of the cost of home care by a nurse and necessary equipment. There was no question of the need for skilled nursing care with TPN in use. The coordinator tentatively set up a time for a "team" meeting for planning the next afternoon. The information that had been gathered was relayed to the nurse, who subsequently spoke with the doctor and the patient, who called Russell about the meeting.

Transition Phase: Decision Making and Planning

At the appointed time the team, consisting of the primary care nurse, discharge planning coordinator, social worker, patient, and her stepson (Russell), assembled to share information that had been gathered, talk through the alternatives available to the patient, decide on one of them if possible, and begin planning for the implementation phase. The meeting took about an hour, during which the coordinator and social worker presented the pros and cons of nursing home care, returning to the patient's own home with a live-in nursing aide, or accepting Brian's invitation to come and stay with him. The financial consequences and potential medical and nursing care problems were included in the discussion. In the midst of the session, the internist joined the group briefly and listened to their progress so far.

Had Mrs. Stewart not been so determined to go ahead with a decision, the team would have adjourned at that point while the family compared notes and reached consensus. It became clear, however, that the patient had already made up her mind that the move to Brian's was the best choice. When she found out that she could have daily home care and good medical support there, that decided it for her. The team then made up a list of what had to be done before discharge and assigned tasks to team members. (See Figure 4–6.)

As the meeting was breaking up, Russell telephoned his brother to report to him about the situation. Brian and his wife had made tentative plans to come up to the hospital the next weekend. This would give them the opportunity to review the plan and learn some of the basics of Mrs. Stewart's care.

The PATIENT would:
— continue to learn about various aspects of her care including how to manage the morphine pump;
— talk with Brian to work out details about the move; and
— coach Russell about what personal belongings she would want to take with her.

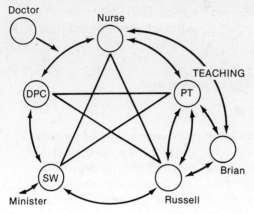

Figure 4–6. *Communication patterns during planning.*

RUSSELL would:
— organize neighbors to keep an eye on Mrs. Stewart's house;
— gather together his stepmother's belongings; and
— arrange with a nurse friend of his wife's to accompany them on the transfer to Brian's.

The NURSE would:
— talk with the doctor about referral to medical care near Brian's home;
— prepare written instructions for the patient's care for the home care nurse and a schedule of medications for Mrs. Stewart;
— continue to supervise Mrs. Stewart's use of the morphine pump; and
— continue patient teaching about medications, personal care, and signs of complications during TPN, arranging to include Brian and his wife in at least two intensive sessions on the weekend.

The DISCHARGE PLANNING COORDINATOR would:
— locate a home care agency, find out who would be visiting Mrs. Stewart, give them a list of equipment needed, and find out what home pharmacist they would prefer working with;
— organize a consultation with physical and occupational therapists to assess mobility and plan energy conservation. They would then do the relevant patient teach-

ing on transfer techniques, etc., and advise the doctor and nurse of any needed equipment for home use.

The SOCIAL WORKER would:
— continue to see Mrs. Stewart for emotional support during the transition and help her make financial and personal arrangements for the move;
— contact the minister of Mrs. Stewart's church to let him know about her condition and the discharge plan.

As these various tasks were completed, each of the professionals involved gave informal feedback to the patient about them.

Transition Phase: Implementation

As the patient neared discharge, the team met briefly at her bedside to confirm transfer plans, answer questions, and be sure that important items had not escaped their notice. Brian's and his wife's visit over the weekend and their participation in teaching sessions made Mrs. Stewart feel much more confident about the decision to go to their home. Brian had been in touch with the doctor she was referred to, and plans were made to see him the day after she arrived. Discharge was organized for the next day. The nurse telephoned the home care agency and spoke with the nurse who would be caring for Mrs. Stewart.

On the day of discharge, enough TPN supplies and medications to last for a few days were readied. Instructions and orders were sent with the patient.

Over the next few days the hospital pharmacist and the coordinator followed up on the situation. The primary care nurse in the hospital spoke with the home care nurse several times. The transfer had been made smoothly, and the patient's care continued uninterrupted.

Analysis of Example 4.1. In this case example, a number of criteria for a successful discharge plan were met.

• The patient and her family were able to use the expertise of available resource people in constructive ways;
• The professionals involved coordinated their efforts, cooperated in sharing tasks and responsibilities, and communicated both formally and informally; and

• The patient and her family were active in the planning process and retained their sense of control and personal power.

Although very complex in terms of the number of professionals involved and the need to coordinate intensive home care in a distant community, discharge planning proceeded efficiently as well as effectively. Physician and nurse initially identified discharge planning needs that would take Mrs. Stewart's emotional and social well-being into account as well as her physical care. As planning progressed, the major vehicle for intra-disciplinary cooperation was the core team that was able to identify and assign tasks (Figure 4–5). The team members each became the leader of extended communication patterns as more resources were involved (Figure 4–6).

Complex planning and sharing large quantities of information is facilitated by a "STAR" team that coordinates communication with the patient.

Team members in the example used a variety of communication patterns to accomplish tasks and consult with other professionals but they consistently returned to Mrs. Stewart with information. The confusion that could have so easily occurred with so many professionals involved was thus avoided, and the patient retained a sense of control and personal power in the situation.

In the next case example, a series of factors complicated the care of an infant, leading to an unsuccessful first discharge attempt.

Example 4.2 Infant with Complicated Care

Jamie's life started precariously when he was born six weeks prematurely. His three-month stay in the neonatal care unit was complicated by pulmonary hypertension, tricuspid regurgitation, right ventricular hypertrophy, and an edematous duodenum. Nevertheless, his development progressed normally, except for his weight.

Jamie's social situation was no less complicated. His mother, Hasun Bea, had emigrated from Korea as a teenager with her mother. Her father and three brothers had been killed in military action. Shortly after arrival in the United States, her mother died, leaving her in the care of distant relatives. Hasun, now 20, was separated from Jamie's father; they had not married.

Jamie required an enormous amount of care. He had to be fed very slowly, and even at that regurgitated much of the feeding. By the time his numerous medications were drawn up and given, and pulmonary treatment done, it was almost time to start over. His mother spent much of every day at the hospital helping with his care. Hasun seemed very devoted to Jamie; she handled him very lovingly, if not confidently. She did not ask many questions but did seem to understand explanations about Jamie and his care. She spoke English well, although she was sometimes difficult to understand because of her heavy accent.

There were a great number of people involved in planning Jamie's continuing care, including several doctors; the primary care nurse; the discharge planner (from a separate, centralized unit); a social worker; and physical, occupational, and respiratory therapists. The discharge planner took the responsibility for coordinating various community agencies and organizing benefits through Medicaid and Crippled Children's Services. Each of the professionals took care to keep Hasun informed of what was being done and to help her learn how to care for Jamie.

The infant was discharged on a cold, rainy day in mid-November with supplies of all medications and a schedule for their administration. Oxygen equipment had already been delivered to the home, and a registered nurse from the Home Care Agency organized to come daily for up to six hours for two weeks. A local pharmacy was to provide Progestimil formula, and a physical therapist would visit twice weekly to do developmental exercises with Jamie and try to improve his head control.

At first, Jamie's care at home went well. The discharge planner, who continued to be in touch with Hasun and the Home Care Agency, reported that the mother was apparently coping well with her infant's care. By the end of the two weeks, the home care nurse had reduced her daily visits to one hour.

Then one night three weeks after Jamie's discharge, he was readmitted through the Emergency Department with diarrhea, fever, and dehydration. He was diagnosed as having pneumonia. The nurse who received Jamie in the Pediatric Unit was one who had previously been involved in his care. When she questioned Hasun about his care at home, she discovered that many of the medications had not been given according to schedule; in fact, one of them had been left forgotten in the refrigerator for almost a week. In her frustration with the mother, the nurse asked her directly: "Can you read English?'' Hasun became very embarrassed and began to cry. "No," she said, "not very well. I tried to remember everything.''

Over the next two weeks of hospitalization, Jamie's condition improved significantly. The doctor tried to reduce the number of medications given to him, and he was gradually weaned off oxygen. A Korean nurse working in another part of the hospital was recruited to help with teaching, and Hasun was encouraged to make her own set of instructions for medication administration and treatments to use at home.

A discharge planning conference was called and included all of the professionals involved in Jamie's care, including the home care nurse. This time tasks were clearly defined and responsibilities assigned so that the approach would be more coordinated. It was decided that the criteria for discharge would be for Hasun to care for Jamie at the hospital for 8 hours on three consecutive days, followed by 24 hours continuously without help. The mother readily agreed to this plan and reported that she was feeling happier because she had just had an abortion. She felt she would be able to concentrate more on Jamie now.

Hasun successfully met the criteria for discharge, and Jamie went home. This time the mother seemed much more confident in his care. The home care nurse was only needed for about a week.

Analysis of Example 4.2. In this case example, discharge planning was initially done using a task assignment pattern among the many professionals involved. This pattern failed in this instance for two reasons. One was that responsibility for tasks was apparently just assumed by professionals without much collaboration or direction; second, there was apparently no one specified as coordinator who was thoroughly familiar with the child's care and his mother's needs. The result was that plans were fragmented among many professionals without the real involvement of the mother. Feeling removed from the planning process and defensive because of the language difficulty, Hasun was unable to make known what she needed to care for Jamie. The planners unintentionally placed the mother in the role of "child" while they played "parents.''

Unfortunately, this is a pattern of interaction that often occurs when the care of non-English speaking patients, people from unfamiliar cultures, or those who are inarticulate in comparison with health professionals is being planned. Anticipating that they will be unable to communicate sufficiently to participate in planning, we simply do it for them, present it as a *fait accompli*, and hope that they understand the plan well enough to implement it. What we fail to recognize in such situations is that we have substantially added to the person's feelings of helplessness and they may not be able even to *hear* our well-intended explanations, much less implement our plans.

In the example, the home care nurse held the key to Hasun's being able to implement the care plan for Jamie. In her own home, the mother may have been less defensive and better able to learn. We do not know what priority the nurse placed on helping Hasun gain the skills she needed. Hasun apparently did not share with the nurse that she could not read English well, nor that she was again pregnant. Anxiety about another pregnancy may well have been so distracting as to make teaching ineffective.

The second attempt at discharge planning was more effective, because it was better coordinated. The conference allowed the professionals involved to share a single goal. Although Hasun was still treated as a "child" in that she was apparently not really included in the planning and was made to pass a "test" before taking Jamie home the second time, her improved mental state following the abortion made it possible for her to take more active control of the child's care.

In summary, these two case examples show the importance of communication, coordination, and collaboration among professionals and with patients and families in the effective planning of continuing care. In the next section we will discuss the practicalities of patient and family involvement in more detail.

4.4 HOW TO INCLUDE PATIENT AND FAMILY AS TEAM MEMBERS

In our discussion of how to improve interdisciplinary communication (Section 4.2), an example was presented listing the functions of health professionals in the discharge planning process (Table 4–1). One way of understanding the importance of including patients and their family members in discharge planning teams is to recognize that professional intervention is successful only when it stimulates appropriate patient or family responses.

> *The functions of health professionals and patients or their representatives in discharge planning are reciprocal: they facilitate and respond to one another.*

For example, a complete assessment of patient needs cannot be carried out unless the professional is given access to information held only by the patient and family. Likewise, teaching is ineffective unless patient and family are willing and able to learn.

Table 4–2 shows the pairing of professional and patient functions. When outlined in this way, it is clear that unless the patient and family are helped to do their part, the discharge plan is at best incomplete and at worst ineffective. Example 4.2 demonstrated what happened when the mother of the patient did not divulge important information, was unable to learn, and did not share in decision-making.

In the following paragraphs, we will review some of the reasons and practical methods for including patients and their family members in each of the three steps of the discharge planning process.

Patient Involvement in Step A: Assessing Needs

Health care providers have no trouble identifying the patient and the family as important sources of information. Anyone who has ever worked in an Emergency Department and been part of the team receiving an unconscious patient by ambulance without any attending witnesses knows how difficult it is to give good care without access to the facts about what happened.

For their part, patients and family members expect to be asked a series of questions and, in response, to share information with health care providers on a wide range of topics. As discussed in Section 2.2, the nurse who is alert to nonverbal aspects of communication often learns about attitudes, values, and beliefs as well as facts by listening carefully to answers.

There is one simple mechanism that changes a person from a passive supplier of information for others to use to an active participant in identifying patient needs.

Table 4–2. *THE RECIPROCAL FUNCTIONS OF PATIENT AND PROFESSIONAL*

Health Professional		Patient or Family Member
Assessment	←——→	Information sharing
Teaching	←——→	Learning
Treatment/personal care	←——→	Informed consent/cooperation
Counseling/support	←——→	Willingness to share feelings/ ability to alter attitudes, behavior
Decision-making support	←——→	Ability to consider alternatives, consequences of decisions
Coordination of resources	←——→	Facilitate involvement of other professionals or agencies
Referral	←——→	Follow-up, implement plan

The person who is told WHY a question is being asked and HOW the information is to be used becomes an active member of the problem solving team.

If people understand the nature and extent of the problems to be solved, they can then use their knowledge and intelligence to be sure that caregivers have all relevant information, not just the answers to specific questions. For example, a patient who is asked: "Where does it hurt right now?" may point to a location in answer. The patient who is first told: "The exact location of your pain is important to your diagnosis" before the specific question is asked may respond: "It hurts here right now, but when the pain began an hour ago, it was further down here." Including the patient in problem solving leads to much better information.

Most people have had the experience of going to a health care provider who asked a series of closed, specific questions but did not really give the patient a chance to tell "his-story." In response, the person can be expected to feel anger, a sense of helplessness, and a lack of confidence in the caregiver's advice. He has been treated like a child who does not have the ability to think for himself. As mentioned in the analysis of Example 4.2, there are a number of groups of people who are vulnerable to such treatment.

Caregivers need to be especially careful not to treat non-English speaking people, those from cultures or socio-economic groups markedly different from that of the caregivers, or the elderly as though they were helpless, unintelligent children.

Recently a woman celebrated her 75th birthday with a large family party. In response to a compliment about her youthful appearance, she was heard to say with a wry smile: "Well, I should *feel* young, too. The older I get, the more I am treated as a mere child!"

Some practical methods of involving the patient and family in information gathering and assessment of needs include the following:

- Offer a brief explanation of *why* information is being sought and how it is to be used before asking questions.
- Whenever possible, start with open questions that encourage the person to think through the problem and contribute feelings as well as facts before focusing narrowly with closed questions (see Section 2.2).
- Listen with C-A-R-E to a person's answers to questions, being sure to communicate both nonverbally and verbally that the information being shared is valued and that the individual is respected.

- Pay attention to nonverbal messages that accompany verbal responses, asking for clarification if they seem incongruent.
- Listen to yourself as you ask a question. Your tone of voice conveys your attitude toward the person and the problem.
- Become aware of the assumptions you make about people belonging to certain categories. Identifying our prejudices is the first step toward overcoming the communication barriers they impose.
- Do not hesitate to ask people what *they* think the problem is or what they think they will need when they leave acute care. People have often developed theories that are sometimes very insightful and always represent beliefs that must be considered as powerful factors in their continuing care.

Contrary to the fantasies of many caregivers and the expectations of many patients, few health professionals are so wise that they are able to obtain full and relevant data by asking a limited number of well phrased questions and then to interpret the information with complete accuracy. Most of us need all the help we can get to reach correct diagnoses and to anticipate future needs. The patient is the most knowledgable person available to us for information about what a problem feels like and what its effects are. Making him or her part of the team greatly improves the "score" of success.

Including the patient and family as partners in gathering information and assessing needs is the first step toward making them full members of the continuing care team.

People who feel that the contributions they are making are valuable and who are kept informed of what is happening and why do not experience the helplessness that is such a barrier to effective discharge planning.

Patient Involvement in Step B: Building a Plan

Teaching, counseling, and support are the major functions of health professionals as patient and family members learn what they need to know to continue care and sort through alternatives. If patients have already formed trusting relationships with caregivers and feel that they have retained a measure of personal power in spite of physical dependence, they will be able to participate in this phase of discharge planning with confidence. It is very important that the nurse, in particular, give clear messages about the "balance of power" in planning continuing care.

It is the patient's right and responsibility to make decisions about continuing health care. It is his or her right to be informed about factors that contribute to those decisions and to use the resources available.

It is the role of health professionals to offer the patient and family the benefit of their knowledge and experience and help them reach the best possible decisions.

There are a number of common scenarios that the nurse encounters that represent problems with the decision-making and planning process.

The Patient or Family Want Others to Decide For Them. When a person begins a conversation about continuing care needs with the statement: "I'm sure you know what is best," the nurse must stop and listen carefully. Such a statement seems to indicate that the person feels helpless, and perhaps even more importantly, that he or she does not anticipate taking control of the situation in the immediate future. If the nurse or others actually do go ahead and decide or plan for the person, they reinforce a sense of helplessness and enter an area of questionable legality and ethics.

Refusing to make decisions or give specific recommendations, however, must be done carefully so that patients do not feel that appropriate care and attention is being withdrawn or that they are being personally rejected. The first step is to *discover more* about why the person does not want to be more actively involved. This is best done through use of open questions and careful listening on the part of the nurse. Inconsistencies between verbal and nonverbal responses are especially meaningful. The most common reasons for this attitude are lack of knowledge about the medical condition and prognosis, fantasies about what will happen after discharge, confusion and uncertainty about how to proceed, depression, or overwhelming anxiety from sources that may be unrelated to the present illness. In Example 4.2, the mother's language problem and anxiety over an unwanted pregnancy may well have explained her passivity in planning her son's care.

The second step is to *offer specific help and support* in addition to pointing out the patient's rights and responsibilities. Nurses will want to use very clear statements about their limitations but also clearly indicate that they and other health professionals will work with the patient to decide about and plan continuing care. They may want to outline what will need to be done in order to reach a decision, or suggest specific contributions that the patient or family members can make, such as reading material about possible alternatives.

People who want others to make decisions for them need *help in learning* how to take control and make use of available emotional supports. They must be able to ask questions without feeling stupid or incompetent. They must be allowed more than the usual amout of time to talk through the consequences of alternatives.

There Is a Manipulative Patient or Family Member. The manipulative person is one who has motives or agendas different from those presented publicly. He or she may withhold information or give conflicting messages to different people in an attempt to steer another's behavior or attitudes. The person who is manipulated feels angry and put down because manipulation is a subversive "power play."

The most common reasons for manipulation of continuing care decisions and plans are that people are attempting to escape from responsibility, they have their minds firmly made up about what is best and want to avoid negotiation, or they are exhibiting patterns of communication that are deeply entrenched. Upon discovering a manipulation attempt, it is not useful for the nurse to "fight fire with fire" and also become manipulative. It is helpful to *try to understand the motive* behind the manipulation. The nurse may need to say something like:

"You seem to feel _____ about this situation (or think _____ ought to be done). Can you tell me a bit more about how you came to this opinion?"

The response should give the nurse added insight about the dynamics of what is going on.

Robert Bramson (1981) gives some very specific advice for coping with difficult people of several types:

"(1) Assess the situation. (2) Stop wishing the Difficult Person were different. (3) Get some distance between you and the difficult behavior. (4) Formulate a coping plan. (5) Implement the plan. (6) Monitor the effectiveness of your coping strategy, modifying it where appropriate." (p. 130)

An important aspect of his advice is that people who feel manipulated need to distance themselves from the emotions of the immediate situation and objectively label or "diagnose" the disturbing behavior. As one nurse said on trying to cope with the highly manipulative wife of a patient: "Once I imagined her as a cat, I could see that she hissed and spat at everyone who didn't scratch her ears." That perception allowed the nurse not to feel personally attacked, but not to give in to "ear scratching" either.

The Patient Makes the "Wrong" Decision. A frequent problem in working closely with patients and their families as they plan continuing care is that nurses develop ideas about what they would like to see happen. If they try to impose these ideas on others, it is the nurses who have become manipulative. Nurses must even be careful about expressing strong opinions, since such expressions may be interpreted by patients as attempts to take over decision making. Confronted by situations in which the "wrong" plans are favored by patients or family members, nurses can do a number of things. One of these is to try to understand themselves better: where do these strong opinions come from? Are there experiences in their past that influence their view of the present situation? Are their opinions based on strongly liking or disliking some of the people involved?

Sometimes nurses feel uncomfortable about patients' decisions, because it seems to them that not all of the contributing factors or all the potential consequences are being considered. A calm and rational explanation of the nurse's reasons for feeling this way will at least help others understand the nurse's views, and perhaps encourage them to think through their own views more clearly.

Finally, nurses can try to understand the "rules" that govern the patient's or family's decision making (Satir, 1972). Some of the more important rules for continuing care decisions involve how money is used, who is responsible for making financial decisions, how household chores are managed, what subjects can be discussed freely and which are taboo, and how feelings are expressed. Such rules reflect values about the quality of life, beliefs about solving problems, and the personalities of the people involved (see Section 3.2). They affect how information is processed and therefore how decisions are made.

Nurses have a responsibility to ensure that all relevant information is available to patients and their families as they make continuing care decisions. Nurses then have a responsibility to respect those decisions even when they do not agree with them.

Better understanding of themselves and of family dynamics helps nurses do this. Awareness of the state of threat or crisis in which decisions are being made also helps nurses encourage families to develop back-up plans and make connections with community sources of help and information so that plans can be modified as needs emerge.

Patient Involvement in Step C: Confirming and Implementing the Plan

Once the basic decisions are made about the nature of continuing care, e.g., nursing home placement, home care, or self-care, preparation for the transition can begin in earnest. Due to early discharges from acute care, there is often only limited time for the teaching/learning and final coordination that must be done in this interval.

Although it takes more time for the nurse to organize, patient teaching should include at least one other person significant to the patient.

The most obvious reason for this is the improved chance that knowledge will be retained or a skill learned by at least one of the participants. Patients are seldom totally free of pain, anxiety, or other factors that dull their alertness and interfere with learning.

A second, even more important, reason for involving other people in the learning process is that any change in behavior will affect those in the patients' immediate social world. Having someone close to them understand the change and support patients' efforts to alter their behavior are critical to their success. Exercise programs, weight loss, special diets, and stopping smoking are all examples of behavior changes that require the support of the entire family in order to be successful. Nurses are encouraged to develop their teaching skills and become adept at helping patients and family members develop motivation for bringing about positive changes in health behaviors. In Example 4.2 the limitation of written material was demonstrated, but in most situations, suitable written support for teaching is very valuable to the patient. Also important is continued contact with caregivers who can reinforce teaching done in the acute setting. We will further explore the practical aspects of coordination with community services in Section 5.3.

In summary, the activities and functions of health professionals involved in discharge planning are matched by reciprocal patient and family functions; one set is ineffective without the other. In this section we have discussed how patients and family members can be actively included in each step of planning continuing care. Guidance has been given for making data gathering more effective and handling some problems of decision making.

SUMMARY

In this chapter we have explored several aspects of teamwork, including who can contribute to the discharge planning team and how organizational and communication patterns differ. Two extended case examples demonstrated some principles of teamwork. Finally, the importance of patient and family involvement in planning continuing care has been discussed and practical guidance given for accomplishing this. The knowledge and skills of a wide range of health care professionals are available to patients and families only when there is teamwork that includes effective communication, trusting coordination of effort, and active cooperation.

FURTHER READING

Rakich, J. S., B. B. Longest, and K. Darr. *Managing Health Services Organizations.* Philadelphia: W. B. Saunders, 1985.
> *This is the second edition of a favorite management text first published in 1977. Part 4: "Managing Human Resources in Health Services Organizations" contains material with particular relevance to this chapter, as does the chapter on organization theory and concepts. There is also an excellent chapter on ethical and legal issues.*

Bramson, Robert. *Coping With Difficult People.* New York: Ballantine Books, 1981.
> *This paperback falls in the category of "pop" psychology but is highly readable and does have helpful advice on handling—and more importantly, preventing— the breakdown of communication between people.*

Satir, Virginia. *Peoplemaking.* Palo Alto, Calif.: Science and Behavior Books, 1972.
> *This very readable and thought-provoking book is now a classic and still probably the best there is on family dynamics. Dr. Satir was world-famous for her seminars for health professionals demonstrating family therapy techniques. This book is highly recommended for all caregivers, especially those who attempt to help families with decision making.*

5

How Community Resources Contribute Care and Support

SUMMARY

FURTHER READING

The objective of discharge planning is to ensure the continuity of care for patients making a transition from one level of care to another. For the patient leaving the hospital, discharge plans that are made within the walls of an acute care facility have little purpose unless they are effectively coordinated with services in the community. This chapter focuses on these critical community "pieces" of the discharge planning puzzle. We begin by looking at how nurses can obtain information about sources of care and support for their patients. We then categorize the many community resources that may be available and briefly outline their services. Practical aspects of making referrals and coordinating services for maximum continuity are then discussed. Finally, the psychosocial implications of accepting help outside of acute care are explored. Throughout the chapter, the importance of setting clear goals for continuing care is emphasized.

This chapter is intended to give the nurse guidance for locating and making contact with community services that will be helpful to patients and their families. For this reason, the content is general in nature and can be applied to any community.

5.1 HOW TO SURVEY COMMUNITIES

The hospital is identified in the minds of many people as the center of the health care community. In fact, it has a limited role to play in the care of community members, a last resort when other approaches to health problems fail. The vast majority of medical and health care takes place in doctor's offices, medical clinics, and pharmacies. The challenge for the nurse in planning the discharges of hospitalized patients is to return them to family and community care. Community care must:

- provide high quality care to meet patients' medical goals and continue what was begun in the hospital;
- make optimum use of community health resources as well as patients' own care and support systems; and
- give appropriate help without undermining the patients' physical and emotional independence.

In order to do this, the nurse must first become familiar with the kinds of services offered in the community and discover how people solve health problems there. In this section, we will explore steps that can be taken by the nurse to identify and investigate the health resources in the community.

Identifying Goal-Oriented Communities

The first problem the nurse encounters in undertaking an analysis of health care resources is to define the word "community." Like "health," it is a term used so frequently that it would seem not to need definition. On closer look, however, we find that its use may create more confusion than clarity. "Community" is used to mean both neighborhood and town, to represent both people and buildings, and as an adjective to modify other words like "services" and "health." Some within the health professions use it to mean any service or person outside hospital walls.

A community has both geographical and interactional components. It is people in interaction bound together by common needs and resources.

A person or family may belong to several communities relating to the ways in which they solve a variety of problems or meet a number of goals (Waring and McLennan, 1979). For example, they may be involved in an educational community, a consumers' community, and a recreational community as well as a health care community (Figure 5–1). In a rural area, these goal-oriented communities may overlap substantially; in a large urban area, each community may have a separate set of participants.

The size of a person's community for solving a particular problem and the number of resources it contains are determined by three factors: *availability, access,* and *time.* For example, the size of the community one relates to for food purchase is determined first by the availability of markets, then by whether one has transportation to get to them, and by the amount of time one can devote to meeting this goal. A frail elderly person may have time, but limited transportation; a single working mother may have little time to pursue bargains in several stores. Both live in small food purchase communities although the resources of the geographical area may be vast.

In investigating a patient's communities, the nurse must ask:

1. What resources are AVAILABLE?

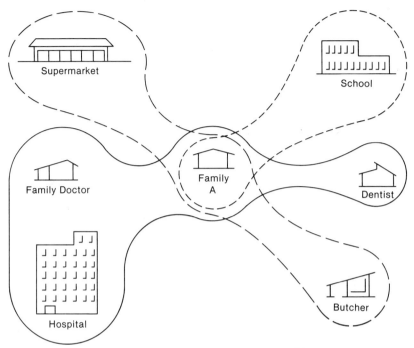

Figure 5–1. *Goal-oriented communities.*

2. *To which of these resources does the person have ACCESS? and*
3. *In what ways does TIME influence the selection of resources?*

The answers to these three questions will allow the nurse to anticipate how well a patient will be able to implement continuing care.

Making a Resource File

In order to make effective plans for patients' continuing care, nurses need detailed and reliable information about the community's sources of help. The best way to assemble such information is for nurses to investigate them themselves. There is no substitute for personal communication with caregivers and visits to the facilities provided for community members.

Investigation of community resources provides the nurse with valuable information upon which to base referrals, ask relevant questions, and measure other services.

The collection of such information will undoubtedly occur over a period of time, motivated by the needs of particular patients. The contacts made and information learned about each resource will help the nurse make more effective referrals for other patients. It also will provide a basis of information for evaluating similar services in more distant communities. For example, a visit to a local senior center will help develop communication with center leaders and an appreciation for the services offered. It also makes the nurse aware that similar services may exist in other communities. Presented with a patient from another area needing such services, the nurse has an idea what to look for and what questions to ask even though the only contact may be by telephone.

Many nurses we have worked with have found that a simple *resource file* is an extremely valuable tool. Collected over a period of time, it can be a card file or loose-leaf notebook with details about each available resource. It is not necessarily limited to medical and health care resources, although this is a good beginning. A sample card for such a file is shown in Figure 5–2.

Aside from the basic information, nurses have found the "comments" section the most helpful. We suggest writing notes here in pencil so they may be updated periodically. For example, one nurse had made the notation "Ms. Peters (Sr. Caseworker) has evening app'ts. for working women" for a mental health agency. This fact greatly increased access for some patients.

There are two basic discoveries involved in locating health care and support services: one is finding out what exists, and the other is

NAME: SERVICE CATEGORY:

ADDRESS: TELEPHONE:

CONTACT PERSON (and position):

SERVICES OFFERED:

ELIGIBILITY:

REFERRAL PROCEDURE:

COMMENTS (about organizational structure, informal communication patterns and priorities, response time in acting on referrals, willingness to coordinate services with others, etc.):

Figure 5–2. *Sample data card for resource file.*

discovering the geographical location of their office and service area. Before beginning an extensive resource file, nurses are encouraged to look at the geographical area of concern as though they were sociologists. Most likely the area can be divided into segments based on socioeconomic factors, dominance of one age or racial group, types of housing, or divisive physical features such as major highways or railroad tracks.

Coding resource file entries according to geographical segments of a community allows the nurse to quickly identify which services might be accessible to a particular patient.

Information about public transportation is especially important in identifying community segments. Some of the implications of such data are demonstrated in Example 5.1.

Example 5.1 Isolation Within a City

Sheila MacIntyre had recently been appointed nursing supervisor for the Emergency Department of a large metropolitan university teaching hospital. Even in the short time she had been there, Sheila was aware that there was growing concern among staff about the numbers of medically indigent patients who used the Emergency facilities inappropriately for minor problems. After some investigation, she learned that most of these patients came from one area of town, quite some distance away.

Interested in trying to understand why this pattern had developed, Sheila contacted the supervisor of the Public Health Nursing office that served the area for an appointment. During the conference, Sheila learned the following about this segment of the larger community:

— Most residents of the low-cost housing in the area were from minority groups, and many were recent immigrants to the country;

— The area was geographically isolated by major freeways that bordered it on three sides;

— Public transportation consisted of a single bus line whose destination was the downtown city terminal, which was within two blocks of the university hospital;

— Transportation to the county hospital that provided free services involved two bus transfers and a cost of $4.50; and

— Recent funding cutbacks had limited staff and increased waiting times for patients of up to two hours in the outpatient clinics at the county hospital.

With this information, it was clear to Sheila that access to more appropriate medical care was very limited for this population.

This kind of understanding of the problems that segments of the population face in meeting continuing care needs helps the nurse plan more realistically with patients. For a patient from the area described in the example, alternative transportation to medical follow-up would need to be considered as well as the availability of local, more convenient services.

Having established what health care and support resources are available and their geographic location, the nurse is ready to telephone or visit them and *ask specific questions* about their services and accessibility. This information will be collected over a period of time as the nurse has reason to be interested in particular services. Recording findings in a resource file saves a great deal of time later.

It has been our experience that nurses often hesitate to ask other health professionals for details of the services they offer. Perhaps they feel defensive about admitting that they do not already know. In most cases, however, health professionals are only too eager to clarify for others just what they do and what kinds of patients or clients they prefer. The following questions are presented as models of what a nurse might ask to obtain information relevant to planning continuing care.

- What kinds of *services* do you provide? What kinds of health problems are of greatest interest to you? Are there services in which you specialize?
- How do people become *eligible* for your services? What kinds of referral procedures do you follow? How does a patient/client initiate contact with you? What information will they need to share with you? Is there a particular person they should ask for? What length of time can be expected before services begin for a new patient/client?
- What *financial* arrangements do patients make for services? What is a typical service fee? Do you accept Medicare assignment? (See Appendix B.) What portion of the service fee is usually covered by private insurance?
- Exactly where are your offices *located*? (Get building and suite location as well as address.) What kinds of transportation are available to patients? What geographical area do you serve?

• Is there anything else I should know about your services that would help me in telling patients about you?

These kinds of questions cover the major areas of information a nurse needs for making referrals to a service and can be easily adapted to various kinds of resources. Asking them will lead to other specific follow-up questions. For example: "Is that on the second floor?" "Is there an elevator?" "Is there wheelchair access?" (See Section 2.2 for a description of the CONE interview, a procedure adaptable to the investigation of community services.)

In summary, surveying community resources for health care and support not only gives the nurse information to use in making referrals but also provides an important perspective on how people in that geographical area solve problems and meet goals. Such insight allows the nurse to ask more discerning questions and to establish rapport with community caregivers more quickly. Well balanced knowledge of a service's availability, access, and time features permit the nurse to more effectively teach patients and their families about services that may meet their needs.

5.2 SOURCES OF CARE AND SUPPORT

In this section, major categories of community resources will be summarized. We have included notes on what kinds of services might be expected from each category and how the nurse might make contact with them. Although far from comprehensive, this listing should provide ideas about how to find out what services exist "out there" in nurses' own communities and stimulate them to ask questions and request information. Resources have been divided into health care services and support services.

Medical and Health Care Services

Every member of the community has health and medical care needs that include health maintenance and health promotion information or services, and access to diagnostic and emergency services when required. For those just discharged from the hospital, medical follow-up is added to this list. In addition, patients may need other services that allow them to regain their health or compensate for disability. Medical and health care services have been divided into three categories for ease of discussion: episodic care, home care, and residential facilities. Some of the major characteristics of each are described below.

Episodic Medical and Health Care Services. Medical and health care services that offer episodic care range from outpatient clinics and private practitioner's offices to day care centers, health education or screening programs, and alternative medicine clinics.

Episodic care is appropriate for persons whose health goals are health maintenance or promotion, diagnosis and entry to care, and continuing medical supervision of a wide variety of disorders, including chronic disease. This form of care makes up the bulk of medical and health care services.

Although service depends on the patient coming to the practitioner, service centers are usually widely distributed in populated areas and are therefore easily *accessible* in a physical sense.

A major factor limiting access to services is *cost;* for those with insurance, part of visit cost may be covered, but patients without such coverage may find their choices for low-cost care limited. With the exception of "drop-in" clinics, episodic care generally requires an appointment. While this takes a telephone and some pre-planning, reasonably *prompt* service is generally given. Busy metropolitan out-patient clinics are an exception, however, and can involve lengthy waits.

In investigating what *sources* of episodic care exist in an area, the telephone Yellow Pages are a good beginning. Local governments or community centers often publish directories of services, as do special groups such as senior citizen's centers and disabled person's associations. Some of the categories of services and their distribution that the nurse might look for include:

- Family physicians and medical specialists;
- Dentists and dental specialists;
- Neighborhood medical clinics (often called Urgent Care, Emergency Care, or Community Care Clinics);
- Outpatient services operated by hospitals or large group practices;
- Specialized clinics such as Well Child Clinics, Planned Parenthood, or Adolescent Clinics;
- Immunization and screening services for children;
- Alternative medicine practitioners (chiropractors, acupuncturists, and herbalists, for example);
- Mental health services operated by government bodies or Family Service Agencies;
- Counselors in private practice;
- Diagnostic screening programs (X-rays, blood pressure, cholesterol, and AIDS testing, for example);

- Day-care programs for seniors, the disabled, or ill or handicapped children;
- Pharmacies and medical equipment suppliers; and
- Health education and promotion programs in schools or colleges or sponsored by local health authorities.

The diversity of episodic care services is great, but all share the goal of providing services to meet specific health needs for those who come to them.

Home Care Services. These are services that come to the patient/client in his or her own living environment. Although visits from caregivers are usually short, they are likely to recur at regular intervals over a period of time.

Home care is appropriate for those with continuing care goals of rehabilitation, chronic illness management, or terminal care whenever their condition prevents them going to the caregiver.

Home care can provide a viable alternative to institutional care when community resources are adequate and patients are able to manage activities of daily living themselves or with the help available from friends, relatives, or a caregiver employed for that purpose.

Home care agencies and visiting nurse associations provide skilled nursing care and physical, speech, and/or occupational therapy. Their services are *accessible* in most metropolitan areas. Rural areas may be served by the Public Health Department. Some of the same agencies provide non-skilled or custodial services.

Some people find it preferable to privately employ a registered nurse or attendant on a part-time or full-time basis. Caregivers may be located through a Nurses' Registry. Potential employees should be interviewed, their qualifications and experience checked, and references contacted. Employment should be for a trial period initially and then a formal employment contract entered that specifies the responsibilities and obligations of all parties. While all these procedures may seem unnecessary at the time, it is well worth the time and effort required to ensure against future misunderstandings or legal complications.

The *cost* of home care is a major consideration. Skilled nursing care given under a doctor's supervision may qualify for partial payment from Medicare, Medicaid, or private insurers. Non-skilled or custodial care generally is not covered. Some agencies have a sliding scale of charges based on patient finances. Due to periodic changes in federal regulations, it is appropriate for the nurse to inquire of agencies or hospital social workers about just what financial arrangements are appropriate for a particular patient.

Home care agencies may be located by looking under "Nursing" in the telephone directory. Pamphlets outlining services and costs for various organizations are often made available to hospital discharge planning departments or social services. The *services* provided by an agency may include:

- Nursing care by registered nurses for adults or children (some offer clinical specialists);
- Home health aids to help with personal care and activities of daily living;
- Physical and occupational therapy and speech pathology;
- Consultation by medical social workers;
- Housekeeping services;
- Live-in attendants or companions; and/or
- Hospice care for the terminally ill.

The advantage of home care is that it allows patients to remain within their own social world and familiar physical surroundings. Some people, however, find it very difficult to adjust to being dependent on family members and close friends. The psycho-social as well as physical aspects of care within the home need to be considered as part of the discharge plan.

Residential Facilities. When a person is unable to manage care at home for physical or social reasons, a residential facility may be appropriate. While *skilled nursing facilities* or "convalescent" homes are the most widely accessible within this category, there are a number of other options for people who cannot stay in their own home. Many communities have licensed *board and care* homes for a limited number of residents. This kind of accommodation is expensive and is not covered by either Medicare, Medicaid, or private insurances, but the quality of life for the frail aged person may be much better than if he or she were placed in a nursing home among ill patients.

Rehabilitation units are sometimes attached to hospital complexes and offer intensive therapy on a short-term, residential basis and, occasionally, job retraining or sheltered workshops. The Veterans Administration hospitals often have such rehabilitation programs. They also may offer "respite" care to families who normally take responsibility for care of a patient; the patient is admitted for a short time, allowing the family to take a vacation. Facilities for psychiatric patients and the developmentally disabled also usually offer a range of care intensity levels depending on patient need.

As the number of elderly increases so, too, do *"retirement" facilities* and senior housing complexes. They can be a useful alternative to living with family members when the person no longer wants to look after a large house or garden or cook his or her own meals. Such facilities always have programs of social activities and outings to keep residents socially involved. They usually provide transportation to medical appointments and shopping. Some facilities offer nursing care and medical supervision as well as housekeeping services. Again, they are generally expensive, but may be less so than a nursing home. Some have an initial "buy-in" fee that can be sizable.

It is important that potential residents or their representatives actually visit the facilities under consideration. An initial appointment should be made with the administrator and followed up with an unannounced visit. Good times to visit are at meal times, late afternoon or evening (to observe adequacy of staffing), or weekends. In assessing whether a facility meets the needs of a particular patient or when generally investigating what is available, the following items bear consideration.

- Location: convenience to family, available public transportation, nearby medical services;
- Common facilities: cleanliness, size, appointments, and lighting in lobby, lounges, hallways, dining areas;
- Residents' rooms: effective use of space, pleasant/comfortable appointments, degree of personalization encouraged, easy access to bathroom, closets/storage available;
- Kitchen (a tour should be requested of administrator): cleanliness, organization, adequate food preparation space, refrigeration, dish-handling equipment, and attitude of staff toward visitors;
- Food (arrange to have a meal): presentation, size of portions, temperature, choice, alternatives for special diets, taste;
- Activities: frequency of events, variety of activities, goals of activity program, attitude of activity director/volunteers, availability of equipment and supplies (books, craft materials, vehicles for transport, exercise equipment), level of activity required to remain in facility;
- Personal and medical care: services available, qualifications of caregivers, level of preparation for medical emergencies, equipment available, therapy programs offered, access to physician consultation and acute care;
- Selection of residents and finances: criteria for entry to facility as resident, licensing for Medicare/Medicaid, expected payment schedule, attitude of management toward financial obligations of residents;
- Atmosphere and attitude of residents: cheerfulness and comfort of surroundings, grooming and responsiveness of other residents, degree of physical activity and verbal interaction by residents, attitudes expressed toward visitors; and

• Attitudes of staff: staff turnover, stated goals, criteria used for encouraging residents to participate in activities and interact with others, positive and negative attitudes expressed by staff, most important problems they experience, and how they respond to these.

Used as a checklist, these factors will stimulate the visitor to a residential facility to ask other questions relevant to the level of care and goals of the patient.

Choosing a residential facility involves paying attention to what services are offered, what criteria are used for offering them, who provides them, what advantages and disadvantages there are in the physical environment, and how people treat one another.

The informal information about attitudes gained in conversation with staff, management, and other residents is as important as the physical environment.

Support Services

In most communities there is a range of support services available that help people solve particular problems or avoid certain difficulties. These services are divided into general categories and described briefly in the paragraphs below. Notes are included as to how the nurse might gather information for a resource file.

Financial Services. The Social Services Department of the local county or shire is a good place to begin to research financial services. It will provide information about state and federal aid programs and special kinds of financial help, such as discount programs and tax counselors. Departmental staff will either offer, or put a person in touch with, financial counseling that includes budget planning.

For the older person, senior centers and the nearest office of the Council on Aging will be able to supply information about financial aid and discount programs. Many now provide health insurance counseling (see Appendix B).

Legal Services. A telephone call to the local Legal Aid Society is a good starting point for finding out about legal services. These societies are federally funded to provide legal advice and aid to those unable to pay for the private services of an attorney. Their services may be limited due to funding or staffing, but generally they will accept defense of a civil suit, bankruptcy proceedings, or administrative law cases (involving Medicare, Medicaid, various welfare programs, etc.).

Local Bar Associations will provide referrals to legal services and verify the qualifications of local attorneys. Sometimes they also offer free, brief legal consultations that help potential clients identify their rights and obligations under the law.

The Social Services Department can also give information about legal services for low-income persons, seniors, and special legal concerns.

Community Groups. Local support groups, the regional offices of national societies, and disease-specific charitable organizations offer a range of valuable services. Because the general community is often unaware of them, the nurse can make an important contribution to continuing care by including them in a resource file and referring patients appropriately. The nurse can find out about such local groups by consulting:

- Other health and social service professionals;
- Telephone directories and directories furnished by senior centers, community centers, or local governments;
- Family service agencies (especially for mental health services);
- The Veterans Administration;
- Adult and child protective services;
- Regional centers for the developmentally disabled; and
- Local newpapers, for stories about service groups (especially church or youth groups and local chapters of larger charitable organizations).

The services offered are so diverse that it is difficult to generalize about them. Some examples of services include Meals-on-Wheels, grocery delivery, transportation, and home repair.

Peer support groups provide a special kind of service in a community. They are groups of people with a similar concern or problem who meet together on a regular basis to share information and their own experiences. The emotional support provided by others who have the same kinds of problems or who have weathered the same kinds of experiences is extremely powerful. In some groups such as Alcoholics Anonymous, new behavior patterns are motivated, encouraged, and supported. Other groups in this category include weight-loss groups, those focusing on substance abuse including smoking, and some mental health groups.

Other peer support groups are established around diagnostic groups or special handicaps. They also share information, problem solving, and emotional support. Socializing in a supportive, accepting environment is an especially important aspect of many groups' activities. Examples include diabetic support groups, post-coronary groups, parents of deaf or blind children, stroke patients, and bereavement groups. Some of these groups are sponsored by national organizations that provide a meeting place, group leadership, and sometimes transportation. Other support groups have grown out of local concerns, meet in available community buildings or churches, and have no professional leadership.

Recreation and Education. Opportunities for recreation and education add greatly to the quality of life for everyone and have special meaning for the person with physical handicaps or chronic diseases.

Community centers often have exercise programs for groups with special needs and a schedule of adult education classes. Seniors with mobility problems due to arthritis, for example, may especially enjoy and benefit from aquatic exercises. Hobby and special interest groups provide socialization as well as recreation. Centers in areas with a large senior population sometimes sponsor events such as sightseeing bus trips or excursions to local attractions.

Discounts for the handicapped or for seniors are available at most recreational and entertainment events, from museums to concerts, from theaters to charitable events, to local festivals and celebrations.

Community colleges often offer special courses for seniors and the handicapped, have discounted tuition for seniors attending regular classes, and provide transportation services. Catalogs are available on request. Colleges also have special entertainment events and hobby skill classes (e.g., ceramics and woodworking) that are appropriate and fulfilling for those with limited physical abilities but a desire for social contacts and mental stimulation.

Libraries are an important community resource not only for books, but also for videotapes and phonograph records. Many have "talking books" or large-print books and periodicals for the handicapped or visually impaired. Those in larger communities often hold literature discussion groups and have special educational programs for children and seniors. Book-mobiles may visit retirement facilities and other selected community locations to make library services more accessible.

In summary, a wide range of health and support services are available in most communities. They are not, however, obvious to the casual observer. The nurse can make a very large contribution to patients' well-being by exploring services in the area and keeping an updated file of information on them. The investment of time and effort made in obtaining details about accessibility, eligibility, cost, and time factors will be rewarded by being able to make more effective and comprehensive discharge plans.

5.3 HOW TO MAKE REFERRALS

Anticipating what the patient will *need* after discharge based on a thorough assessment is a major piece of the discharge planning puzzle.

Knowing what *services* exist in the community and which of them is relevant to the patient's needs is another piece. Making a referral is the most common way to start fitting these two pieces together. The referral process is more than just filling out a form with cursory information and telling the patient a referral has been made.

The roles of the nurse in making referrals include those of teacher, communicator, and coordinator.

A referral that effectively brings community services together with patient needs includes:

- helping patient and family learn what services are available in the community;
- helping them learn how to coordinate the patient's continuing care; and
- helping the relevant community services learn what is needed, why, and for how long.

In this section we will especially focus on the role of the nurse in communicating information. We begin by discussing the importance of initiating this process early in the patient's care. Practical aspects of effectively transmitting a "picture" of the patient to community services are then explored. Finally, we consider the communication skills necessary in receiving a referral and giving useful feedback to other professionals.

Introducing Community Assistance to Patient and Family

One of the first challenges faced by the nurse in giving excellent patient care is to help the patient learn about the nature and cause of the medical problem. This is the basis on which informed consent is given for treatment. Early patient teaching needs to be carefully planned and the patient's responses carefully monitored because it is the first step in helping the patient begin to consider his or her future well-being. The physical stress of illness, complicated by what the patient imagines is going to happen, can escalate into a crisis if information given is only half understood or is so detailed that it is overwhelming (see Section 3.1). If there is an opportunity to have the patient and family members tell the nurse what their previous experience with medical care have been, the nurse will be in a better position to guide them toward an understanding of reality without causing undue stress (see Section 2.3).

Confronted with a diagnosis that has serious implications for the future, the patient typically feels apprehensive and very alone. This is an appropriate time for the nurse to begin to introduce the idea that there is help available in the community. This early information does not need to be very specific, nor should the patient be led to believe that she or he is to have no responsibility for continuing care, but the fact that the patient will not be left alone without assistance in coping should be made clear. Some examples of early information about community resources that served to reassure patients while still helping them cope with reality are briefly described as follows.

Example 5.2 Giving Early Information About Resources

- A 16-year-old girl is discovered to be a diabetic. She imagines that she is the "only one in the whole world" with a problem like this. The nurse gives her a pamphlet describing American Diabetes Association services to young diabetics and tells her that the hospital sponsors a group for young patients with this disease that meets monthly.
- A 48-year-old male executive is admitted with a severe myocardial infarct. He knows he has had a heart attack and imagines that, if he survives, he will be unable to continue work, and his family will be destitute. The nurse sits down with him and calmly describes the cardiac rehabilitation program in his community, discusses with him some ways in which stress can be reduced, and lets him know that he will have the help and support of professionals throughout his recovery.
- A Spanish-speaking woman has a simple mastectomy. In broken English, she tells the nurse that she is worried about her husband's response to her surgery and thinks she will now be an invalid. The nurse gives her a booklet called "Reach To Recovery" with basic information about mastectomy written in Spanish, tells her she will soon be able to return to her normal activities, and makes a mental note to check to see whether there is a Spanish-speaking social worker or counselor on the hospital staff.

In each of these cases, fears about the future added greatly to the patient's state of stress. Discovering the nature of these powerful fears and anxieties allows the nurse greater depth of understanding in anticipating needs. If the nurse's response indicates to the patient and family that such fears are silly, they will become defensive as well as stressed. If, instead, the nurse helps them understand that their fears are unfounded BECAUSE help is available to solve their particular problems, then they can let go of the fears and begin to deal with reality.

> *Helping the patient and family identify sources of community assistance early in care reduces the stress caused by unrealistic fantasies and allows the patient to develop awareness of the kind of support that will be offered.*

This is patient teaching whose goals are at a simple level, that is, *understanding* that help is available and *recognition* that caregivers are concerned about the future and will assist the patient in planning for it (see Table 2–2). As care progresses, this early teaching becomes the basis for more complex goals such as *evaluation* of specific needs in comparison with services offered, *utilization* of appropriate community help, and *performance* of learned self-help procedures.

General information and reassurance offered early in care gives the patient and family the important messages that they will not be abandoned to cope by themselves and that caregivers expect them to be involved in the planning and implementation of continuing care. More detailed information will be required about community resources as they begin to sort through their options, clarify continuing care goals, and come to terms with realistic expectations of the patient's progress and others' help.

> *The ideal result of teaching focused on community resources is that the patient adopt an attitude of "supported self-reliance": an acceptance of appropriate help while maintaining control of the direction and goals of continuing care.*

The issues surrounding the development of supported self-reliance will be further discussed in Section 5.4.

Transmitting Information to Community Services

Making a referral to a caregiver in the community requires that the nurse or referral source "paint a picture" of the patient, his or her needs, and the context within which care will be given. While there are many variations of referral forms, few are ideally suited to every patient. Therefore, the nurse will want to consider the problem of transmitting appropriate and useful information as a whole without being restricted by a particular form. The nurse may choose to modify the available form or supplement it with verbal or additional written material. Some ideas about the kinds of information that complete the picture for the recipient caregiver follow.

Information about the *patient as a person,* in addition to the usual vital statistics, will include:

- level of knowledge and understanding about the medical problem;
- attitudes toward the prognosis and continuing care;
- involvement in decision-making and problem solving; and
- physical and emotional responses to treatment.

Information about the patient's *needs for care,* in addition to specific medical orders and current physical data, will include:

- identification of both major and minor problems and their importance to the patient;
- clear definition of continuing care goals;
- barriers such as stress or lack of personal resources that may influence progress toward these goals; and
- specific procedures or elements of care with which help is needed.

Information about the *context* within which community care is to be given might include:

- what is known about the patient's experiences and perceptions that will affect further learning;
- the makeup of the patient's primary and secondary social groups and the nature of support they provide;
- the degree of involvement of family members in patient teaching and decision making;
- the attitudes of family members toward the patient, diagnosis, and prognosis; and
- relevant physical features of the patient's living situation at discharge.

These items of information would, of course, supplement the usual data that give name, address, doctor, arrangements for other supportive services, and financial information. The information suggested above is heavily weighted toward subjective judgments by the caregiver about attitudes, beliefs, and values that have not been directly observed. The "Detailed Needs Identification" form that is part of Step B in the second part of this text is suggested as a starting point for collecting this kind of information. While professional ethics require that nurses be careful about stating such judgments as though they were confirmed facts, these items provide information about the patient as a whole person, not just as a diabetic who needs insulin injections, for example.

Just as color is an important part of any picture, so

> *information about a person's attitudes and feelings, while subjectively reported by the nurse, help to complete the "picture" given in an effective referral.*

Nurses may feel more comfortable sharing subjective information verbally rather than in writing. They may thus informally include what led to their judgments and how events may have affected patient responses. Verbal communication has the advantage of allowing the community caregiver to assess the attitudes of the informant as well as the validity of the information.

Objective information presented as such in referrals must, of course, be checked carefully for accuracy.

One area that often causes unnecessary confusion is the transfer from hospital to community of specific *medical procedures;* few agencies follow exactly the same protocol. In addition to giving the new caregiver a copy of the hospital procedure, the most effective method for eliminating confusion and patient distress is to invite the community caregiver to observe the hospital procedure. This also serves the purpose of introducing the patient to the new person and allowing their relationship to begin developing before care is transferred. When the procedures are life-sustaining, such as total parenteral nutrition, the transfer of trust is as important as the protocol.

Another area of potential confusion and unnecessary interruption in patient care is the *timing* of referrals. Hospital personnel who are used to 24-hour services sometime fail to realize the impact on community care of sending off a referral on a Friday or the day before a holiday. Not only is it often very difficult for a home care agency, for example, to provide good care to a new patient on a weekend, but attempting to meet such a demand may generate a great deal of anger at hospital staff perceived as being inconsiderate. The legacy of that kind of anger is much more difficult relationships in the future—all the more reason to start the discharge planning process early in patient care and prepare both patient and community services for transitions. As a last resort, a quick telephone call to a community caregiver by the nurse giving warning that the patient is likely to be discharged within a day or so will improve the possibility of continuity.

Receiving Referrals and Giving Feedback

Although referrals from community agencies to acute care facilities are not as common as referrals from hospital to community, they certainly do occur and provide the opportunity for acute care staff to reciprocate with continuity of patient care and good feedback. In most instances, referrals of patients to acute care come from services in the community that receive referrals. It is unfortunate that these referrals often become swallowed up in the hospital record system and, due to the number of caregivers, do not receive a personal response.

If a community-based health professional has taken the time to write a referral, he or she deserves a timely, personal response.

The reason for a referral is to ensure continuity of care. In most cases the patient will return to the care of the referring community caregiver following an acute episode. A simple telephone call to the initiator of a referral to let her or him know that it has been received and read is not only polite, professional behavior, but it also secures a working relationship from which the patient will benefit.

For both community and acute care health professionals, the reception of a referral brings with it the responsibility to give some feedback. Ideally, this feedback begins immediately. Recognizing that referral information is useful only if its messages are clear and unambiguous, nurses will want to be sure they understand the "picture" presented.

It is important to clarify referral information and resolve any apparent contradictions very early in a patient's care.

This should be done with an open, cooperative manner rather than an aggressive, challenging one. A working relationship can develop out of an inquiry that begins: "I wonder whether you can tell me a bit more about Mrs. Bloggs. . . . " On the other hand, one that begins: "What on earth did you mean by . . . " will be heard as the challenge it is and will result only in defensive, uncooperative responses.

Implicit in an inquiry to clarify information is the opportunity to help the person making the referral learn what the recipient needs. Every conversation like this can contribute to a better understanding of what is important to the receiving service and, therefore, to better referrals. As noted earlier, the verbal exchange of information not only allows the transmission of subjective judgments and opinions but also allows the professionals involved to get to know one another better.

In summary, the transmission of information at referrals between services is most effective when approached as a "picture" of the patient provided by one caregiver for another. Both objective and subjective information is appropriate to a full picture. Patient care greatly benefits from the coordination made possible through good referrals. Patients also benefit from knowing early in their care that acute care and community professionals will work together to meet their continuing health care needs.

5.4 PATIENT ACCEPTANCE OF COMMUNITY HELP

Those who work routinely in acute care and have become used to cooperative patients are sometimes surprised when families are less than enthusiastic about having a caregiver come into their homes, when patients refuse nursing home placement although in need of nursing care, or when patients fail to keep follow-up appointments with their physicians. Superficially, these behaviors would appear to be self-defeating and illogical, and these patients are sometimes labeled "non-compliant." In this section, we will try to help the nurse make sense of such resistance to accepting help. Our initial discussion will be of the factors that contribute to acceptance or rejection of help. We then will consider how to anticipate patients' level of acceptance and how to help them steer the narrow course toward supported self-reliance.

Factors In Accepting Help

The anxiety generated by a medical crisis is usually enough to overcome people's natural resistance to asking for help and giving up some measure of personal control over events. Their anticipation of an uncomfortable experience is usually balanced by relief that something is being done about the problem. In seeking care from a hospital or clinic, they enter the "foreign" social system of medical care (see Section 3.3). Most expect that the encounter will be temporary and therefore are willing to expend energy learning the "rules" of behavior that apply to this situation. Like a visitor to a foreign country, they try to adapt so that their presence is accepted and they do not attract criticism and hostility from the "natives."

Upon discharge from acute care, the tables are turned, however. Now caregivers may come as visitors to patients' own social worlds, patients may be expected to interrupt their daily routines to keep appointments, or, in the case of residential care, they may be "immigrating" permanently to the foreign world of being cared for. Each of these situations requires different kinds of acceptance and coping mechanisms from those required to enter acute care.

To accept the help of others requires an admission that one is unable to care independently for oneself.

In the following paragraphs, some of the psychological and socio-cultural factors contributing to resistance to follow-up care are explored.

Resistance to Episodic Care. In the vast majority of cases, patients leaving a hospital after acute care are referred to one or several kinds of episodic follow-up. They may be told by their doctor that they should come to the office within a certain interval, an appointment may be made for them with an outpatient clinic, or they may be instructed to get in touch with various health professionals in the community. Patients seldom announce that they have no intention of following such recommendations, but a surprising number fail to make appointments or fail to keep them when made for them. In one study, only 55% of discharged patients had made follow-up appointments within six weeks (Rorden, 1986, pp. 146–147).

There seem to be at least three factors at work in such follow-up failures. Perhaps the most significant is the *psychological* factor mentioned above. Continuing episodic treatment requires that the patient acknowledge that the health problem that precipitated hospitalization has not been "fixed" and that, like a child, he or she continues to need help. The patient who has not been helped to understand the nature of the problem and its implications for future health is particularly vulnerable to resisting follow-up. So are the independent souls who find the child-like role of "patient" degrading and frustrating. High quality patient education and an attitude of patient–caregiver equality are necessary to remove this psychological factor as a barrier to care.

There is also a significant *social* factor involved in resisting follow-up care. Not only must patients admit to themselves that they continue to need care and are not totally independent, but they must admit this "weakness" to their primary social group. A supportive family that encourages continuing efforts to fully resolve the medical problem without treating the patient as an invalid or martyr is less common than might be imagined. Usually family members have been frightened by a medical crisis and recover their pre-illness view of the patient slowly, unless there is teaching intervention by a health professional. It may also be difficult for them to accept and support changes in patient behaviors such as altered diets or exercise programs without special help. (See Section 6.2 for a discussion of motivation and change.)

Finally, there is a *financial* factor. Usually there is not much choice about hospitalization when a medical crisis occurs, in spite of fears about the meaning of it to family finances. Many people do, however, choose to avoid episodic community care because of financial concerns. Indeed, Medicare and private insurance plans often cover only a small portion of community care. Such additional expenses after a hospital stay may seem insupportable to the elderly and to low-income families.

These three factors are evident in the following case example.

Example 5.3 Resistance to Investigation of Heart Murmur

Rose Tyler was a 64-year-old retired schoolteacher. Each of the previous three or four winters, Mrs. Tyler had come down with a bad cold that had turned into bronchitis. The problem had always responded to medical treatment. Her husband was retiring in a few months, and they would be moving to Arizona the following spring. She hoped that the drier climate would put a permanent end to this problem. This winter, however, she had again developed symptoms and so made an appointment with her internist. His examination revealed a systolic heart murmur that had not been noted before. In addition to treating Mrs. Tyler's bronchitis, he recommended that she see a cardiologist with offices in the same building.

Rose was not particularly eager to cope with a new medical problem, but she did make an appointment with the cardiologist as instructed. Her arrival for that appointment was met with some confusion; it seemed that the office staff could not locate the information that was supposed to have been transferred from the internist. She waited while they telephoned him and then sent someone down to pick up a duplicate copy. Once in an examining room, she again waited a long time. She could hear two men talking and laughing in an adjoining room and assumed that one was the doctor.

When the doctor finally did appear, he seemed in a great hurry. He barely greeted her, so intent was he upon reading the chart. He listened briefly to her heart, took her blood pressure, and then said: "I don't think it's anything too serious but I want you to get some tests done. Tell the receptionist that I want to see you in two weeks." He had been in the room not quite five minutes. Mrs. Tyler left the office feeling a mixture of anger and dismay.

Once home, a telephone call to her private insurance company revealed that her out-of-pocket expenses for the ECG, stress test, and blood tests that had been ordered would be over $400—a lot of money to a couple saving every possible dollar for their retirement. It did not take her long to decide that she would not follow up on the tests or go back to the cardiologist. She wondered whether she would have the courage to go back to the internist, since she was not following his advice. When her husband asked Rose what the cardiologist had found, she just said: "Oh, he said it was nothing to worry about."

In this case example, the patient's anger about the impersonal manner in which she was treated by the cardiologist and his staff and the social implications of a medical problem interfering with the couple's planned retirement move, combined with concern over the cost of tests, led Mrs. Tyler to decide against further follow-up of the heart murmur. That decision also created a barrier to her continued care by the internist, since she now felt defensive.

A combination of psychological, social, and financial factors frequently influences patients to ignore symptoms, deny medical needs, or resist continuing care. Telling people what caregivers think they *should* do is not enough to motivate the desired behavior in most instances.

> *Caregivers who find out how the patient feels about recommendations and how he or she interprets the consequences of seeking further medical help are in a good position to help the patient follow through on continuing care plans.*

Obtaining information about feelings and interpretations requires careful listening to the answers to open questions (see Section 2.2). Early identification of a patient's concerns about and potential resistance to continuing care plans allows for modification of those plans before a follow-up failure occurs and anger and defensiveness complicate relationships.

Resistance to Home Care. From the caregiver's point of view, the easiest kind of follow-up care for patients to accept ought to be home care; they remain in their own physical and social environments while care is given. Yet many people experience care at home as an invasion of privacy and a severe social disruption.

One way of understanding these negative responses to an apparently ideal solution to continuing care needs has been described by sociologist Erving Goffman (1971). He sees people as actively and purposefully choosing "selves" to present to others during social interaction. The choice of a particular "self" is based on:

- an estimate of the nature of the social situation;
- the "rules" that seem to govern acceptable behavior; and
- knowledge of and attitudes toward the other people involved.

All "selves" that are presented to others come from a person's own self-image or identity and the desire to have that identity maintained in interaction with others. One may, within quick succession, talk with a friend, discipline a child, and discuss a business transaction, for example. In each instance a different "self" represents facets of one's personal identity.

When a presented self (for example, "capable mother") is challenged deliberately or unwittingly by caregivers (for example, a pediatric nurse), the person experiences *threat*, which may be mild or severe depending on how closely the presented self is tied to personal identity. Defense against such a threat may lead to withdrawal from the interaction, withholding further information (as did the young mother in Example 4.2), or altering the person's view of the supposed helpers by devaluing their importance, knowledge, or skills or inferring hostility in their approach.

> *The caregiver in the community works within the patient's immediate social world; the "selves" encountered are those that are appropriate to intimate social relationships.*

These selves characteristically reflect the most valued aspects of personal identity and are vulnerable to threat by a caregiver's overt, or even implied, lack of acceptance.

An example was presented to a nurse recently. As a staff member of a school for "exceptional" children, she had reason to contact the mother of a severely retarded child. From other sources, she knew that the woman presented herself to social acquaintances as a concerned mother with a child who was "slow." The nurse was not entirely surprised, therefore, when the mother responded with some hostility and considerable resistance to her telephone attempt to set up a home visit. The nurse was aware of the threat that her visit could present when the degree of the child's retardation was obvious. During the home visit she took care to preserve some social distance by addressing the mother formally and asking open questions that allowed the mother to divulge only as much information as was comfortable for her.

Because receiving help implies lack of competence in some aspect of one's life situation, a self-image of independence and strength may be severely threatened by well-intentioned health professionals. The following case example demonstrates this point.

Example 5.4 Independence Threatened by Care

Both Lester and Dorothy Riggs were in their mid-eighties. Until very recently they had been totally independent, living in the small farmhouse they had occupied for 45 years. Over the years they had sold off pieces of the property to supplement their retirement pensions, but they prided themselves on never having had to ask either their children or strangers for physical or financial help.

In 1985, Lester had suffered a slight stroke that had left him with some residual weakness on the right side. Almost exactly two years later, Dorothy had a similar stroke. She recovered use of her limbs quickly, but at discharge was still incontinent. She went home with a Foley catheter, a bedside commode, and a referral to the Community Nursing Service.

Betty Allen had practiced as a visiting nurse in this farm community for several years. She knew of a number of people like the Riggses who struggled to stay in their old home. Dorothy seemed to be managing pretty well at home; she was able to get around by using a walker for stability and could now use the commode regularly. Betty saw her three times a week to irrigate or change the catheter and do strengthening exercises with her.

One day Betty's visit coincided with the beginning of the midday meal preparations. Although it was only 10 A.M., Lester was laboriously getting out pots and pans and awkwardly chopping vegetables for some stew. He reported, with obvious pride, that he had learned to cook several years ago when Dorothy's hands and feet had started to bother her so much (from arthritis). Except for a period right after his stroke, he had cooked a "good hearty meal" for the two of them every day. It took him three to four hours of exertion, and he got "awful tired" but, he said, "If I wasn't doin' that, I'd just be sittin' starin' out the window." One of their neighbors frequently gave him new recipes to try out, and another friend did their shopping every week.

Betty suggested to them that Meals-on-Wheels services were available to them if they ever felt they needed it, but didn't push the subject.

Dorothy made good progress with bladder training after the catheter was removed, and Betty stopped visiting the Riggses. One day almost a year later she happened to be in their neighborhood and dropped in to see them. Dorothy was doing well, although her eyesight was now so poor that she could barely read. It was Lester who had changed. He was sitting half-asleep in his chair and seemed much more frail. Dorothy reported that he had burned his hand while cooking one day, and someone at the hospital had ordered Meals-on-Wheels for them. Lester had never gone back to cooking because people at the hospital had told him he was too old to do that anymore. He mostly just sat in his chair.

In this case example Mr. Riggs's social interactions had revolved around his role as family cook, a role that was very important to his self-image as an independent person capable of looking after and providing for his wife and himself. When a service replaced him in this role and health professionals seemed to view him as old and incompetent, his self-image was threatened and eventually eroded as he came to think of himself in these terms as well; he quickly "learned" to be helpless (see Section 3.2). This kind of situation presents a real dilemma for caregivers: if patients are able to reject or discontinue services, although upsetting to caregivers, they may be exhibiting strength rather than weakness.

The best-intentioned help, provided inappropriately, may do significant damage to self-esteem and independence.

Resistance to accepting home care can also be caused by financial concerns. Patients and their family members are often confused about what their entitlements and insurance benefits are. The legal language of insurance policies and the limited scope of news items about changes in federal and state programs fuel anxieties about the financial consequences of allowing care to begin. For example, patients covered by Medicare and Medicaid are eligible only for home care that involves "skilled nursing care," but even health professionals are sometimes unclear about exactly how "skilled" is defined. Private insurances often provide home care, but only for a limited number of visits, implying that the patient must keep track of visits made and be sure to terminate services accordingly. Housekeeping assistance, meal preparation, and other non-medical needs are rarely included in insurance plans. Since paid help in one's own home is very expensive, patients often must rely on charitable groups for these kinds of services. The psychological implications of accepting "charity" can be an insurmountable barrier to accepting care.

Accepting Residential Care. An alternative to at-home care when finances or community services are limited, or the physical condition of the patient demands it, is residential care. This option is regarded by virtually everyone as a "last resort," yet it may be the only way to ensure continuing care (Wachtel *et al.,* 1987, p. 98). In addition to serious financial consequences (see Section 3.4), the "immigration" of a person to the "foreign" world of residential care has monumental psychological and social implications.

From the *patient's* point of view, long-term, residential care means confronting the fact that he or she is no longer independent and cannot be cared for in familiar surroundings. Even if a stay in a convalescent home is planned as a short stay, the patient's sense of helplessness is emphasized. Elderly or seriously ill people may become quite confused and disoriented by this kind of move. No matter how reassuring family members are about their continued concern and involvement, moving out of one's own social world into a world in which personal belongings and familiar relationships are necessarily limited feels like abandonment. Patients can be expected to grieve over these losses during a transition period; without supportive help and effective listening, they may become permanently depressed. These kinds of psychological and social issues, combined with worry about death and financial hardship, result in the strenuous resistance that many patients mount against residential placement.

From the *family members'* point of view, the decision for residential care is often tinged with a sense of failure at not having been able to provide adequate care at home. For many families this decision represents a moral dilemma: to what extent should children and/or careers be jeopardized by a commitment to care for a sick or elderly parent? While feeling guilty about abandoning a family member to strangers, they also may feel a sense of relief at relinquishing the burden of care. Fears about financial liability typically complicate the desire to arrange high-quality care.

> *Unless family members receive help in dealing with the conflicting emotions and difficult decisions surrounding residential care, continued relationships with the patient will suffer greatly, and with them, the patient's mental and physical health.*

From the *caregiver's* point of view, helping a patient and family decide whether residential care is an appropriate form of continuing care is also fraught with conflicting emotions. It is instinctive for the nurse to want to protect the patient: from further injury to health, from aggressive or unconcerned relatives, from financial ruin, from feelings of alienation or abandonment, and from continued acute care that is no longer appropriate. Balancing those conflicts sometimes leads nurses to falsely reassure the patient and family (hoping that the situation turns out better than is feared), to refuse to become involved in the decision making, or to become coldly clinical or very directive in their approach. None of these alternatives is very satisfying for the nurse, nor do they help patients or families resolve the problems they face. It is a narrow path that the nurse walks in presenting accurate, unbiased information to patients about residential care while meeting their emotional needs during decision making.

How to Encourage Supported Self-reliance

The first step toward helping patients and their families make sound decisions about continuing care plans is for the nurse to be aware of the psychological, social, and financial issues outlined above. In the following paragraphs a number of specific guidelines for the nurse will be discussed. They have as their practical goal encouraging patients to accept appropriate care while maintaining their sense of integrity, control, and personal identity.

Guideline #1: Anticipate the factors that will influence the patient's and family's decisions.

As nurses interact with patients and visiting family members on a daily basis during acute care, they can begin to anticipate not only patients' physical needs for continuing care, but also their approaches to decision making. Some clues that will help nurses anticipate how decisions will be handled include:

- the openness with which individuals express their feelings and concerns;
- the depth and ease of communication apparent between patient and family members;
- information about the social roles played by the patient and the importance of family members to those roles; and
- the degree to which insightful questions are asked regarding continuing care needs, the decision process, and the consequences of selecting various options.

With these clues in mind, the nurse is able to share subjective, but valuable, data with colleagues involved in the discharge planning process. These data will go a long way toward avoiding time-consuming mistakes, such as failing to involve key decision makers in the process, assuming a level of involvement by the patient that is in error, or failing to give complete information about a favored option.

Guideline #2: Start early to give complete information about continuing care options, taking time to be sure that information is understood.

As discussed in Section 2.3, people often do not know enough about continuing care needs or options to formulate good questions. It is up to the nurse to give information over a period of time so that knowledge and awareness can develop. Whenever a question is asked or a concern expressed, it should be viewed by the nurse as an opportunity to teach. Making use of such an opportunity includes efforts to make sure that information is understood and allowing time for the expression of the feelings that surround facts.

Again, we emphasize that it is *not* the nurse's responsibility to know everything or to be able to respond completely to every request for information. Rather, it *is* the nurse's responsibility to respond as fully as possible, acknowledge limits openly, and be sure that a resource for further information is provided.

> *Guideline #3: Expect expressions of confusion and uncertainty when needs are being identified or options introduced.*

Uncertainty about one's own needs and confusion about the consequences of selecting any particular option are to be expected when decisions involve such a complex combination of feelings, facts, and social meanings. Described in the counseling literature by Robert Carkhuff (1973), this period of uncertainty precedes the beginning of real problem solving. Rather than giving advice or overwhelming people with new information or more detailed descriptions, it is best to encourage them to talk through their thoughts and feelings. By hearing themselves, they begin to establish priorities and come to terms with the problems to be solved. The nurse need not have formed an opinion of what decision OUGHT to be made—in fact, the nurse is a much more effective helper if that has not happened. Instead, the nurse can use this period to build trust through active listening, clarification of issues as they arise, and acceptance of the feelings expressed (see Section 2.2).

> *Guideline #4: Encourage the patient's and family's sense of involvement and control in the decision-making process by helping them develop appropriate interpersonal skills.*

A patient and family immersed in the demands of acute care may find it difficult to resume active involvement in decision making and adjust their self-image to include control over post-hospital events. One very powerful way the nurse can help them make this transition is to recognize, encourage, and give positive support for signs of interpersonal skills such as negotiation and expressions of self-interest. Added to whatever self-care skills can be developed in patients, these kinds of skills that allow people to assertively pursue their needs, desires, and rights are the basis for self-reliance once they return to the community.

One of the more effective methods for encouraging these kinds of skills is what teachers and counselors call "behavior rehearsal." This is a kind of role-play in which patient or family members pretend that the nurse is the person to be questioned or confronted. The person tries out words and approaches and gets feedback from the nurse about what the response might be. Behavior rehearsal helps people work through some of their fantasies about others' response to a particular approach and gives them a strong sense of support and approval. Some examples of situations in which this kind of method may be used effectively follow.

- A patient needs to tell a family member that he does not want to go to live with her following discharge.
- A daughter needs to open a discussion with her mother about the possibility of nursing home care.
- A patient needs to tell a doctor that he does not want to undergo further tests or surgery.

In order to be able to practice approaches to these kinds of situations, people must have worked through some of their own feelings about the situation, have organized their own priorities, and trust the person helping them in the rehearsal.

Behavior rehearsal helps people put theory, ideals, and opinions into practice with the best chance of having them accepted by others and ultimately feeling in control of their own decisions and destiny.

This kind of skill building is an excellent basis for accepting appropriate community support for health care while maintaining self-reliance.

In summary, in this section we have explored some of the psychological and social factors involved in accepting health care in the community. While the issues raised by these factors are complex, the nurse needs an awareness of that complexity before being able to usefully help people make continuing care decisions. The goal of "supported self-reliance" has been introduced and a number of guidelines presented for use by the nurse in helping patients and families toward this target.

SUMMARY

This chapter has been devoted to helping nurses more clearly understand what kinds of health care services exist in the community and how they can effectively work with those services in planning continuing care. We have emphasized the role of the patient in taking responsibility for continuing care decision making. This role is facilitated by patient teaching, which begins early in care, and by awareness of the impact of psychological and social, as well as financial, factors on acceptance of care. The more nurses know about the health and medical care services in their communities, the better able they are to prepare patients for continuing care and coordinate services in their behalf.

FURTHER READING

Archer, S. E., and R. Fleshman. *Community Health Nursing: Patterns and Practice.* North Scituate, Mass.: Duxbury Press, 1975.
   This text, like most others devoted to Community Health Nursing, includes information about how to contact community sources of help and support and chapters about nurse-patient relationships in the home. Nurses who have not had community experience will benefit from reading sections in this and other such texts on community approaches to nursing and then comparing this with their own hospital-oriented approaches.

Shield Healthcare Centers. *Health Care at Home: A Resource Guide.* Soneko Press Inc., 1984.
   Shield is a maker of health care products and they clearly have a commercial intent in producing this book, but it does give valuable information to patients, families, and health professionals unfamiliar with practical details of care in the home. It includes information about sources of help and a section on finances as well as product details. Available from Shield Healthcare Centers, Inc., 50 Industrial Road, Berkeley Heights, New Jersey, 08873.

Martinson, I. M., and A. Widmer (eds.). *Home Health Care Nursing.* Philadelphia: W. B. Saunders, 1989.
   This text focuses on the provision of nursing care to individuals in the community. The first part of the book discusses the place of home care in the general context of medical and health care. A chapter on discharge planning is included. Subsequent parts of the book detail the nurse's roles in relation to home care, general approaches to various categories of care, and guidance for caring for patients with specific disorders. In addition to being a textbook for those immediately involved in home care, this book serves as a thorough introduction to home care approaches for hospital nurses.

6

Putting the Pieces Together for an Effective Plan

Arranging Details of Transitional Care
Example 6.3 A Wrong Address Delays
Transition Home

6.4 HOW TO EVALUATE DISCHARGE PLANNING
Using Discharge Planning Audits
Evaluating Patient Goal Attainment
Discharge Planning Program Evaluation

SUMMARY

FURTHER READING

In the foregoing chapters, we have examined the major pieces of
the discharge planning puzzle. In this chapter, our aim is to show how
they can be brought together to form a coherent and coordinated plan
for continuing care. Our emphasis is on the practical application of
concepts and principles. We begin with the three basic steps of the
discharge planning process (see Figure 1–2 in Section 1.3) and identify
two important decisions about goals that are part of this process. These
decisions and the factors that go into making them are discussed in the
first section. This is followed by an exploration of the role that
motivation plays in the success of the discharge plan. We include
guidance for the nurse in encouraging positive motivation in patients
and families. We then look at what needs to be done just prior to a
patient's discharge to ensure continuity of care. Finally, the evaluation
of continuing care and its importance to nurses for improving skills and
putting experiences into perspective are explored.

Figure 6–1 shows the three basic steps toward continuing care.
Step A occurs during the acute phase of a patient's care. It involves
using data collected during admission screening and medical and nursing
assessment procedures to determine realistic goals of patient care. Step
B follows from this first decision: based on the intensity of discharge
planning services implied by the goals of care, goals of intervention are
determined. Step C occurs as the patient prepares to enter the continuing care phase and implement the plan made. It involves evaluating
the patient's present level of strengths and resources and deciding
whether these will adequately balance needs and the stressors that will
affect the patient in the forseeable future. These three steps form the
basis of the worksheets that are presented in Part II of this text.

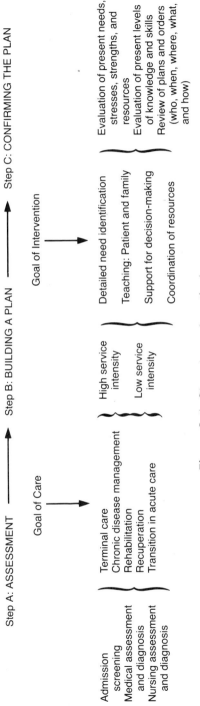

Figure 6—1. *Steps toward continuing care.*

6.1 MAKING DECISIONS THAT GUIDE
DISCHARGE PLANNING

At the time that a patient is admitted for acute care, a number of procedures are completed in quick succession. These generally include the collection of basic personal and financial information and initial assessments by medical and nursing staff. Both doctor and nurse collect data from patient examination, observation of behavior, and patient and family interviews and from these data make initial diagnoses. Medical management and nursing care plans are formulated based on these diagnoses. The same data can also be used to take the first step in discharge planning, namely, the identification of patient care goals. While these goals may be general at first, they provide a focus for discharge planning intervention and answer the questions of how much and what kind of help is needed. In this section we will explore the first two steps toward discharge planning. We look first at the kinds of data that are relevant to the discharge planning process and at what kinds of goals may be identified for patient care, then at how to build a plan for intervention.

Collecting Data Relevant to Discharge Planning

The most intense activity of the admission phase of acute care is devoted to the collection of information about the patient and his or her condition.

The more quickly a complete "picture" of the person is assembled, the more appropriate and effective will be the medical and nursing care intervention.

While data collected initially has as its principal objective the identification of present problems and immediate needs, this same information can also be used to determine future needs for continuing care.

Generally, there are three major sources of initial patient data: an admission screening procedure, a medical assessment, and a nursing assessment. Shorter hospital stays have encouraged hospitals to collect information from patients even prior to admission and to include questions beyond the usual medical history and financial data. Diagnostic tests and medical examinations may also be done prior to elective hospital admissions. These data, combined with interviews, examinations, and observations of behavior, all contribute to an overall picture of the patient and his needs.

In the following paragraphs, we will review the items of data that have particular relevance for determining continuing care needs. Some institutions have established a set of criteria using these data points to trigger referral of patients with a high risk of complex continuing care needs for special assistance. It is important to note that no one item by itself has been shown to be a good predictor of specific continuing care needs, but in combination they give important clues to caregivers on which to base planned intervention (Wachtel *et al.*, 1987).

Age. The age of the patient has long been an important criterion for identifying "risk." The very young and the very old have an identifiable, although not quantifiable, risk of suffering long-term negative effects from an incidence of illness. Yet the nature of the risk is really less associated with specific age than it is with other factors such as degree of physical and financial dependency, extent of supportive social relationships, and adequacy of nutrition (Lamont *et al.*, 1983). Twenty years ago children under the age of two and adults over the age of 65 were widely referred for discharge planning services on the basis of age alone. Today, with increasing numbers of elderly persons in the population and decreased hospital stays and staff resources, it is common practice not to refer due to age alone unless the person is 85 years old or more. Medicare regulations, however, require that discharge planning services "be available" to hospitalized Medicare recipients. Those over 65 are therefore screened to determine whether risk factors other than age signify the need for special services.

Medical Diagnosis. Of primary importance to both acute and continuing care is the diagnosis made by the physician on the basis of history, physical examination, and corroborating tests. The following aspects of diagnosis are especially relevant to early discharge planning activities:

- the state of the patient's *health* prior to the onset of acute distress;
- the *extent* of organ system involvement in a disease process;
- the relative *severity* of the present episode;
- the patient's early *responses* to treatment; and
- the *prognosis* for recovery.

As the patient's care progresses and each of these aspects become more thoroughly known, their contribution to continuing care goals is more significant.

> On admission to acute care, the diagnosis in combination with other data helps to define general goals of patient care; later on, increasing information about how the patient has been affected and the responses to treatment help to "fine tune" specific objectives of care.

Activities of Daily Living. A useful measure of a patient's functional abilities and, therefore, the amount of assistance that will be required following hospitalization was proposed by Katz *et al.* in 1963. This index rated level of dependency on the following activities:

- feeding,
- dressing,
- bathing,
- using the toilet,
- transferring (from bed to chair and back), and
- continence.

Other authors include instrumental activities in this list such as ability to do housework, climb stairs, shop, ambulate, and cook (Wachtel *et al.*, 1987). In Part II of this text, the reader will find a somewhat more extensive list of items included under the general topic of activities of daily living. Whatever list is used, the intent is to discover whether the person is able to manage everyday activities alone or needs the help of others. Although a patient may be more dependent while in the hospital, the level of abilities prior to hospitalization is at least a good starting point for determining the patient's needs afterward. There is little justification for waiting until a patient's condition has stabilized to begin making plans for continuing care (Davis *et al.*, 1984). To do so is likely to delay discharge or strand the patient with incompletely organized assistance.

Mental Ability. Another dimension of a person's relative independence in functioning is an assessment of mental abilities. The most commonly used factors are *memory, orientation,* and *judgment.* These data are, of course, highly subjective and inferential. Elderly persons may say they forget things easily and yet be quite able to function independently with the help of simple memory aids for such things as medication. Others may suffer disorientation due to the medications they are receiving or unfamiliarity with the hospital and the expectations of caregivers (Smith, 1986).

Social Background. Aside from age and diagnosis, the social support and resources available to patients are powerful determinants of long-term patient care goals. There are a number of factors at work here, perhaps best summarized by the Health Balance Model discussed in Section 2.1.

Generally speaking, the more out of balance a person's social strengths and resources are in meeting his or her physical and emotional needs, the more intensive will be the discharge planning intervention that is needed.

Those without a spouse available to give care and those to whom home care services are inaccessible are at much greater risk than others with disabling illnesses of needing nursing home or other residential placement (Watchtel *et al.*, 1987). If they had previously been living independently, they will need very intensive help to make the transition in care smoothly. Glass *et al.* (1977) and others show that previous nursing home residents almost always (97%) return to a nursing home (see Figure 6–2). There is evidence, however, that more should be able to return to community care, but they become victims to a series of "self-fulfilling" prophecies by family members, caregivers, and even themselves who *expect* that this will be their destination after discharge, and therefore they fail to investigate other options.

The social factors that most dramatically influence the amount of discharge planning help needed will seldom be completely known at admission unless a careful and sensitive interview procedure is followed. The nurse needs to know how extensive the patient's primary social group is and how involved they have been or are likely to want to be in the patient's care; the breadth of the patient's social group reflecting interests, hobbies, and leisure activities; and how much both patient and family know about available community sources of medical and health care. Financial factors cannot really be separated from social ones, in that accessibility to community care is so often financially determined (see Section 3.4).

Other Patient Data. Other data of relevance for determining goals of patient care include a patient's eating and sleeping patterns, ability to communicate verbally as well as to read and write, and attitudes toward his or her present illness. In this latter category the nurse needs to know the degree to which the patient is aware of the diagnosis and its consequences for the future, cooperates with care procedures and caregivers, and is interested in learning about self-care and doing things independently. Finding out how and why the patient sought care for the present illness and whether there is a doctor in the community who is consulted regularly may give the nurse clues about the patient's attitudes toward medical follow-up.

In combination, these kinds of data give a picture of the person, indicate how dependent she or he will be on the help of others after discharge, narrow the realistic options for planned continuing care, and guide the nurse in planning teaching and coordination activities.

It is important that both objective and subjective data be recorded as they come to light so that the "picture" of the patient can be readily shared with all caregivers.

This, together with a clear statement of patient care goals, will help to coordinate the efforts of everyone involved in guiding the patient who is preparing for discharge.

Deciding on Goals of Patient Care

There are two basic stages in reaching a decision about patient care goals. The first of these, discussed in the preceding paragraphs, is to piece together as complete a picture as possible of patients and their needs. The second is to focus attention beyond present problems and physical care imperatives to anticipated outcomes and goals.

Since discharge planning is a future-oriented activity, it is essential that caregivers look forward toward potential patient needs.

Nurses are practiced at making educated professional judgments about patients' physical nursing care needs, even when their condition is changing rapidly. In order to make similar judgments about needs following discharge, nurses use their skills of observation to anticipate the outcome of the present acute episode of illness. The nurse who has been able to form a relationship of trust with a patient is in an excellent position not only to observe the degree to which the patient can perform activities of daily living but also to become aware of the patient's attitudes and mental abilities. While the nurse may feel appropriately uncomfortable guessing exactly how much help will be needed in another six months, enough information is available to determine a general goal toward which to work. This kind of "forward thinking" is only dangerous if done with inadequate information or in isolation from other decision-makers, including the patient and other caregivers.

Participation by both patient and family in determining goals of care after discharge allows them to begin to anticipate their needs and make realistic plans.

The nurse holds the key to their involvement because of ongoing interaction with them. The challenge is to initiate the transfer of responsibility for health care that will be the patient's and the family's after discharge. Their motivation to implement a plan and reach health care goals begins with their early involvement in the planning process.

In the following paragraphs we will review the major categories of post-discharge goals of care.

Transitions in Acute Care. For many patients who enter acute care, it is clear that they will be progressing to different care units during their hospitalization. For example, a patient may move from intensive care to a medical or surgical unit, between specialist and generalist services, or from acute care to minimum care units as a reflection of changing needs for care. Caregivers who admit the patient therefore have two kinds of continuing care activities to plan: one of gathering relevant data to help in determining post-hospitalization goals, and the second of deciding how to coordinate the smooth transition of the patient's care to another in-hospital unit.

While the decision of when and where to transfer is made largely on medical grounds, the patient's attitudes toward self and caregivers, the amount of psycho-social support being received, and the present level of dependence on help to do activities of daily living all determine the patient's needs during the transfer process. At the very least, both patient and family will need to know what to expect of caregivers in the new situation. If hospitalization is like visiting a foreign country to many people, transfer to a new unit within the hospital is equivalent to traveling to an unknown city in that foreign land. The nurse's familiarity with other hospital units allows him or her to begin early patient teaching that will encourage rapid readjustment once the transfer occurs.

For the patient who is especially dependent on others for physical care or emotional encouragement and support, the nurse can help to transfer trust to new caregivers by introducing them to the patient prior to transfer and by providing them a full picture of the patient and his or her needs.

Patients with strokes or spinal injuries, those with sight, hearing, or speech impairments, and the parents of sick children are examples of people who especially benefit from careful attention to transitions in care.

Recuperation. The vast majority of patients admitted for acute care will return home to recuperate. Due to shortened hospital stays, however, few of these will not need some special help if they are to fully regain their health. Reaching the goal of recuperation means that patients must become aware of the nature of their acute problems and understand activity, diet, medication, and medical follow-up instructions. It is difficult for many people to accept a "sick role," that is, allowing others to wait on them, having diminished responsibility for work and decision making, and less involvement in family activities once they return to familiar surroundings. The nurse can help patients with this transition by encouraging them to talk about their feelings and any problems that they anticipate during the recuperation period. Sometimes practicing responses to questions or demands from others with patients help them plan more realistically. In addition to other kinds of patient and family teaching, nurses have the opportunity to help recuperating patients learn more about their bodies and how to better protect their health.

Rehabilitation. The goal of rehabilitation is appropriate for those who have lost some normal bodily function as a result of an acute episode but have a reasonable chance of regaining it or learning to compensate for its loss. It may not be immediately clear, especially in the early days of hospitalization, whether rehabilitation will be short-(less than six months) or long-term. As the patient progresses and caregivers observe the responses to treatment, they will have a better idea about what to plan for.

The needs of a patient in rehabilitation will change during the course of recovery. Discharge planning is usually focused on the first one to three months of this process. It is most important that the patient be helped to learn how to modify this plan as needs change.

The patient also needs help in enlisting the support and encouragement of family and friends and in preparing for the inevitable ups and downs of any rehabilitative process.

Whether a person's continuing care goal is short- or long-term, rehabilitation depends on the diagnosis, level of health prior to the acute episode, degree of physical impairment, and motivation to work through discomfort and frustration to accomplish specific objectives. The availability of professional help in the community to monitor progress and guide the patient's efforts is crucial to success. Whatever the nurse can do to help the patient transfer trust to community caregivers before discharge will enhance motivation.

A high level of patient motivation for reaching rehabilitation goals demands excellent communication and coordination between hospital and community.

Any gap in time that occurs between discharge and the start of a community rehabilitation program may allow patient motivation to sag, bad habits to become established that will need to be broken later, or inappropriate dependencies to develop. The nurse will want to especially note the patient's personality characteristics (see Section 3.2) and use these as a guide in planning an appropriate rehabilitation program.

Chronic Disease Care. For the patient with a chronic condition that will continue to warrant post-hospital attention, there are two basic concerns: continued medical supervision and personal care. A wide range of care options may be selected depending on the patient's condition, physical limitations and abilities, and the availability of community care and support. If the patient is to be discharged to community care, the nurse's concerns include answers to the following questions:

• What help will the patient need for activities of daily living and for how long?

- How will shopping, cleaning, and food preparation be handled and by whom?
- What kind of medical treatment or supervision is needed, and how will it be provided?
- Does the patient need special equipment or devices, how will they be used, and who will take responsibility for them?
- What are the patient's financial resources and how will they be managed?

If placement in a residential care facility seems the best option, the nurse's concerns include answers to these questions:

- How and by whom is the decision to be made about placement?
- What kinds of emotional and social issues surround institutional placement for this patient?
- What can be done before and during the transitional period to protect the patient's physical independence and mental and emotional health?
- What are the financial realities of the level of care anticipated, and how are resources to be managed?

For the patient with a diagnosis of a chronic disorder, discharge planning must begin at admission with a thorough assessment of abilities and strengths as well as deficits.

The complexities of planning for continuing care of patients with chronic conditions often demand the involvement of several specialist health professionals in the hospital and the community. Coordination of effort through good communication is essential.

The nurse will need excellent communication and teaching skills to meet the challenges presented by this kind of discharge planning.

While it is dangerous to make assumptions about individual patient needs based on statistical surveys, the chart presented in Figure 6–2 serves to alert the nurse to some of the major factors affecting discharge decisions. It is based on a study of 337 persons over age 65 who were admitted to the hospital. As can be seen, the most significant factor in determining that a patient will be discharged to nursing home care was found to be previous residence in such a facility. For other patients, an accumulation of factors led to decisions about destination at discharge. Those who were basically able to take care of themselves, including the performance of heavy household chores, or who had someone at home to supplement their abilities were much more likely to return home. The researchers note that the patient's age and mental state also correlate with discharge destination. Criteria such as those

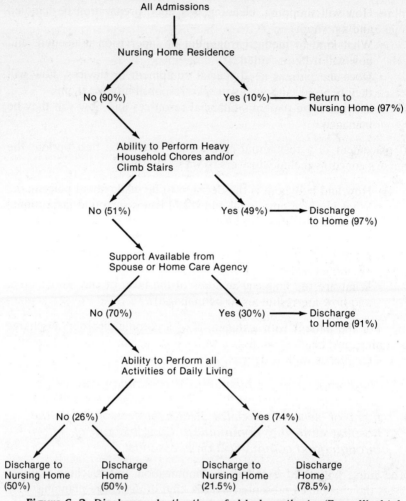

Figure 6–2. *Discharge destination of elderly patients. (From Wachtel, T. J., Fulton, J. P, and Goldfarb, J.: Early prediction of discharge disposition after hospitalization. The Gerontologist 27:1, 98–103, 1987. Used with permission of the Gerontological Society of America.)*

shown in Figure 6–2 help to identify patients who will need intensive help in planning their discharge.

This information, added to the patient's diagnosis of one or more chronic conditions, will lead the nurse to make an early assessment of probable discharge planning needs and alert specialist team members to the findings.

Care During Terminal Illness. In recent years caregivers have become much more aware of the rights of a patient with a terminal illness to know about his or her condition and participate in decision making about how care is to be handled. The growth of home-based hospice services has improved the quality of care and support for those who are able to choose non-institutional care.

There are a number of stages in the planning of this patient's discharge. The first is the medical determination of the most likely prognosis, made on the basis of the patient's history and the doctor's judgment, supported by clinical findings.

The second stage is the most difficult emotionally: giving information to the patient and family members about the disease and the patient's prognosis. Because of continuing interaction with them, the nurse usually has a very intense teaching and support role during this period of awareness and beginning grief process. It is critically important to effective discharge planning that this stage begin as early as possible, because the participation of patient and family in decision making must usually wait until the initial grief responses of denial and anger have been worked through (Kübler-Ross, 1969).

The third stage is the examination of options available for continuing care. Most families are unacquainted with the care and support services in their communities. The appropriateness and accessibility of these to the patient must be explored before rational decisions can be made about discharge. During this stage, philosophical issues surrounding the quality versus quantity of life will need to be explored as well. In their distress over their ill member, families are often very unrealistic about what they can offer in terms of 24-hour care. They need gentle guidance in assessing their priorities, energy, and the potential effect of stress on their own health before committing to a plan.

Finally, there is the stage of planning, teaching, and coordinating the patient's discharge. The nurse's concerns include that the patient and family have:

- Knowledge of the disease and its most likely progress;
- Plans for pain control;
- Access to appropriate equipment and know how to use it;
- Access to emotional support from friends, counseling, or bereavement groups;
- Plans for dealing with legal and financial issues; and
- Physical care skills if the patient is to return home.

In addition, they need to know how to identify crisis points in the disease process and how to get approriate help. Knowing how death is likely to occur is an important part of this.

Planning continuing care for the terminally ill and those
with life-threatening chronic disease presents an emo-

*tional challenge for nurses but also a rewarding oppor-
tunity to use the full range of their personal and professional skills.*

None of their patients benefit more than these do from nurses' abilities
to assess need, communicate well, teach effectively, and organize
efficiently.

Building a Plan for Intervention

Having determined the general goal of continuing patient care,
the nurse is now in a position to decide what can be done to make a
viable and realistic plan and move toward implementation. The patient
care goal provides a rough estimate of how intensely the nurse will
need to be involved. The patient transferring from one unit to another
will need information, reassurance, and coordination between caregivers; this represents a simple and quickly completed involvement in
discharge planning. In contrast, the patient going home to be cared for
by his or her family during the last days of a terminal illness will require
a very high level of involvement by the nurse.

In many institutions where a specialist discharge planning team is
available, patients with the goals of long-term rehabilitation, care of
disabling chronic disease, or terminal illness are referred for team
services as soon as the goal is identified. For those hospitals where
access to a specialist team is limited, the social work department may
be able to offer consultation or casework if it is alerted to the kinds of
emotional and financial issues of concern to these patients.

In the following paragraphs the major contributions to be made
by the nurse in building a discharge plan are discussed.

*The aim of the nurse's intervention is to give patient and
family the knowledge, attitudes, and skills necessary for
implementation of the discharge plan.*

Detailed Need Identification. One of the most important aspects
of effective discharge planning is to identify exactly what kinds of
continuing care will be needed. The patient who has undergone
intensive care in the hospital will have had technologically complex
care. Before rational decisions can be made about a discharge plan, it
must be determined which procedures will need to be continued
routinely, which might need to be carried out in an emergency, what
equipment will be needed, how it will be maintained, how dependent
the patient will be on others for care, and who will provide this care.
Consultation with the patient's doctor(s) is the first step for the nurse

in identifying continuing care needs. Consultation with home care nurses may also be valuable if the nurse is not thoroughly familiar with how hospital procedures are "translated" to home care. These kinds of consultation will also help identify just what the patient and home caregivers need to learn before leaving the hospital. A determination of what will be needed after discharge provides the nurse with a framework for beginning coordination activities and evaluating learning progress.

Patient and Family Teaching. One of the most important skill areas that the nurse brings to discharge planning is in helping others learn (see Section 2.3). In order for a plan to be made and implemented, both the patient and family need to learn new knowledge, attitudes, and skills, or be able to effectively modify and apply previous learning. No matter what other team members are involved in the discharge planning process, the nurse will be the primary teacher. For the patient going home to *recuperate,* discharge teaching may involve only instruction in taking medications and medical follow-up, along with instruction in protecting and improving future health. For the patient going home to *manage a disabling chronic disease,* teaching involvement by the nurse is intensive and time-consuming, but is the critical difference between the patient remaining in the community or having to be institutionalized. This kind of teaching is made more complex because of the number of family and professional caregivers who must be coached on how to coordinate their efforts.

The nurse is constantly teaching through word and deed. Attention to how learning can be used following discharge allows the nurse to incorporate teaching into many of the interactions with patient and family members.

The following case example demonstrates a teaching approach by the nurse that was integrated into all aspects of a child's nursing care.

Example 6.1 Teaching Intervention with Parents

Tommy Bakke had an uncertain start in life. Born with airway instability, he now had a permanent tracheostomy. In spite of the complex care involved, his parents were eager to take him home. Although young and inexperienced with child care, especially the management of a fragile infant, they were intelligent and willing to learn. Both parents had visited Tommy every day of the 8 weeks since his birth, and his mother, Susan, usually spent several hours at his bedside.

Kathy Frank had recently taken over as Tommy's primary

care nurse. She had developed a good relationship with Susan and felt she could handle the child's care at home, given the right preparation and support. Kathy began her planning by making a list of the skills the parents would need to master before discharge. They included suctioning, chest physiotherapy, CPR, and equipment maintenance, in addition to being able to assess Tommy's condition and identify his needs quickly and accurately. With the exception of CPR, there were no resources for learning these skills except Tommy's bedside. Kathy began by going over her list of skills needed with the doctor and with both parents. Together they organized a schedule that would allow the parents to be present during the most active periods of Tommy's care. Now whenever Kathy prepared to suction, for example, she explained exactly what she was doing and why: why she wore gloves, how she checked the pressure on the machine before using it, how she determined how far to insert the catheter, and why she turned Tommy's head to one side and then the other. By using every caregiving activity as an opportunity to teach, Kathy helped the Bakkes develop the understanding they would need for procedures done at home. This took extra thought and planning but not much extra time. Gradually she had them do portions of the procedures under her supervision and began pointing out what modifications might be made in the home setting.

In this case example, the nurse used her time efficiently to instruct the parents in the procedures they would need to carry out after discharge. By making a detailed plan of what needed to be learned, she was able to guide them through the levels of learning complexity (see Section 2.3), and by allowing them to do elements of care under her supervision, she helped them develop practical skills and confidence.

Patient and family teaching is like building a fortress out of building blocks: one starts with a foundation of understanding and then builds on each layer until the goal is reached. The goal of discharge planning intervention involving teaching is to give the patient and family a well-grounded fortress of knowledge, attitudes, and skills that allow them to meet challenges and take effective action to protect the patient's health.

Support for Decision Making. A great deal of emphasis has been placed on the role of the nurse in establishing relationships of trust with patient and family (Section 2.2) and in helping them participate as discharge planning team members (Section 4.4). In the next section the subject of motivation and its effect on decision making will be discussed. The nurse's willingness to listen, to inform, and to guide provides important aspects of support to patients and families struggling to determine what course of action to take. The nurse must be prepared for an evolution of ideas and opinions as decision makers learn more about the patient's needs and come to terms with the realities of trying to meet them. The nurse must also be prepared to accept decisions that are different from those she or he might make. Instead of advising or directing, the nurse will represent reality by helping patients and their families carefully think through as many of the consequences of a decision as possible before discharge.

Coordination of Resources. The essence of coordination is communication. It has to do with placing the pieces of the discharge planning puzzle in a working configuration. The specific communication skills the nurse contributes to coordination of the discharge plan are discussed in Section 2.2. The nurse's intervention in this area may range from a few simple telephone calls and some short explanations, to taking a major role in setting up and leading team conferences (see Section 4.3), meeting with community caregivers, and transmitting detailed medical and social information. Every discharge plan will need some level of coordination if it is to be implemented effectively.

In summary, we have explored each of the elements of the first two steps toward continuing care shown in Figure 6–1 in this section. We have looked at the kinds of information that are important to identifying the general goals of continuing care. The goal then determines the intensity of discharge planning services needed. Finally we have reviewed the major kinds of intervention that the nurse might choose in helping patient and family implement the plan.

6.2 MOTIVATION FOR SUCCESS OF THE PLAN

Motivation is a mental state of readiness that propels one forward to seek, to learn, and to change. Motivation is expressed as interest in a subject or activity, eager anticipation of change, or recognition of the importance of an incentive or goal. The development of motivation by the patient and family to implement a discharge plan is important because, whether a plan succeeds or fails is up to them. Caregivers in the acute care setting can provide the tools that allow a plan to work in the form of knowledge, skills, equipment, and support services, but its implementation is basically out of their hands. How often nurses and others say to a patient preparing for discharge: "It's up to you!" And indeed it is.

The subject of motivation has been mentioned frequently within these pages. In this section we will draw these discussions together and offer some guidance to the nurse for encouraging positive motivation.

Principles of Motivation for Change

In the mid-1940s Kurt Lewin, psychologist and educator, proposed a simple model for understanding the process of change. He saw it as having three phases that he called "unfreezing," "moving," and "refreezing." If one imagines an ice cube, the meaning of these phases becomes clear. Faced with a need to change one's attitudes or behavior, the person must first "unfreeze," that is, become aware of the need to change, be willing to think through the consequences of the resulting circumstances or behavior, and respond positively to an incentive. The person must develop *motivation* to change.

It is not by chance that the model implies that a greater expenditure of energy is required for thawing and reforming than for moving. Lewin was especially aware that those taking the role of helper— teachers, parents, or nurses, for example—are often so focused on the "moving" aspects of change that they fail to give appropriate attention to the other two phases. Many health education programs provide examples of what Lewin meant. We are often eager to tell people that they ought to lose weight, reduce cholesterol intake, or stop smoking, but we devote little time or energy to helping them understand *why* they need to change their behaviors, and we provide few appropriate incentives or motivation for other aspects of "unfreezing." Likewise, we often fail to follow up and give support to change efforts or positive feedback for progress toward a goal.

> *One of the most powerful motivators is a person's perception that his or her need can be met.*

Abraham Maslow (1943, 1962, 1970) pioneered in the identification of needs and their relationship to motivation. His work, which spanned three decades, made an outstanding contribution to the understanding of human behavior. The ideas he presented are easily understood and readily applied to patient care situations.

Maslow suggested that everyone has some general needs that they seek to fulfill. These *unmet needs* motivate behavior. Maslow saw these general human needs as arranged in a hierarchy of complexity, with the simpler, more elementary needs at the base, progressing through a number of successive steps to the higher, more complex needs, as shown in Figure 6–3. Once a particular need is fulfilled, another, higher need takes its place as a motivator. Each level of fulfilled need provides

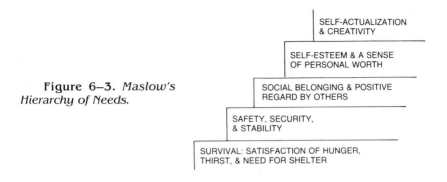

Figure 6–3. *Maslow's Hierarchy of Needs.*

the vantage point from which one can perceive that more is available and within reach.

The behavioral stages of human development provide an example of this model. During infancy children are totally dependent on others for *survival*. Their behavior reflects their needs for food, water, warmth, and physical protection. As their awareness increases, the need for a stable, close, nurturing relationship becomes paramount. They need to feel *safe and secure* in their environment. Then, during the school years, their personal world expands; they need *social belonging* and acceptance by others. Although they do not stop needing food and safety, their behavior reflects more concern for this emerging and as yet unfulfilled need. School-aged children, for example, are particularly interested in learning something new if their friends are also involved. As children move toward the adolescent years, they need to develop feelings of *self-worth* so that they have the confidence to take on adult responsibilities. Finally, adults need to feel that their contribution to life is *unique and creative;* they strive toward fulfilling the level of their greatest potential.

In addition to describing the maturational sequence of behavior changes, Maslow's theory of a needs hierarchy contains some important concepts affecting the motivation of adults. These are summarized as follows:

- Unmet needs are reflected in people's interests and concerns, and in perceived problems and goals.
- People are motivated to fulfill the highest unmet needs within their perception as long as more basic needs are met at a satisfactory level.
- People whose dominant needs are self-esteem and self-actualization continue to be motivated by these throughout life; they are never completely fulfilled.
- At a time of high stress or personal reverses, such as during ill health, people experience needs in more basic areas, such as

survival or safety. The higher needs that motivated them before their illness continue to concern them, but the majority of their energy will be used to meet the more urgent, elementary needs.

This last point is of special significance to discharge planning. Even while concerned about how very basic needs are being met at present, the patient and family are called upon to make decisions about future care. It is not surprising that they often lack motivation to do this anticipatory decision-making. In their present state of crisis or threat, the future may seem unreal and the problem of continuing care relatively unimportant (see Section 3.1).

Factors Affecting Motivation

In order to more fully understand what promotes or blocks motivation, an overview of how people solve or manage problems is useful. There have been many models or lists of steps proposed as attempts to clarify the problem solving process. The problems of continuing care have three characteristics that have led us to use a counseling model as a basis for our discussion about motivation. These are:

- Continuing care problems are multi-dimensional involving both facts and feelings;
- In order to be implemented, continuing care decisions often demand that consensus be reached between several decision-makers; and
- The behavior changes that result from continuing care decisions will affect all aspects of a person's life.

The work of Robert Carkhuff (1980) suggests a model that has been helpful in drawing attention to the different kinds of motivation that are required to implement a discharge plan (Figure 6–4). His focus, like ours, is on "goals" rather than on problems with discrete solutions. Carkhuff lists three such goals: awareness, understanding, and constructive action. Before the person is able to reach the first goal, however, he or she experiences a stage of uncertainty and confusion owing to the mixture of ideas, beliefs, facts, and possibly conflicting emotions surrounding any "personal" problem. Medical problems and health crises are not only very "personal," they are also potentially complex to solve and pervade all aspects of one's life.

In Chapter 3 we discussed in detail some of the factors that contribute to a person's state of uncertainty and confusion. These include:

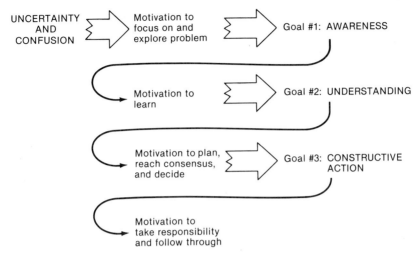

Figure 6–4. *Goals to be reached in solving problems.*

- a state of stress, which is likely to be very high due to the person's illness and the circumstances surrounding it,
- the person's beliefs about what is happening,
- the degree of control or personal power he or she feels in the situation, and
- the social and cultural factors that represent conflict or offer support.

In order to resolve this state and begin to approach the first problem solving goal of "awareness," people must be motivated to focus on the situation in which they find themselves and begin to explore its implications for their future. We have mentioned many reasons why they may find this difficult to do. These include a sense of helplessness (see Section 3.2), a state of crisis (see Section 3.1), and the effects of medication and the disease process itself that may dull the ability to focus attention.

Once patients or family members have reached an awareness of the problems posed by the need for continuing care, they can begin to work toward goal number two: "understanding." In order to do this they must be motivated to learn in greater depth what the patient's needs will be after discharge, what options are available, what the most likely consequences are of taking each of them, and what needs to be learned before discharge.

Learning what needs to be learned is one of the most important aspects of reaching the goal of understanding.

Examples of people who have reached this point are those who understand that insulin can be self-administered and that they will be helped to learn this skill before leaving the hospital, or those who understand that they can make use of support services in their struggle to cope with a terminal illness. Coming to terms with what knowledge, skills, and attitudes need yet to be learned signifies that the person is beginning to anticipate the kinds of behavior changes that will be required if continuing care is to be successfully implemented. It also is the first step toward taking over responsibility for coordinating care from acute caregivers.

The third goal, "constructive action," requires motivation to reach consensus between patient, family members, and caregivers, and to make decisions. This is the stage during which specific plans are made and responsibilities following discharge clarified.

> *Consensus implies mutual trust between the parties to decision-making and a mutual understanding of the problems faced.*

In Chapter 4, many aspects of teamwork and group decision-making were discussed. The reader is especially encouraged to review Section 4.4 on how to involve the family and patient in decision-making.

Once a plan is made and constructive action has been taken in learning appropriate skills and coordinating relevant resources, motivation of yet another kind is needed in order to actually carry out the discharge plan.

> *Implementation requires the motivation to accept responsibility, to act on the learning that has taken place, and accept the consequences of ongoing decision-making.*

Diabetics must actually give themselves insulin every day and deal with the consequences of a decision to eat some candy offered to them. The family of the terminally ill patient must follow through on coordinating continuing care, cope with their own as well as the patient's grief responses, and prepare to make decisions about the level of intervention that will be requested when death is near.

Motivation is the energy to progress, to grow, to change. Motivation is not automatic, nor can it be "switched on" when needed. The motivations required to reach the goals of problem solving and then to implement a plan of continuing care are complex and involve patient, family members, and caregivers in an intense communication process.

How to Encourage Positive Motivation

In the paragraphs above we have described some theoretical approaches to motivation in order to help the reader more fully understand what motivation is and how it develops. We then discussed the process of problem solving and the kinds of motivation required to reach each goal. We now want to look at the practical aspects of what the nurse can do to encourage problem solving and promote the kinds of motivation needed.

The first aspect of encouraging the motivation of others is the nurse's own level of motivation to help with solving the problems of continuing care.

Motivation is contagious; the nurse's willingness to explore problems, to find out about and explain options, and enthusiasm for making realistic plans will help patient and family also become motivated.

There certainly are instances in which patients and families make discharge plans without the help of caregivers. Seldom do these plans consider all available options, and they often result in feelings of anger and frustration from trying to get information from reluctant informants or coordinate services with groups that use their own language for communication. In these circumstances the quality of patient care suffers immeasurably. It is much more helpful to have motivated nursing staff on their "side" to guide, encourage, and coordinate their planning efforts.

A much better situation is one in which the nurse takes the lead in inspiring motivation to think through and ultimately plan the discharge of the patient. Families are often so overwhelmed by existing circumstances that they are unable to focus on the future without enthusiastic leadership from the nurse.

Reaching Awareness. Helping the patient and family focus on the problem of continuing care and begin to explore their thoughts and feelings about it can and should begin very early in the patient's care. Even as they share the information collected during medical and nursing assessments, the patient and family can be helped to see that caregivers are interested in all of a person's health care, not just his or her hospitalization. The nurse's use of good communication skills to encourage exploration of both the facts and feelings surrounding the acute episode are an important step toward the first goal of problem solving (see Section 2.1 and 2.2).

The development of trust between patient, family, and caregivers is an essential ingredient for being able to reach consensus on decisions later.

As the patient's physical condition and likely needs in the future become more clear, the nurse's ability to share information and express a professional view of the nature of the continuing care problem helps move the family and patient toward increasing awareness of the tasks and decisions that lie ahead. It is especially important that any predictions about the future emphasize what *can* be accomplished rather than what can *not*. As Mader (1988) points out, there is a fine but critical line between encouraging unrealistic hopes and giving a patient permission to try to overcome the effects of an illness. Hope and motivation are closely linked; the destruction of hope not only produces an emotional crisis but also ends motivation to plan for the future in all but the most determined patients.

Reaching Understanding. Once awareness has been reached, the next step is to help patient and family learn about their options for continuing care and about what they will need to know and be able to do in order to take over responsibility from caregivers. In Section 2.3 we discussed the role of the nurse as teacher in detail.

> *"Readiness" or motivation to learn is determined by a person's perception of a need that can be met and a basis of experience on which to build new learning.*

The nurse encourages motivation to learn ("unfreezing" in Lewin's terms) by helping the learner identify the need clearly, giving information about how it might be met, and exploring what other experiences can be used as the foundation for new knowledge, attitudes, and skills. Nurses use their communication skills and resources to bring patients' perceptions and experiences together with opportunities that nurses themselves provide for learning (see Figure 2–3).

Reaching Constructive Action. Motivation to reach consensus and make decisions is perhaps the most difficult to develop because it is clearly future oriented. Patients and families embroiled in the realities of acute care often cannot see how they can possibly succeed in reaching the goal of constructive action. The nurse's role in helping with this kind of motivation is to show them how they can build on their understanding of the problem and clear the way for using the communication channels that exist. In practical terms, the nurse can:

- arrange that doctors and continuing care specialists be available for meeting with patient and family,
- coach patient and family on what questions to ask and how to obtain information,
- give family members telephone numbers and the names of contact people who can give them specific information about community sources of help,
- help the family set up a meeting with a financial advisor or social worker,
- make time for in-depth discussions about available options, and

• set up a schedule of learning that has short-term goals.

The nurse's assessment of the personalities of the people involved in decision-making are very useful in encouraging motivation to decide and plan (see Section 3.2). For example, the non-closure person will need more help and encouragement than the closure one.

The goal of the nurse in moving people toward constructive action is to help them experience personal power and a sense of control over their future.

All that the nurse has done to include the patient and family in caregiving, to provide information to them, and to help them avoid feelings of helplessness will now help them progress toward constructive action.

Continuing care decisions belong to a category that management experts term "open." That is, the aim is to reach decisions that are "good," even though all aspects of the problem and the exact consequences of any chosen action are presently unknown. Other examples of open decisions are job and relationship choices. We cannot know, except in hindsight, just how good our decisions are; we do the best we can and modify our behavior later as the need arises. Realizing that their goal is to find a "good" decision about continuing care options is helpful to people who are experiencing some apprehension about making a choice. Emphasis should be placed on problem "management" rather than on solutions. They should be encouraged to approach decisions as ones made for a relatively short term (one to three months, for example), to build re-evaluation and consultation with others into their plan, and to realistically consider what kinds of changes in the patient's condition will require modification of the plan.

The more complex the continuing care of a patient will be, the more important it is for both patient and family to feel that they have access to help and consultation after discharge and for them to anticipate changes in the discharge plan without a sense of failure.

The patient who leaves acute care knowing there is support in the community and expecting modifications of the original plan, is motivated to implement the plan and follow through on care.

In the following case study, some examples of responses by a nurse that stimulate patient motivation are shown, along with an analysis of these responses.

Example 6.2 Helping to Motivate an Accident Victim

Bob Snyder, age 38, and his wife were on vacation in a large city when the accident happened. They were hit by an

204 • DISCHARGE PLANNING GUIDE FOR NURSES

out-of-control car as they waited on the median strip of a divided street. Bob's wife suffered only minor injuries, but Bob sustained severe damage to his left leg and hip, including two breaks in the femur and a partly shattered acetabulum. Following surgery, he was transferred to a hospital in his home community for treatment and rehabilitation. The following are excerpts of dialogue between Bob and his primary care nurse as his care progressed.

Just after the patient arrived at the community hospital, his primary care nurse completed a nursing assessment.

Nurse: "I'm going to ask you a series of questions about your health before the accident. Your answers will help with planning your care after you leave the hospital."

Analysis: Very early in the patient's care the nurse introduces the idea of discharge planning and lets him see that she is interested in his health generally and not just in his injury.

A few days later.
Patient: "I'm really getting worried. I just can't see how I'm going to manage."

Nurse: "Progress must seem pretty slow to you right now. Can you tell me a bit more about what it is that's especially worrying you?"

Analysis: In response to the patient's expression of confusion and uncertainty, the nurse invites exploration of his feelings.

Patient: "I think the therapist expects that I'll always need crutches."

Nurse: "You've made tremendous progress in a short time. How do you feel about what you've accomplished so far?"

Analysis: The nurse helps the patient focus on the positive and encourages motivation to continue to improve.

Another few days later.
Patient: "I can see that I'm going to have to do a lot of things differently for as long as I need crutches."

Nurse: "Have you thought specifically about what those things are? Let's make a list and see what we have to work on before you go home."

Analysis: The nurse encourages him in his motivation to think about the practical aspects of his life after discharge. The list will provide some short-term learning goals that patient and caregivers can work toward.

Now anticipating
discharge.

Patient: "It's going to be awful to just have to lie around the house. I'd much rather be working."	*Nurse:* "Have you talked with your boss about your recuperation? Are there parts of your job that you might be able to do at home?"	*Analysis:* The nurse realizes that his job is a major motivator for the patient and encourages him to take responsibility for starting some negotiations with his company.
Patient: "Because they did x-rays yesterday, I missed therapy, and I can really notice the difference. I'm weaker today."	*Nurse:* "It's going to be just as important that you keep up exercises and therapy at home. Just in one day you learned something terribly important."	*Analysis:* The nurse reinforces the patient's awareness of the need for consistency in the therapy program and points out the relevance for his continuing care.

In this case example the nurse was alert to the stages through which the motivation of the patient progressed. Her communication with him emphasized positive progress and awareness of continuing care needs while not losing sight of reality.

In summary, in this section we have explored both theoretical and practical aspects of motivation. Our goal has been to help the reader develop an awareness of the importance of patient motivation for discharge planning and implementation of continuing care, an understanding of the different kinds of motivation needed, and some insight into practical ways in which the nurse can encourage patient motivation. The goal will have been reached if the nurse-reader makes encouragement of positive patient motivation an integral part of the care that is provided.

6.3 STEPS TOWARD IMPLEMENTATION

As the patient nears discharge, there are several actions by caregivers that improve the chances of effective implementation of the discharge plan. These involve communication activities whose general goal is to survey the whole discharge planning puzzle and whose specific objectives are to clarify the transfer of responsibilities for care, to review the entire plan to be sure nothing important has been overlooked, and to make last-minute arrangements for the immediate transition period. Each of these activities is discussed in this section.

Together, they confirm the plan for continuing care which is Step C of the process shown in Figure 6–1.

Communication and the Transfer of Caregiving Responsibility

By the time the patient is ready for discharge, communication links will have been established between caregivers of various disciplines, concerned family members and friends, and those in the community who will play roles in the patient's continuing care. Most importantly, a basis of communication will have been established with the patient. All these kinds of communication will have contributed to the nurse's impression of what kind of person the patient is and what kind of world he or she has been living in.

> *As the patient prepares to leave acute care, it is appropriate to ask: "In what ways have this person and his or her needs changed?" and "What kind of world will the person be returning to?"*

Just as the nurse examined the patient's health balance in the initial assessment to determine what was needed to begin the discharge planning process (see Section 2.1), a re-examination of that balance just before discharge serves to ensure that the patient's present needs will be met by the plan. It will also serve to guide the transiton to community care.

Information about changes in the patient's health balance will have been collected as discharge plans were made and teaching progressed. Other information will have been gathered in conversations with both patient and family and in observing their behavior. In the following paragraphs we will briefly review the patient's needs, demands, strengths, and resources and discuss how these four elements of the health balance influence the transfer of responsibility for health care.

Needs or Deficits. The early discharge of patients has led to greater attention to physical needs and knowledge deficits by discharge planners. Throughout the acute phase of treatment, caregivers must constantly ask themselves: "Is this treatment or procedure going to be continued after discharge?" If the answer is "yes," then preparations need to be started immediately to give the patient or community caregivers the information and skills they will need. Prior to discharge, the patient's continuing needs or deficits must be realistically measured against strengths and resources so that the transition in responsibility for care can be made smoothly. A patient may, for example, have been taught to irrigate a colostomy and may have done so flawlessly for several days before discharge. Yet confidence may evaporate when the patient thinks about all the things that could go wrong when instant access to expert help is no longer available. The patient will at least need reassurance and probably further teaching to fill in any deficit of knowledge in how to handle complications.

Other kinds of needs or deficits that the nurse must identify before discharge are how the patient is going to refill medication or supplies and maintain equipment, and how he is going to accomplish the instrumental activities of daily living such as shopping, preparing meals, and washing clothes. If others are going to lend a hand, this is the time to be sure that solid arrangements have been made for this help and that they are aware of the nature and extent of their responsibilities. The checklist presented in Part II, Step C will help both nurse, patient, and family identify needs or deficits, ask appropriate questions, and anticipate the realities of continuing care.

Demands or Stressors. The transitional period just after discharge is a time of risk due to physical, emotional, social, and sometimes cultural stressors. It is a time when physical problems can exacerbate, interpersonal tensions can escalate into battles, and the presence or absence of social acceptance makes the difference between positive motivation to recover or depression. In Section 3.1 we discussed the anxiety and stress caused by relinquishing control to caregivers when a person becomes a patient. The stress of taking back control is also very significant. Even in the most simple case, a patient going home to recover faces changes in social roles and the ability to meet the demands of others to be an "employee," "parent," or "spouse," for example. Lingering physical disabilities mean that the patient will have to strike a balance between allowing others to do some elements of care and insisting on independent self-care. There are some distinct psychological differences between "waiting to get better" and "trying hard to get better."

The nurse can make a major contribution to the effective implementation of continuing care by helping both patient and family explore the stresses that will occur during the transition period and take steps to reduce their negative impact. As discussed in Section 6.2 and shown in Figure 6–4, the first step in motivation to solve a problem or prevent its development is awareness. Caregivers who are immersed in the hospital or clinic environment may find it very difficult to visualize just what it will be like for the patient after discharge and, consequently, equally difficult to give specific guidance. Therefore, taking the time to ask "open" questions that help patients themselves explore potential stressors are especially important (see Section 2.2). The nurse might ask: "What do you think your biggest problem is going to be during the first two or three days after leaving here?" and "What do you look forward to most in going home?" The answers will help the nurse learn what the patient's priorities are and how to make the transition more smooth.

Strengths. The physical, intellectual, motor, and emotional strengths that the person brings to acute care are a powerful influence on response to treatment and plans for continuing care. The effects of a disease process and medical or surgical intervention may leave patients without great physical strengths when they are discharged, but the knowledge they have gained about themselves, the skills they have acquired, and the positive attitudes they have been helped to develop about continuing care all make major contributions to their health balance. These mental and emotional strengths are the result of learning from planned teaching, from on-the-spot explanations and answers to questions, and from the examples provided by caregivers. The potential that good teaching has for steadying the health balance and improving the patient's chances of successfully managing continuing care cannot be overestimated.

Resources. Appropriateness, availability, and access are the three basic guidelines in determining which resources in the community should be involved in a person's continuing care. It takes careful attention to all forms of communication with patient and family to accurately assess what resources of time, money, skills, and motivation they have to help with continuing care. The skills of a social worker or discharge planning coordinator will be helpful in making this assessment, especially in complex situations. In addition to their availability and accessibility, community caregivers ranging from the physician to home care and social welfare agencies must also be assessed for what they have to offer that is appropriate to patient continuing care goals. (See Section 5.1 for guidance on how to survey community resources.)

There are two major ways in which plans that depend on community resources are open to failure. The first occurs when the resources of the family to provide care on a long term basis are overestimated. The time that it takes to give personal care and the fatigue that overtakes even very committed family caregivers can undermine the most carefully made plan. Another kind of failure can occur when the practical details of access to community services or agencies are not considered. The need to transfer buses on the way to an appointment or the need to fill out a lengthy financial form can be enough to destroy motivation to follow through with a plan if these setbacks occur unexpectedly. See Section 5.4 for further discussion of factors in patient acceptance of community help.

The health balance provides a framework for looking at how a patient's needs may have changed during acute care and what kind of personal world they will be discharged into. This awareness, along with good communication skills, allow the nurse to better help prepare patients and their families for the realities of continuing care.

Review of Detailed Continuing Care Plans with Patient and Family

Reviewing all the details of the continuing care plan with the patient and all family members who will share responsibility for its implementation serves three basic purposes. One is to be sure that nothing important has escaped attention. More than one unfortunate patient has been sent home without anyone remembering that a supply of groceries would be needed, for example. A second reason for review is that it gives the patient the chance to consolidate learning and ask questions, at the same time allowing the nurse to confirm that the patient's level of knowledge, attitudes, and skills are adequate for the tasks ahead. This is the time when "what if . . ." situations can be explored and unrealistic fantasies laid to rest. Finally, a review helps clarify exactly what responsibilities each individual has and what can be expected to happen. For each subject area within the discharge plan, one asks **who** is responsible, **when** is action to be taken, **where** is this to take place, **what** is to be done, and **how** is it to be accomplished—the key questions abbreviated to "4W-H."

The review of discharge plans just before the patient leaves acute care is the time to reinforce learning, not the time to do major teaching.

Unless knowledge and skills are well advanced and learning goals substantially met by this time, the review will be confusing, demoralizing, and counter-productive. (See Section 2.3 for guidance on effective patient teaching.) Written instructions are an excellent device for ensuring compliance with instructions and are generally reassuring for patients, but their intent should be to augment other teaching methods, not to replace them. Careful guidance as to who, when, and how to call if questions or problems arise is an important part of the review.

Whether a checklist such as that presented in Step C of Part II of this text is used or not, the areas that are generally included in the plan review are as follows:

- Medical follow-up
- Medications
- Treatments and procedures
- Activities
- Nutrition and diet

- Identification and management of complications
- Health maintenance and promotion
- Community services and resources

A useful approach to this review makes use of the principles of the CONE interview described in Section 2.2, with each subject area representing a CONE. The content introduction may simply be: "Let's talk about your medications. . . ," followed by an open question such as: "Tell me about the medications you will be taking at home." This kind of open invitation allows the patient the opportunity to tell the nurse all that has been learned in the subject area without feeling as though as though a quiz is being given. It also allows the nurse to judge at what level learning has occurred and how adequately prepared the patient is to handle problems that may occur at home. The open invitation to discuss a subject can be followed up with a question of narrower focus such as: "You said you will count your pulse before taking your Digitalis. What if your pulse is 48?"

Finally, whichever of the "4W-H" questions have not been mentioned within the context of the open discussion can be explored specifically and in detail.

> *The knowledge and skills that will be the basis of discharge plan implementation must be reviewed prior to discharge in a reassuring and confidence-building, rather than threatening, way.*

The CONE approach allows the patient to discover how much has been learned and invites clarification of anything he or she is still uncertain about. It also allows the nurse to evaluate the results of teaching efforts. The quality of information is critical to the plan's success. If the nurse asks a series of "closed" questions such as: "Do you know how to take your medications?", little or no useful information will be received because patients under pressure generally will say "Yes." It is better to discover gaps in knowledge while plans can be adjusted. The patient may need more explicit written instructions or a family member may have to learn to check the patient's pulse, for example. Although the patient cannot be expected to do additional learning while entering the transitional phase of care, the organization of information into "rules" or "steps" can help make better use of what has already been learned.

Arranging Details of Transitional Care

The three steps discussed as part of "Confirming the Discharge Plan" (Step C, Fig. 6–1) have a narrowing focus. In the first, the patient's present needs and health balance are re-examined. In the second, details of the continuing care plan are reviewed and the patient's knowledge and skills evaluated in the light of the patient's own responsibility for plan implementation. This final step has the narrowest and most time-limited focus: arranging details of what is to happen in the few hours between the time the patient physically leaves the acute care facility and the time the plan begins to function and community caregivers take up their responsibilities. This is always a period of anxiety and some discomfort; the most minor details that have been overlooked can seem monumental. If, for example, the family has not brought appropriate clothing to the patient, there can be delays, frustration, and anger complicating an already tense situation. If the billing office has not been notified of the patient's departure, there can be annoyance, delays, and unnecessary confusion.

A checklist of questions appropriate for the nurse to ask in anticipation of the patient's transition out of the hospital include:

- What does the patient or a family member need to have or do before the patient can leave?
- How will the patient get to the required destination and who will be there to receive him or her?
- What does the patient need to have in hand at the time of departure?
- Who in the hospital needs to be notified and by whom?
- Who will take responsibility for getting implementation of the continuing care plan started, and what do they have to do?

While the specific content of each question may vary according to the kind of acute care facility, the intent is to ensure that those first hours go smoothly and allow the patient the chance to adjust to a new environment without undue stress. By this time, referrals will have been made and information to other services and agencies already transferred, so that the problem in these latter stages of acute care is to activate the plan. One would like to avoid the kind of situation described in the following case example.

Example 6.3 A Wrong Address Delays Transition Home

A discharge planning coordinator recently told of an incident that occurred early in her career. A patient was discharged from the hospital to his home by ambulance. Shortly after his departure, the nurse received a call from a very annoyed ambulance driver. It seems that the house whose address he had been given did not exist; there was only a vacant lot on that corner. Investigation revealed that the address on the medical record was an old one transferred to the patient's chart from an admission several years before. No one had verified that address or found out that the patient had moved. His former home had been torn down to make way for a freeway.

While this kind of situation is certainly a learning experience for all concerned, it would be much better to avoid such distress, even once, through wise planning and careful checking of details.

In summary, three aspects of the final step of the discharge planning process have been discussed, those that confirm the plan just prior to the patient's discharge. The goals of this step are to re-examine the patient's immediate physical and emotional needs, clarify continuing care responsibilities, evaluate the adequacy of the patient's knowledge and skills, and review specific details of the transitional period. Taking the time and making the effort to confirm the discharge plan greatly increase the probability of the plan's effective implementation; it is the follow-through that ensures that the goal is met.

6.4 HOW TO EVALUATE DISCHARGE PLANNING

In this section we reach the concluding step of the discharge planning process by evaluating what has been accomplished. In Section 1.3 we described discharge planning as a process whose long-term goal is continuity of health care for patients. We emphasized the dynamic, interactive, and patient-centered nature of that process. Throughout this text, our focus has been on identifying changing patient needs and helping patients and their families gain the knowledge, skills, and contacts with community resources that will allow them to take over responsibility for continuing care. Evaluating such a complex, individualized process is not a simple matter. Some of the evaluative questions that might reasonably be asked include the following:

- Were patient needs and risks identified early in the patient's acute care?
- Were patient learning goals identified and teaching documented?
- Were referrals complete and made in a timely fashion?

- Was the patient able to verbalize continuing care goals and the steps to take to reach them?
- Was the patient satisfied with his role in the discharge planning process and the decisions made as part of it?

- Did the patient comply with medical advice and follow through on continuing care plans?

- Is responsibility for initiating discharge planning and accountability for the completed process clear in the policies of the institution?
- Does the reporting system used support discharge planning need identification and patient teaching documentation?
- Are in-service education programs in place that give staff members discharge planning knowledge and skills?

The above questions have been divided into three groups, suggesting three different approaches to evaluation. In the following pages we will explore each of these: the use of audits of the discharge planning process, patient goal attainment, and program evaluation.

Using Discharge Planning Audits

Well-run and financially viable organizations have always used a range of measures that help administrators evaluate whether staff members are complying with policies and procedures, whether problems exist in how organizational goals are met, and where improvements might be made. In recent years these kinds of measures, combined with performance appraisals and the setting of standards, have been termed "Quality Assurance" (Wilson, 1987).

One of the primary methods used to assure quality in medical care institutions is the review or "audit" of medical records. The retrospective review of nursing records to determine compliance with standards of quality care in general and discharge planning services in particular have been required by the Joint Commission on Accreditation of Hospitals for more than a decade (Burkey, 1979).

Retrospective audits have the advantage that they deal with "hard" data. A patient record either has a discharge summary that meets a set of standards or it does not; either discharge teaching is documented or it is not. Audit procedures have often been combined with "peer" review, meaning that a group of nurses reviews the records of their peers, evaluates their performance on that basis, and suggests specific improvements. Increasingly, discharge planning audits have focused on early identification of discharge needs or risks (within 48 hours of admission), evidence of discharge teaching, and planning for posthospital needs that involves the patient and/or family in information and decision-making (American Hospital Association, 1987).

The legal requirement that discharge planning serves to

> *"prevent reasonably foreseeable harm"* after discharge means that the hospital, and by implication the nurse, has an obligation to assess needs, teach, and communicate effectively.

A review of records is the most straight-forward and objective way of ensuring that these steps are being taken. Although many nurses regard the review of their records defensively, audit procedures act to their direct benefit in two ways: they help protect nurses legally, and they uncover areas in which they may need help in improving skills and meeting standards.

Retrospective audits are effective in demonstrating whether record-keeping standards have been met, but they occur too late to have any effect on the process for those patients whose records are being reviewed. Theoretically, the concurrent audit of records should be even better, because behavior on the part of caregivers could be guided and altered rather than just judged later. As a practical alternative, however, concurrent audit will not be widespread until and unless nursing care is recorded on computer files and computer programs are designed that alert nurses to time requirements and help them document care completely. One attempt at doing this is a software computer program based on Part II of this text now being developed.

While audits are a useful tool for evaluating the extent of discharge planning services to patients, they have distinct limitations in helping to judge whether patients actually implement plans or meet continuing care goals. An audit shows, for example, that teaching has been done, but not whether learning has occurred. It can evaluate the process and the procedures, but not the outcome of discharge planning; it is an excellent "first few chapters," but not the full story.

Evaluating Patient Goal Attainment

Whenever a nurse has worked intensively with a patient and family on identifying continuing care needs, teaching them about options and alternatives, and helping them develop skills and make realistic decisions, the *outcome* of these efforts are of special significance to the nurse.

There are three basic dimensions to the evaluation of outcomes of discharge planning: failure to meet goals, patient satisfaction, and positive goal attainment.

Failure to Meet Goals. While this is certainly a negative outcome, it is the one caregivers are most likely to hear about. Patients readmitted to the hospital within 14 days are monitored by Utilization Review

Committees or Professional Standards Review Organizations (PSROs). For these patients, it must be asked whether discharge planning was adequate and appropriate. Aside from those readmitted, nurses often get feedback from community agencies or the families of patients when things do not go well and additional information or services are needed. In Section 7.2 we discuss some of the ethical issues surrounding continuing care decision-making and the problem of "allowing" people to fail.

Patient Satisfaction. This dimension of evaluation is very subjective in nature. People are generally satisfied with services if their positive expectations are met and their goals parallel those of caregivers. They are more likely to be satisfied if they *like* the people who are giving them care. They are more inclined to follow the advice and pursue the suggestions of caregivers whom they trust and respect. Determining satisfaction, of course, requires feedback, and mechanisms for this are relatively rare (Muenchow and Carlson, 1985). In other industries, questionnaires are sent to recipients of services to determine customer satisfaction. There is certainly some potential for this approach within medical care. Usually, however, caregivers do informal surveys of former patients by telephoning them to find out how things are going.

Positive Goal Attainment. Whether the details of a particular plan worked well or not is part of a larger evaluation concern: were continuing care services provided as planned, and was the patient placed at the most independent level of care possible? As Muenchow and Carlson (1985) found in their review of discharge planning programs, methods for obtaining feedback usually do not include information on these two outcomes of services. Prospective payment systems may put pressure on hospitals and community agencies to obtain this kind of data, but there is also a legal barrier in the way. The American Hospital Association's report on legal issues in discharge planning (1987, p. 61) notes that if a hospital representative contacts a patient to find out how appropriate the discharge plan was, it opens the door for the person to inform the hospital that in some way the plan has failed. Having been informed of a problem, the hospital may be expected to rectify it, and failing this, may be legally liable for any injury that results. It is very difficult to construct a feedback mechanism that gives only good news, but hospitals have reason to avoid knowing about the bad news! In all probability, information about whether planned goals have been attained will continue to be largely informal; community caregivers will mention to nurses how patients are doing or patients will return to the hospital for social visits to report their progress.

These dimensions of evaluating the outcomes of discharge planning highlight the importance of identifying *goals* as well as problems or risks within the planning process. It is only against goals that progress can be measured. Goals also point to the need for effective *communication* between patients and caregivers so that appropriate learning occurs and expectations of progress and the services of others is realistic. At issue are patient satisfaction and the ability of families to make a plan work even in the face of temporary reverses.

Discharge Planning Program Evaluation

The increasing number and extent of regulations regarding discharge planning activities have led medical care organizations to review their policies and procedures in this area.

Establishing, conducting, and evaluating a well-coordinated program of discharge planning demands the cooperation and involvement of all departments within the institution.

It means that policies must support agreed-upon goals and objectives. It means that record-keeping procedures must support the level of information and communication needed to meet those objectives. And it means that staff members must be educated in the skills of need identification, patient teaching, and community coordination and receive valid feedback about their performance in these areas. While this is a complex recipe for success, the need for such well-organized and consistent programs becomes more evident as health care personnel work with the realities of prospective payment and shorter hospital stays. Some of the ethical issues for institutions in providing high quality care while containing costs are discussed in Section 7.2.

Evaluating discharge plans in terms of their process and outcome can be rewarding for nurses and other professional staff. A good and complete plan demands that they make full use of their assessment, teaching, and communication skills. To be prevented from seeing the results is a little like striving to prepare a gourmet meal but not having a chance to taste it. Aside from the sense of incompletion that might follow such an experience, the people involved in the preparation cannot learn and improve their skills unless they know the outcome. The challenge for nurses and the institutions that employ them is to find ways to help discharge planners enjoy the process and derive satisfaction from the outcome of their labor. Only then will they be motivated to document completely, refer intelligently, and use their considerable talents to improve the continuity of care for patients and the quality of their lives, as well as reduce costs.

In summary, we have reviewed three approaches to discharge planning evaluation in this section by discussing audit procedures, outcome information, and program evaluation. Each has both benefits and limitations. The evaluation process is made more difficult because responsibility for health care is transferred once the patient leaves acute care. Yet evaluation is an essential step if discharge planning is to improve and caregivers are to develop their skills.

SUMMARY

Our goal in this chapter has been to bring together the concepts and principles discussed throughout this book and show how they can be applied to the practical process of discharge planning. We have done this by exploring both the factors to be considered and the resulting decisions in each of three steps toward continuing care: assessment, building a plan, and confirming the plan—the A-B-Cs of discharge planning. We have also examined the subject of motivation and given the nurse some guidance on how to stimulate positive motivation and prepare patients for assuming responsibility for implementing plans. Finally we have discussed aspects of discharge planning evaluation and its importance to the nurse, the patient, and the acute care institution. We again emphasize that involvement in discharge planning offers nurses the opportunity to develop and use skills in assessment, teaching and communication for the benefit of patient's future health as well as for their own professional satisfaction in a job well done.

FURTHER READING

Baulch, Evelyn. *Home Care: A Practical Alternative to Extended Hospitalization.* Millbrae, Calif.: Celestial Arts, 1980.
Written by a caretaker for other caretakers, this book is a practical guide on how to provide home care. It includes chapters on the care of children, the elderly, and the terminally ill. It discusses "burnout" and how family members can care for themselves.

Mace, Nancy L., and Peter Rabens. *The 36 Hour Day: A Family Guide to Caring for Persons with Alzheimer's Disease, Related Dementing Illnesses and Memory Loss in Later Life.* Balitmore: Johns Hopkins University Press, 1981.
This book focuses on families of persons with incurable dementing illnesses giving them clearly written, practical advice. It is a valuable resource for both caretakers and professionals.

Muenchow, Judith, and Barbara Carlson. "Evaluating Programs of Discharge Planning." In McClelland, E., K. Kelly, and K. Buckwalter (eds.). *Continuity of Care: Advancing the Concept of Discharge Planning.* Orlando: Grune & Stratton, 1985.
The authors of this chapter review a number of discharge planning programs and show how evaluation works in practice. They include a list of "common elements"

in all the programs that are helpful to people involved in setting up an evaluation system. Their focus is on the outcome of planning.

Rovinski, C. A., and D. K. Zastocki. *Home Care: A Technical Manual for the Professional Nurse.* Philadelphia: W. B. Saunders, 1989.
After a brief introduction, this book is indeed a technical manual, outlining specific procedures in each of a very comprehensive list of bodily systems and other categories of nursing care. Following each set of procedures is a set of resource data including normal values, methods for evaluating patient status, etc. This would be a valuable book in the clinical setting as a reference and also as a means of communication with community caregivers.

Smith, Barbara A. "When is 'Confusion' Translocation Syndrome?" *American Journal of Nursing* 86(11) Nov. 1986; 1280–81.
This short article is worth reviewing periodically by all nurses. It is a cautionary tale about how an abrupt change in environment can distort mental functioning and result in derogatory labels and ineffective communication, especially with the elderly. It has special significance for assessing mental abilities as part of discharge planning.

Stoddard, Sandal. *The Hospice Movement: A Better Way of Caring for the Dying.* New York: Vintage Books, 1978.
This book is a classic in the field of caring for the terminally ill. It provides an historical view of the hospice concept and its development in America.

Task Force on Legal Issues in Discharge Planning. *Discharging Hospital Patients: Legal Implications for Institutional Providers and Health Care Professionals.* Legal Memorandum Number 9, Chicago: American Hospital Association, 1987.
This document is the report of the Task Force on Legal Issues in Discharge Planning. It is well organized and surprisingly readable. Its table of contents is sufficiently detailed to allow the reader to immediately find sections relevant to them. It should be readily available as a resource to all professionals involved in discharge planning.

Wilson, Christopher R. M. *Hospital-wide Quality Assurance.* Toronto: W. B. Saunders, Canada Ltd., 1987.
This Canadian book gives a clear overview of the increasingly complex subject of quality assurance. It can help any nurse better understand the goals and organization of Q.A. in hospitals and some of its limitations.

7

How Ethical Issues Influence Discharge Planning

Most nurses perceive a recent increase in situations where a choice of what is "good" or "right" is unclear. Rapid changes in health and medical care delivery have raised questions of ethics for individual health professionals, for institutions, and for patients. Discharge planning is one area of patient care that seems especially surrounded by controversy. Our objective in including this chapter is not to resolve

219

the controversy, but rather to address some of the issues involved in discharge planning. Our hope is that this discussion will help nurses formulate questions to ask themselves, their organizations' administrators, and their legal advisors and thereby help them resolve some of these dilemmas for themselves.

In this chapter we will briefly examine three facets of the ethics of discharge planning. All have economic and legal implications as well as ethical ones. If any generalization can be made about these ethical issues, it is that "what is right" is often not congruent with "what is economically sound" or "what is legally defensible."

The three sections of this chapter have been constructed around a series of case examples. In the first section we ask: "Who makes decisions about discharges?" We then go on to consider the issue of quality versus quantity as it applies to continuing care. Finally, we present some ideas about the nurse's dilemma of time and effort versus personal and professional satisfaction.

7.1 WHO MAKES DECISIONS ABOUT PATIENT DISCHARGES?

Throughout this book we have emphasized the involvement of patient and family in decisions concerning discharge plans. The need for trust-building communication, for well-planned teaching, and for coordinated approaches by caregiving professionals as the means for reaching the goal of self-determination by patients have been discussed at length. The ability of nurses and other caregivers to influence progress toward that goal is, however, admittedly dependent on some stability in staff assignments that allows a group of professionals to become acquainted with a patient's needs. In many hospitals, lack of stable staffing patterns and the involvement of representatives of third-party payers with their own agendas add up to discharge plans that are imposed on patients or that fail to meet even their physical needs, much less their social and emotional needs. The case examples that follow demonstrate some aspects of a more general problem.

Example 7.1 A Case of Too Many Discharge Planners

Mr. Carlton was admitted to Eastside Hospital following a stroke. Although he initially had almost complete paralysis of the right side, he began to recover some function with intensive physical and speech therapy. At age 67, his chances of rehabilitation seemed good and his physician, neurologist, and primary care nurse encouraged him to think in this direction. The patient belonged to a Health Maintenance Organization (HMO) with headquarters in another city.

As the patient's medical condition stabilized, his physician recommended that he be discharged to a nearby rehabilitation unit. His wife, however, wanted him to come home. She and their daughter had worked out an elaborate plan for looking after Mr. Carlton's physical needs. They asked the nurse a number of questions about home care services in the area. Knowing that finances were a problem for the family and being uncertain about the HMO's policies, the nurse referred the family to the hospital's discharge planning coordinator. The coordinator was familiar with the coverage offered by the HMO but had recently experienced a series of negative incidents involving the HMO's discharge planner. She went immediately to introduce herself to the patient and his wife, gave them some basic information about her department's services, and planned to meet with them the next afternoon.

The following morning a young woman arrived at Mr. Carlton's bedside and introduced herself as the discharge planner. He was confused about just who she was but thought she was from the same department as the lady he had met yesterday. She informed him that arrangements had been made for his transfer to a nursing home in a neighboring city about 25 miles away. He would be taken there by ambulance the next day. The patient told her that he didn't want to go to a nursing home, but his speech handicap made it very difficult to communicate the strength of his feelings.

A great deal of confusion ensued in the next few hours. The second discharge planner had been from the HMO. She had had no conversation with the hospital's coordinator and did not know of the family's plans. As it turned out, the family lived in an outlying area that was not covered by the home care agency with which the HMO had a contract. The nearest nursing homes under contract with the HMO had no beds available. The family could not afford to pay for care in the rehabilitation unit on their own and, angry with the HMO, decided to refuse the nursing home placement. Mr. Carlton went home to a highly stressed family and without a realistic plan for follow-up care or rehabilitation.

This case example is representative of an unfortunate number of situations in which the "players" on the "stage" of discharge planning have their own "scripts" that are not well coordinated with one another. The doctors, family, hospital discharge planning coordinator, and HMO all thought that they had the patient's best interests in mind. Each had a vision of what "ought" to happen. It is easy to blame the HMO's discharge planner for making a plan without consultation, or the doctor for not finding out that the cost of rehabilitation was not covered. One can even imagine that the "bad blood" that may have developed between the hospital's and HMO's discharge planning departments was at the root of the lack of communication. Whatever caused this kind of problem to develop, the patient and his family were the ones who suffered its effect. Some of the questions arising out of this example are:

- How could this situation have been avoided?
- Whose responsibility is it to communicate with whom?
- What might the nurse have done differently?
- Were the patient's rights upheld?
- What responsibility do doctors and hospital discharge planners have to intervene with HMOs or other such "outside" organizations?
- Does the HMO have the right to send its representative to examine a patient's record or to discuss plans with a patient? Under what conditions?
- What are the provisions of the contracts your hospital has with third-party payers?
- What are your hospital's policies regarding discharge planning services, utilization review, and quality assurance?

Third-party payers will continue to have a rapidly increasing impact on hospital care for the foreseeable future; they are the source of reimbursement for institutions. Their major priority can be expected to be cost containment, if not cost reduction. At the same time, the hospital is responsible for the quality of the care it provides even while remaining financially viable. The individual nurse is responsible for meeting professional standards of patient care. In an increasing number of cases these concerns and priorities conflict with one another. The feature article of the American Hospital Association's *Discharge Planning Update* (1987, p. 9) concluded with the following statement:

"Without exception, the discharge planners interviewed agreed . . . that third-party discharge planning will become a very serious consideration in the near future. And it will take knowledge, expertise, and consummate management skills to work out mutually acceptable arrangements—arrangements that will not leave the patient and his family out of the picture."

Today's rising medical care costs will undoubtedly lead to an increase in the influence that economic issues have on care planning. How should patient access to limited resources and services be determined?

Ethical questions about who should decide the destination of a discharge are not limited to the intervention of third-party payers. In the next case example the nurse finds herself caught in the emotional tug-of-war between the patient, his doctor, and his family.

Example 7.2 Emotional Issues Complicate a Discharge

Glen Adams was admitted to the hospital two days before his 29th birthday with *Pneumocystis carinii* secondary to acquired immune deficiency syndrome (AIDS). He had known of his AIDS diagnosis for about six weeks. Glen's parents were aware of his homosexuality and had invited his lover to their home on two occasions, but his perception was that they really did not accept his life-style. His sister had been more open and supportive and had visited him regularly. Glen had nearly told his sister of the AIDS diagnosis but instead just alluded to his being sick a few times recently. The present physical crisis presented him with an emotional crisis as well.

Linda Benson had cared for a number of AIDS patients in the past year and was well aware of the emotional struggle that many faced. She quickly developed a rapport with Glen, who seemed to relate to her as a trusted older sister. Linda encouraged him to talk about his disease, his fears, and his family. At first he made comments like: "Maybe I'll just die quietly and nobody will have to know about this (the AIDS)." Linda accepted these statements but encouraged him to think about how he might include his family now that he really needed their support. Gradually Glen developed a plan for confronting his family; they were unaware that he was hospitalized. Meanwhile, Glen's doctor was aggressively treating the pneumonia with intravenous Penamidine, although some side-effects were occurring. Glen telephoned his parents and sister and all arrived at his bedside within a few hours. Linda made herself available to them to answer questions and provide support for Glen. The encounter went pretty well, with the family trying hard to control their sense of shock and at the same time reassure Glen of their love and concern.

Over the next few days, the patient's physical condition began to improve, and he felt relieved that he had been able to talk to his family. Everyone began to focus on Glen's discharge. One morning Linda came on duty to find Glen tearfully collapsed in a chair. He said that his parents had come the evening before to tell him that they had arranged for him to be admitted to a "treatment center" in Arizona for AIDS patients. Glen said he wasn't sure whether this plan was a way of removing him far from the family or reflected their irrational hopes for his recovery or both. When asked what HE wanted, Glen replied that he just wanted to go home to his apartment and spend whatever time he had with his friends.

The next day Glen was again feverish and showed symptoms of a fungal infection in his mouth and throat. Within a very short time he was experiencing violent diarrhea and vomiting as side-effects of medication. When his doctor next visited, Glen told him that he did not wish to have his disease treated aggressively; in fact, he would prefer that all treatment be withdrawn. The doctor received this request as though it was a personal attack and gave Glen a lecture about the necessity of putting up with a little discomfort. Linda walked into the room in the middle of the lecture and suspected what had happened. She made sure that she stopped the doctor on his way out. After a brief discussion with her, the doctor calmed down and suggested that the staff psychiatrist be called for a consultation with Glen to determine his mental state. The patient readily agreed. The psychiatrist found Glen to be somewhat depressed, but mentally competent to make his own decisions.

In this case example, the emotional issues surrounding a diagnosis of AIDS added substantially to the patient's distress. He seemed to accept his prognosis and wanted limited medical intervention. The family's fantasies about a "cure" clouded their ability to see Glen's need to be with those who could give him love and support. Glen felt understandably trapped by the family's attempt to make decisions for him. His sense of loss of control was increased by his perception that the doctor was attempting to force aggressive treatment on him. Each of the people involved felt they were behaving ethically and with Glen's best interest in mind. The nurse found herself caught up in Glen's tug-of-war with his family and his doctor while wanting to give him support and be an advocate for his wishes.

Three ethical principles were involved here: *autonomy*, or the preservation of self-determination; *beneficence*, or the duty to give help and preserve life; and *nonmaleficence*, or the requirement to relieve suffering and do no harm (see Young, 1988, Ch. 2). Some of the questions that arise out of this example are:

- What are the patient's rights in this situation? Are those rights changed at all because of his "depression" and emotional distress?
- What are the family's rights? Was telling them of Glen's AIDS a "good" thing to do?
- What are the doctor's duties and responsibilities? How is it possible to separate personal and professional beliefs about "proper" treatment methods?
- What are the nurse's duties and responsibilities? How can she act ethically in this situation?
- What would you now do if you were the nurse?

In summary, the number of people involved in modern medical care leads to some ethical dilemmas about who should make decisions about continuing care. The recent imposition of financial issues as a driving force for decisions often seems to compromise either the patient's rights, ethical principles, or both. Nurses have been encouraged to examine their own behavior in the light of their own ethical system and to clarify legal and economic facts surrounding discharge planning issues.

The reader may wish to know the outcome of Example 7.2. After considerable discussion with all parties, Glen's autonomy was upheld, and he went home to his apartment supported by a home-based hospice program. He died peacefully two months later with his sister and friends present.

7.2 HOW CAN ISSUES OF QUALITY VERSUS QUANTITY OF CARE BE RESOLVED?

Legal and economic issues are also at the heart of quality versus quantity dilemmas. All caregivers are familiar with the questions now being raised about the distribution of scarce medical resources. Examples of such questions are:

- What criteria should be used for organ transplants, and how should those who do not qualify be cared for?
- Under what circumstances is cardiac surgery justified, and what are the legal and economic implications of doing unnecessary surgery?
- To what extent should the lives of deformed or seriously impaired infants be preserved and by what means?
- How can the rights of patients who want limited medical intervention or "no code" status be protected while offering them quality palliative treatment?

- Should terminally ill patients be admitted to Intensive Care Units?
- Is the preservation of life at all cost in all circumstances still a valid ethical stand for medical professionals? What are the realistic legal liabilities of pursuing any other philosophies?

There are two basic quality versus quantity issues: one has to do with whether the physical, emotional, or economic costs of extending the life of an individual is balanced by the available quality of life. The second seeks to answer how limited, high quality resources are to be distributed fairly among the people within a community or society.

In his excellent book *Alpha and Omega: Ethics at the Frontiers of Life and Death,* Ernle Young (1988, Ch. 9) presents a clear and highly readable discussion of the ethical interplay between the principles of *beneficence* and *nonmaleficence.* Given the sophistication of today's medical care, a choice must frequently be made between prolonging "meaningful" life and extending the dying process. Deciding which of these two principles has precedence in a particular case can be an agonizing decision often based not on medical fact, but on judgment and intuition.

Young also discusses the potential conflicts between *beneficence and justice,* particularly "distributive" justice, that demands fairness in the allocation of resources. In economic terms, this conflict is often referred to as the "cost-benefit ratio": does the cost of a particular treatment or procedure match its benefits to the patient? The following case example is the report of an actual court case decided in 1986 in California.

Example 7.3 Wickline Versus State of California

The patient involved in this case was admitted in 1977 to a California hospital with arteriosclerosis and occlusion of the vessels of the right leg. Since surgery was indicated, authorization was sought from the state's Medicaid (Medi-Cal) program. Ten days of in-patient care were approved. Complications occurred during the post-surgery period requiring two additional surgeries. The patient's physicians requested that an additional eight days of hospitalization be approved. Only four were authorized by Medi-Cal. The patient was discharged after the fourth day without further requests for an extension by the doctor.

Subsequently, the patient developed pain and color changes in her right leg. She was re-admitted nine days later and over the next three weeks underwent a below-the-knee amputation followed by an above-the-knee amputation when her condition failed to resolve. Suit was filed against the State of California alleging that the patient's leg would not have been lost if an adequate number of acute care days had been authorized. While the jury held in her favor, the State Court of Appeals disagreed. It found that Medi-Cal was not liable, since it is the physician's responsibility to decide when a patient should be discharged. The court went on to make a statement that will have wide implications for future legal actions:

> ". . . *third party payors of health care services can be held legally accountable when medically inappropriate decisions result from defects in the design or implementation of cost containment mechanisms. . . . However, the physician who complies without protest with the limitations imposed by a third party payor, when his medical judgment dictates otherwise, cannot avoid his ultimate responsibility for his patient's care.*" (228 Cal. Rptr., p. 671)

In the above case, the patient argued that by not allocating her a greater *quantity* of medical resources (days in hospital), the *quality* of her care was compromised and resulted in amputation. Aside from the legal issues, the example raises the following questions:

- How can medical documents be made to accurately reflect the needs of patients so that better decisions can be made about allocating costly or scarce resources?
- What can nurses do when they disagree with a patient's physician about the timing of a discharge or when they feel an appeal should be made for an extension from the third-party payer?
- What input do nurses have in your institution to the Utilization Review and Quality Assurance procedures?
- What policies of your hospital determine allocation of resources (e.g., what criteria is used in offering Intensive Care or rehabilitation services)?
- What standards of nursing care are recognized in your insitution, and how are they used to assess quality of care?

In the next case example, a quantity of services were offered to the patient, but it was difficult to determine whether they improved the quality of her life.

Example 7.4 Family Environment Works Against Handicapped Child

Peter and Emily Reed desperately wanted a child of their own. Both had been ·married previously and had teenage children. When Emily conceived, she was 42 years old. The pregnancy progressed normally, but Emily's doctor suggested that she have an amniocentesis. The Reeds did not believe in abortion under any conditions and very much wanted the child, so they did not bother with the test.

Emily delivered a five-pound girl, whom they called Kelly. The baby had clear symptoms of Down's syndrome and severe kyllosis that would have to be corrected surgically if she was ever to walk. With support from family and friends, the Reeds approached Kelly's care optimistically.

Things went reasonably well for the first few months, although it became evident that Kelly was probably seriously retarded. Emily had quit her job to care for Kelly and was very patient with the feeding problems that were the major focus of the infant's care. A public health nurse visited regularly to supervise the situation and give support to the mother. She arranged for Crippled Children's services to provide braces for Kelly's feet in the hopes that the kyllosis could be at least partially corrected.

Kelly was about 8 months old when the family situation began to disintegrate. Peter and Emily were having marital problems, and the public health nurse suspected Peter was physically abusing his wife. There were times when she visited that Emily seemed vague and forgetful in contrast with her former intelligent alertness. The nurse attempted to talk with Emily about what was happening to her, but she would not discuss any subject except Kelly and her care.

One day Emily telephoned the nurse to say that she would be out of town visiting relatives for several weeks. Two weeks later, Kelly was admitted to the hospital suffering malnourishment and dehydration. She had been brought in by police who had investigated reports by neighbors of household disturbances and a continuously crying child. It seems that Peter had beat up Emily and then moved out. Both of them apparently had been using cocaine on a regular basis. Emily's response to this crisis was to go on a cocaine "binge."

Shortly after admission, Kelly suffered a cardiac arrest but with intensive effort was resuscitated. Faced with child endangerment charges, Emily fled the state. Kelly was made a ward of the court, and plans were made to institutionalize her. Her life-span prognosis was anticipated to be no more than 12 years. She was profoundly retarded.

In this case example, initially the parents and later the hospital decided in favor of the principle of beneficence—Kelly's life was preserved at all cost. Questions as to the quality of that life can be raised due to her apparent neglect and subsequent institutionalization. For caregivers, this kind of case presents some serious dilemmas:

- Should the obstetrician caring for Emily during her pregnancy have insisted on an amniocentesis? If she had had the test, should he have tried to argue her out of her anti-abortion stand?
- Should the infant's care at home have been more closely supervised, or should more elaborate plans for support of the mother have been made prior to Kelly's discharge?
- Should the public health nurse have intervened more aggressively when she suspected problems in the family? What ethical and legal right would she have had to do so?
- Should the child have been resuscitated when she had a cardiac arrest? Would caregivers have had any ethical right to withhold treatment?
- Kelly's care has already consumed some public expenditure. Should she receive surgical correction of her kyllosis? How can it be determined whether the ability to walk will add substantially to her quality of life?

These kinds of questions are not isolated to rare occurrences for caregivers; rather, they are almost everyday issues. The ethical principles of doing "good" and preserving life are often in conflict with the requirement that we, as caregivers, do no harm. Likewise, the principle of perserving the patient's or his spokesman's autonomy and self-determination often conflict with the fair distribution of social and medical resources. If nurses avoid thinking about these kinds of dilemmas, they risk finding themselves in a legal as well as ethical crisis. Instead, they must become aware of the basis for their selection of personal values and thoughtfully consider the practical consequences. Nurses also need to clarify the policies of their institution, the current legal precedents affecting their nursing practice, and the economic issues influencing care in their area.

In summary, in this section we have examined some of the parameters of the issue of quality versus quantity as it affects caregiving decisions generally and discharge plans specifically. As with most ethical dilemmas, there are few absolute "rights" to be found in the examples and questions we have raised. Individual caregivers have both a professional obligation and a personal responsibility to examine these kinds of issues and compare their own values with those currently predominant in their community.

7.3 DOES INVOLVEMENT IN DISCHARGE PLANNING BENEFIT THE NURSE?

Discharge planning demands time and effort by the nurse. It is appropriate in this final section of a chapter devoted to ethical dilemmas to pose the question of the cost-benefit of discharge planning activities for the nurse. There are three potential benefits that we will propose. Each nurse will have to decide whether these benefits balance the costs of time and effort.

> *The nurse's role is key to patient assessment, documentation of needs, and teaching. Participation in these activities meets a professional standard of care (see JCAH Nursing Services Standard IV).*

In some institutions, the nurse's role in discharge planning is made very specific in job descriptions and/or job performance evaluation documents. In others it is left more open to the individual's discretion to meet formal or suggested nursing care standards. Since hospitals are required to offer discharge planning, this responsibility is usually passed on to the nurse in some form. By participating, the nurse meets professional demands and the requirements of his or her employer. It is clear that good planning and teaching lead to shorter hospital stays for patients and is therefore of economic benefit to the institution. The nurse who performs these roles thoroughly and with skill and enthusiasm will please nursing supervisors and hospital administrators.

> *Discharge planning provides the opportunity for the nurse to improve assessment, communication, and teaching skills and to develop increased awareness of the consequences of acute care.*

Most nurses find that the practice of nursing affords almost constant opportunities to learn and grow. For many, this is one of the intrinsic rewards of the job; improving skills develops self-confidence and a sense of personal worth. Unlike some other aspects of acute care, discharge planning seeks to meet a very specific goal—that of preparing the patient and family for discharge. Not only do the nurse's skills contribute directly to meeting this goal but, by giving attention to discharge planning, the nurse develops a greater awareness of the consequences for patients and families of the acute care experience. This awareness is not limited to physical consequences but extends to emotional, social, and even spiritual areas of functioning. Sometimes nurses feel very isolated from the "real world." Discharge planning allows them to fit their contribution to the patient's well-being into a larger context.

Discharge planning allows the nurse to actively pursue a philosophy that values high quality comprehensive care for patients.

Just as readers like to know what happens to people described in a case study, nurses are usually interested in what happens to patients who have been under their care. Often this interest goes beyond clinical curiosity and extends to genuine emotional caring for the person and family. Involvement with patients in this sense is an outgrowth of a philosophy of nursing that demands that the nurse give each patient the best quality and most comprehensive care possible. The reward for devoting full attention, the most intelligent use of skills, and concern for others is a deep sense of accomplishment and fulfillment. In some instances, patients or their families reward the nurse directly with a "thank you" or a visit to report success. In any case, nurses who participate in discharge planning are soon reassured that their efforts give patients a better chance of meeting their health goals. And for many nurses, this is what nursing is all about.

SUMMARY

In this chapter we have explored some of the ethical considerations that surround discharge planning. We have posed a great many questions related to who makes decisions, how quality and quantity of care are balanced, and what the motives of nurses are in participating in discharge planning activities. It is acknowledged that the ethical issues we have discussed are imbedded in economic and legal concerns. Using a number of case examples, we have described the principles of autonomy, beneficence, nonmaleficence, and justice as guidelines for coming to terms with one's own philosophy of care. While there are no easy answers for the nurse, we believe that at least formulating the questions is an important first step toward a higher standard of quality care.

FURTHER READING

American Hospital Association. "Discharge Planning Update." Chicago, Illinois.
The "Update" is a periodical published six times each year by the Society for Hospital Social Work Directors within the A.H.A. It contains current information on discharge planning issues. The November–December 1987 issue, for example, contains several articles about third-party payers.

DeBellis, Robert, *et al. Continuing Care: For the Dying Patient, Family, and Staff.* New York: Praeger, 1985.

Although this book suffers from some unevenness due to multiple authors, its series of chapters on specific disease entities ranging from various forms of cancer to A.L.S. and irreversible heart disease make it a valuable resource for caregivers. There are also several chapters on dealing with the stresses nurses and physicians experience in caring for terminal patients.

"It's your decision: A practical guide to modern nursing ethics." *RN* Magazine, October 1988.
Under the above general heading, this issue contains a series of articles related to ethics. They include the effects of staff shortages; issues raised by AIDS, abortion, and death and dying; and concerns about witnessing a patient's consent or observing professional incompetence. The series concludes with a very useful "resource file" on ethical issues.

Young, Ernle W. D. *Alpha and Omega: Ethics at the Frontiers of Life and Death.* Menlo Park, Calif.: Addison-Wesley, 1988.
This little book should be on every caregiver's bookshelf. It is a concise, highly readable book by the chaplain to Stanford University Medical Center. He uses case studies to explore the full range of ethical issues that confront everyone involved in medical care. He espouses no particular religious philosophy but shares his own ethics and wisdom developed throughout a career of helping others. This book is also available in soft cover from the Stanford Alumni Association as part of their "Portable Stanford" series.

The reader is encouraged to seek current information about the economics of health care, legal issues, and ethical concerns in professional journals such as the ones listed here and in the popular news media. Quality care demands informed practitioners.

Study Questions and Exercises

These study questions and exercises may be used as part of a class or by individuals wishing to improve their understanding of topics and issues discussed in this book. The maximum learning benefit is derived when answers and experiences are discussed with classmates or colleagues. This kind of sharing helps all participants clarify their thinking, consider alternative ideas, and see issues with a broader perspective.

CHAPTER 1

1. Look for copies of newspapers that are at least 10 years old in your public library. In what ways have the topics of civic concern changed? What health topics were the focus of attention then?

2. Interview a person who is at least 65 years old. Ask them in what ways being ill is different today than it was in their youth.

3. In what ways has the structure of your family affected your health and your medical care?

4. Look for old telephone directories in your public library. Compare listings of long-term care facilities, doctors, and community agencies with a current directory. How might you explain the changes?

5. Interview two or three patients who have received intensive care but are now in a medical or surgical unit. Ask them how they felt when the were first moved out of I.C.U. and what they would most like to have known about their destination. How and when were the patients' questions answered? What implications do the interviews have for how you help patients make transitions in care?

6. Identify discharge planning team members and/or consultants in your institution. Find out how they are contacted, what kind of problems they feel constitute appropriate referrals, and how they prefer to work.

7. Interview a medical social worker. Ask him or her to explain the most common financial problems seen in your community. What resources exist for solving these kinds of problems?

8. Discuss the nursing roles in discharge planning with several nurses who have been on staff for five years or more. How have their roles changed over time?

CHAPTER 2

1. Make a list of factors that are presently affecting your own health balance. Compare these with at least two other people.

2. Review the nursing records of several patients. What information recorded in the nursing assessment is important to that patient's discharge plan? What additional information will be needed before a plan can be made?

3. Analyze recent conversations with two friends. Which of the four qualities (warmth, respect, empathy, genuineness) discussed in Section 2.2 were apparent to you? How were they demonstrated? How did you respond?

4. List ways in which you show respect and empathy to patients. Compare your list with at least two other people.

5. Tell three people about a concern of yours in approximately the same way. How did each person respond to you? How did you feel? What nonverbal messages were given?

6. Prepare 4 or 5 "CONEs" for an assessment interview. (See "Using Questions" in Section 2.2.) Try out at least two of them with colleagues (in a role-play) or with patients.

7. Watch a series of television commercials. What are the sponsors trying to teach? Do they focus on knowledge, attitudes, or skills? How do they attract the attention of the viewer and relate their information to something the viewer finds familiar?

8. Identify three learning needs for a patient. What is the level of readiness for each? Write specific learning objectives. How does the patient's readiness compare with the level of learning needed? How will this influence your teaching plan?

9. Analyze a lesson you have recently attended for the sequence the teacher used. How does it compare with the lesson sequence suggested in Table 2–3?

10. Skills are best learned through trying out a method, evaluating the result, and practicing. Try out the methods suggested in each of the three sections of Chapter 2. Select those that work for you in your

situation and then practice them. Comparing notes with classmates or colleagues is especially helpful.

CHAPTER 3

1. Analyze your own stress levels at the end of a busy day. What events contributed especially to your perception of stress? How did you react to these events? Under different circumstances would you have reacted the same? What do you do to relieve your own high stress level?

2. Analyze the current stress levels of several patients. What events or circumstances in addition to their medical conditions are contributing to these levels? What behavior gives you a clue to their stress levels?

3. Think of two or three situations you have observed in which someone has faced a crisis. Analyze how the situation was handled by other people. What did they do that was helpful? Unhelpful?

4. Complete the following statements:
—I admire more the ability to
   (a) organize and be methodical.
   (b) adapt and make do.
—In reading a textbook or instruction manual I prefer that
   (a) examples are used to show how ideas can be applied.
   (b) general principles are explained before details are added.
What do your answers reveal about your personality characteristics? How is your interaction with others affected by them?

5. Ask two friends to identify something that they know they should do for their health or well-being (such as have a medical checkup, go on a diet, or exercise) but have not yet done. Try to discover why they are unmotivated in terms of their health beliefs, previous experience, or interference from other people.

6. List experiences that you have had in the past year that make you feel good about yourself and increase your self-esteem. List experiences that have made you feel impotent or helpless. What is it about these experiences that make them more or less powerful in your life?

7. Answer the question about your own network of secondary social supports posed in the second part of Section 3.3.

8. What are the major ethnic groups in your community? List what you know of each group's special foods, customs for celebrations, religious customs, and practices surrounding death and dying. Add to the list by talking with others. Listen for positive or negative attitudes toward these groups.

9. How do people in your immediate social world handle discussions about family finances? What financial impact would it have on your family if a parent had a major medical crisis or needed long-term care?

CHAPTER 4

1. List the resource people available for discharge planning in your hospital. What are the major contributions that can be made by each? If possible, ask a representative of each professional group what they would like patients to be told about the services they offer.

2. Diagram the organization of discharge planning services in your facility. What organizational policies and structures have an impact on the way professionals communicate with one another or on services provided?

3. Interview several professionals of different backgrounds asking: "How could communication be improved by those working in discharge planning?" Discuss responses and suggestions at a staff meeting, if possible.

4. Diagram the patterns of communication related to discharge planning for two patients. How did they differ? Why?

5. With a small group of classmates or colleagues, make a table of functions such as that in Table 4–1 showing the contributions of various resource people to discharge planning. In what ways could this information be used to help people communicate better?

6. Interview several patients who are about to be discharged. Find out how they perceive the discharge planning process in their cases. To what degree did they feel a part of that process? Who made the decisions about plans? Do they feel adequately prepared to implement the plans?

CHAPTER 5

1. Make a rough map of your community. Diagram your "goal oriented communities" using Figure 5–1 as a guide. What factors of availability, access, and time influence the shape of each?

2. Using a road map of the area in which you live and/or work, identify segments within it related to socio-economic factors, geographically isolated areas, etc. Identify major transportation routes, especially rail and bus routes, and their access points. How do these factors influence health and medical care in your area?

3. Start your own card file of community resources. Fill out cards

such as that shown in Figure 5–2 for those services or agencies you already know about. Telephone those services to update or complete your information if needed.

4. Using a telephone directory and/or a community resources publication as references, make a master list of all those services or agencies in your community that you would like to investigate. As time and opportunity arise, add these to your file.

5. Visit at least two community services or agencies for information to add to your card file. Use the list of questions at the end of Section 5.1 as a guide.

6. Working with a classmate or colleague, rehearse what you might tell a patient about specific continuing care services. Have your partner give you feedback about how your use of words or non-verbal behavior might influence a patient's acceptance of that information.

7. Talk with a community health nurse or visiting nurse about how people react to home visits or home care. Ask how he or she handles the situation when a person seems resistant to accepting care.

CHAPTER 6

1. How are patients screened for risks that would indicate their need for high-intensity discharge planning services? What criteria are used? Compare the forms used with Form 1 in Part II.

2. Construct several "CONEs" for an interview whose goal is to confirm a discharge plan. (Refer to Section 2.2.) Try out your CONEs in a role-play with a classmate or colleague. Were you able to obtain information about the person's knowledge, attitudes, and skills without them becoming defensive?

3. Observe the discharge of a patient without taking part (if possible). What was done to reinforce learning? What was done to ensure continuity of care? What could have been done better or differently? How?

4. Review the medical record system used in your hospital. In what ways does it support the recording of discharge planning information and discharge plans? What procedure is followed for nursing audits? What feedback do nurses get about the results of audits?

5. What are your hospital's policies about confidentiality of patient information? What guidelines are there for making referrals to community agencies?

6. What continuing education opportunities are offered to help nurses learn assessment, communication, coordination, referral, and discharge planning skills? What is the evaluation of the educational

programs by those who have participated? Are there any barriers to participation?

CHAPTER 7

Throughout this chapter, questions are posed relating to various aspects of nursing ethics. Any of these could be the basis of formal or informal discussions by nurses. Current cases could also provide material for discussion about the dilemmas that are created by ethics, economics, and concerns about legal liability.

TWO

The A-B-Cs of Discharge Planning

The second part of this book has a unique format in that it includes a series of worksheets designed to help the nurse prepare discharge plans for patients. It is organized around the three basic steps of the discharge planning process: **Assessment, Building a Plan, and Confirming the Plan** before discharge. (See Figure 6–1 for a model representing these three steps.) Our goals in presenting this material in this way are to guide the nurse through a simple, step-by-step procedure for constructing discharge plans that meet patients' needs and to offer an ideal. The first is accomplished through the organization of easy-to-use forms on which to record patient information that reflect the progression of the discharge planning process. The second goal is met by offering the reader very comprehensive lists of the kinds of information that can be important to successful continuing care. Nurses with whom we have worked on the development of this material have commented that initially they found the amount of detail we asked for rather daunting, but then two things happened: they quickly adapted the information to their own patients' needs, and they became more alert to a broader range of possibly important patient data. In a sense, they mentally filtered out the things they did not need, but in the process, the "filter" became much more sensitive.

The three steps of constructing discharge plans are organized as follows:

In **Step A: Assessment,** the nurse is asked to record information that will help identify areas of special risk for the patient and serve as a guide in determining the intensity of discharge planning services required and the general goal of continuing care. The data included on the assessment form (Form 1) are based on established criteria for identifying service needs. This initial assessment can be completed quickly, using information available at admission or shortly thereafter.

Step B: Building a Plan is divided into five sections reflecting five major goals for continuing care:

- Step B/1: Recuperation (Forms 2, 3, 4, and 5)
- Step B/2: Rehabilitation (Forms 6, 7, 8, and 9)
- Step B/3: Chronic Disease Management (Forms 10, 11, 12, and 13)
- Step B/4: Residential Care (Forms 14, 15, 16, and 17)
- Step B/5: Terminal Care (Forms 18, 19, 20, and 21)

Each section offers guidance on completing a Discharge Plan Summary appropriate to the selected goal of care. It has been designed to allow flexibility in recording data that reflect patient progress and change. The information contained on the Summary is augmented by a Detailed Needs Identification and associated Definitions and Descriptions, and a Discharge Teaching Plan format. Together, they encourage early collection of information relevant to discharge planning, involvement of patient and family in the process, and communication among caregivers that leads to better coordination of effort.

The fact that it is sometimes difficult to determine even a general goal early in a patient's care has been taken into account; the approaches presented here are easily adaptable to changes in goal. For example, Step B/3 can be used for chronically ill patients whether they go home to manage their disease or go to residential care. When the initial picture of needs and goals is confused, we advise that the nurse choose the most complex approach likely. For example, a patient who has had coronary bypass surgery may be seen as potentially fully recuperating or as having a chronic coronary condition whose management will require some life-style changes. We would recommend using approach B/3 in order to avoid the possibility of skipping over something important in Needs Identification or teaching.

Step C: Confirming the Plan is organized as a checklist (Form 22) to be completed prior to the patient's discharge. It helps the nurse evaluate the patient's knowledge, attitudes, and skills as he or she prepares to leave acute care. It also reminds the nurse of details of coordination that are sometimes overlooked.

We encourage nurses to compare the approaches offered here with the ones used by their institutions. Better patient care will result when professionals knowledgeably evaluate their own goals and the methods used to accomplish them.

How to Assess Goals of Continuing Care

The first step in the discharge planning process, as it is in the nursing process, is to assess the complex of factors that surround the patient who has come for acute care. By looking at the strengths and deficits affecting the patient's physical, emotional, and social status, we can begin to make some judgments about present needs, existing risks, and how we might best help the patient begin the path toward the healthiest and most independent level of which he or she is capable.

Even as the patient is admitted to acute care, the focus of discharge planning is on the future of a whole person whose "world" will be affected by this experience.

We begin by obtaining information about the patient's past level of functioning in various areas of life and combine this with data about the present medical episode to answer the following kinds of questions:

- What are the major characteristics of the "world" the patient has been living in?
- What strengths and deficits does the patient have that will affect the outcome of this acute episode?
- What kind of impact will the patient's medical diagnosis have on future well-being and independence?
- How much and what kind of help is the patient likely to need to reach the highest level of functioning?

Answers to these kinds of questions help us determine the *direction* and *general goal* of our discharge planning efforts.

Hospitals and clinics always collect some patient information at, or even prior to, admission. Much of this information is useful in planning for discharge if its form and content make it accessible to caregivers. In addition, the medical and nursing assessments made within a short time of admission also contribute important data that

243

may be used to help predict the intensity of discharge planning services needed and realistic goals toward which to work. The form that follows (Form 1) is an example of one method of recording information relevant to discharge at or very soon after admission. Its focus is on identifiable areas of "risk" that alert caregivers to a patient's special needs. It makes information accessible by collecting it in concise form in one place. The areas chosen for attention are those shown by research to have special meaning for a patient's discharge plans (see Section 6.1).

Readers are encouraged to compare this form with those used by their institution. They may wish to try out this particular one and evaluate whether it aids them in beginning the discharge planning process earlier and/or in better communicating with their colleagues about patients' needs. Note that space is available for individualized comments that give a more complete picture of the patient.

FORM 1. *STEP A: INITIAL ASSESSMENT OF DISCHARGE NEEDS*

PATIENT IDENTIFICATION No.:   DATE:
NAME: UNIT or ROOM No.:
1. AGE: SEX:
2. MEDICAL DIAGNOSIS (at admission): Admitted on (date):_____

3. SELF-CARE RISK—Note abilities BEFORE admission.

Activities of Daily Living

___independent for ADLs
___unable to feed self
___unable to dress self
___unable to bathe self
___unable to prepare own meals

Toileting

___able to use toilet
___continent
___variable continence
___incontinent bladder
___incontinent bowels

Mobility

___able to walk unaided
___able to transfer unaided
___able to walk with aid
___transfers with help
___confined to bed

4. MENTAL STATE

Memory

___not assessed
___good/normal
___variable
___poor

Orientation

___not assessed
___alert/aware
___variable
___disoriented

5. SOCIAL RISKS

Living situation (before admission)

___with spouse/relative/ friend
___alone
___in residential care facility
___homeless
___cares for dependent

Community involvement

___not assessed
___resident for less than 1 year
___relatives live in area
___no relatives in area
___family not aware of admission

6. ECONOMIC RISKS

Finances

___not assessed
___employed or fully supported
___unemployed or retired
___Social Security recipient
___receiving aid or welfare

Insurance coverage

___insurance for acute care
___belongs to HMO
___Medicare/Medicaid
___no insurance

7. RISK IDENTIFICATION

Areas of special risk identified above or special risk factors that apply to this patient:

8. GOALS OF DISCHARGE PLANNING/CONTINUING CARE

___Uncertain at this time
___Recuperation
___Rehabilitation
___Chronic disease management
___Residential care
___Terminal care

Patient will probably need

___high-intensity discharge planning
___social work assistance
___counseling assistance
___special teaching
___more extensive needs identification

Person who will lead discharge planning:

_____

SIGNED_____ DATE_____

B/1

How to Build a Plan for Recuperation

In days past, the patient who expected to completely recover from an episode requiring acute care was not offered discharge planning intervention. Formal preparation for leaving the hospital was limited to brief instruction about medication, activities, and when to contact the doctor for follow-up. These patients had an advantage that today's patients do not share, however. By the time they were discharged, they had already progressed well into the recovery period.

The patient with the same reason for hospitalization would now be released much sooner and go home still needing some aspects of acute care. Discharge planning services are frequently not offered today, either, but for a different reason: there is too little time to plan. The need, however, is even greater, especially in the area of complication management. An approach that will help the nurse carry out discharge planning activities for the recuperating patient must, therefore, be both effective and very efficient. With today's greater understanding of the roles that diet, exercise, and stress management play in health, there is also a tremendous opportunity to help patients become healthier as well as to avoid illness in the future.

In this section an approach is outlined that includes the use of four separate but coordinated forms. They are:

- the Discharge Plan Summary,
- a Needs Identification and associated Definitions and Descriptions, and
- a Discharge Teaching Plan.

In some instances, the Discharge Plan Summary will be sufficient to report relevant data and organize an approach to patient teaching and referral. In others, where care is more complex, complications have already occurred, or psycho-social factors make comprehensive plan-

246

ning more important, the nurse will want to use any or all of the other forms.

The purposes of using special discharge planning forms are to communicate important information to other caregivers so that efforts can be coordinated, and to help the nurse quickly identify the patient's discharge needs and organize an efficient approach to teaching and referral.

With these goals in mind, we will review the major attributes of each of the forms presented and described here.

A written **Discharge Plan** is a method used for communication and coordination of effort among caregivers. It is also appropriately used to involve patients and their family members in the discharge planning process by including them in the gathering of data and the clarification of objectives and priorities. Form 2 represents a *summary* of information collected from several sources and combined to give an overview of patient needs and professional intervention. It is designed to reflect the progression of needs identification, patient and family teaching, and decision-making about plans for continuing care. It can and should be begun very early in the patient's care and updated as care and condition progress. Such a form might, for example, be started while the patient is in intensive care so that it becomes part of the information that is transferred to the next level of care.

In addition to the summary, guidance is given for completing a **Needs Identification** using the associated **Definitions and Descriptions** (Forms 3 and 4). The detailed information that they contain gives a comprehensive picture of the patient's needs at time of discharge. If nurses have used the comparable forms in other Step B sections, they will be aware that these are more compressed and simplified versions, reflecting the need for concise information obtained quickly. Nurses are encouraged to use the space provided to note individual factors affecting continuing care. An estimate of how long a particular need is likely to persist is especially useful.

The **Teaching Plan** format (Form 5) that we suggest is especially appropriate to situations in which patient or family teaching is complex, language difficulty or lack of relevant experiences on which to base learning are particular problems, or teaching includes a number of subject areas. Such a plan will help the nurse organize learning experiences for patient and family and coordinate the teaching input of several caregivers.

Whatever forms or recording devices are used, the goal is to be sure that the recuperating patient's needs are met so that recovery will be safe and uncomplicated.

FORM 2. *DISCHARGE PLAN SUMMARY FOR:* _____

PATIENT IDENTIFICATION NO.: _____UNIT/ROOM: _____

GENERAL GOAL: Recuperation from acute episode and the recovery and promotion of the patient's health.

A. SPECIAL SERVICES DURING ACUTE CARE:
Note with + those that will/may need to be continued AFTER discharge.

___None   ___Respiratory therapy   ___Patient/family
___Intensive care   ___Physical therapy   counseling
___Isolation   ___Occupational therapy   ___Mental health/
___Surgery   ___Speech therapy   psychiatric
___Blood transfusion   ___Social services   ___Discharge planning
___Other: _____   team
     ___Rehabilitation team

B. IDENTIFICATION OF RISKS/DEFICITS   Patient's age is _____
*Note with * those risks present BEFORE admission.*
Note with ↑ areas in which IMPROVED FUNCTION is expected.

___No special risks   ___Mobility
     identified   ___Communication
___Activities of daily   ___Learning ability
     living   ___Social situation
___Toileting   ___Financial situation

C. TEACHING NEEDED FOR PATIENT OR FAMILY IN SUBJECTS OF:
___No separate teaching plan
Note names and phone numbers of family or others involved in teaching.

___Medical follow-up   ___Activities/Exercises   ___Health Promotion
  ___in progress   ___in progress   ___in progress
  ___completed   ___completed   ___completed

___Medications   ___Nutrition/diet   ___Community services
  ___in progress   ___in progress   ___in progress
  ___completed   ___completed   ___completed

___Treatments/Procedures   ___Complication manag.   ___Other: _____
  ___in progress   ___in progress   ___in progress
  ___completed   ___completed   ___completed

FORM 2 *Continued*

D. POST-HOSPITAL SERVICES: __None needed.
Medical follow-up by:

_____

   Home Care: __Needed   __Decision in progress

Referral made to _____on _____by _____
   Special Equip: __Needed   __Decision in progress

Referral made to _____on _____by _____
   Social Services: __Needed   __Decision in progress

Referral made to _____on _____by _____
   Mental Health/Counseling __Needed   __Decision in progress

Referral made to _____on _____by _____
   Educ./Supp. Serv.   __Needed   __Decision in progress

Referral made to _____on _____by _____

Note details of services needed, options considered, and agencies/caregivers involved. Continue on back of sheet if needed.

E. SPECIFIC OBJECTIVES OF CONTINUING CARE: *Detail plans and goals for up to three months after discharge.*

ANTICIPATED DISCHARGE TO _____
ON OR ABOUT _____WITH CARE COORDINATED BY _____

F. COORDINATION OF INFORMATION: *Note exactly where information can be located (e.g., "Nursing Care Plan" or "Form 111")*
__Initial **assessment** of discharge risks can be found: _____
__Further details of continuing care **needs and plans** can be found: _____
__Details of **teaching** planned and/or completed can be found: _____
__Copies of **referrals** or detailed plans can be found: _____

PLAN INITIATED BY: _____ON: _____.   UPDATED: _____

INTRODUCTION TO NEEDS IDENTIFICATION

When a person experiences a medical episode that requires intensive acute care, many aspects of his or her life are interrupted. For most people, such an episode represents a crisis, even though for caregivers it may not seem especially threatening. As discussed in Section 3.1, there is an opportunity for change at the time of a crisis that may not be motivated otherwise. A person whose very life seems in jeopardy is likely to re-evaluate present life-style and consider changes that will protect him or her from similar episodes in the future or generally improve health. Guidance from the nurse in thinking through such changes and making a realistic plan will greatly improve the chances of successful implementation. Identifying specific needs and learning about values, priorities, and life-style allow the nurse to individualize that guidance and help the patient avoid discouraging reverses.

Information on which to base guidance for health promotion is one reason for special needs identification.

Patients leaving the hospital in these days of early discharges generally experience a period of relative dependency on others before fully recuperating. The longer this period is expected to be, the more important it is that the full range of needs be identified before discharge. Realistic anticipation and planning may make the difference between complications or re-admission and a smoothly progressive recovery.

Anticipation of a period of physical dependence between discharge and full recuperation is also a reason for gathering information about patient needs.

Such a period of dependence has much in common with rehabilitation in terms of planning and helping with realistic expectations. If areas of special risk have been identified such as age, living situation, or finances, the nurse is encouraged to complete the more detailed version of the Needs Identification found in Steps B/2 or B/3.

A suggested format for recording information about post-discharge needs is shown on Form 3, with Form 4 devoted to definitions of each option on Form 3 and a description of specific additional information that may be important to the patient's continuing care. Many aspects of the patient's strengths and resources are included.

In addition to providing details of patient needs for caregivers in the acute care setting so that they might better help both patient and family plan continuing care, a form such as the Needs Identification can become a valuable method of communication with community caregivers who will work with the patient toward health goals. Of course, sharing such information must be with the full consent of the patient, and all aspects of professional confidentiality must be observed.

FORM 3. *NEEDS IDENTIFICATION FOR* _____*I.D.* __

INSTRUCTIONS: Check all appropriate options for each item, indicating the expected level of ability at discharge.

1. SELF-CARE:

A. A.D.Ls *(eating, dressing, bathing)*	B. BLADDER/ BOWELS	C. MOBILITY	D. INSTRUMENTAL A.D.Ls *(meal prep., clothes care)*
___Indep.	___Continent	___Indep. trans.	
___Super.	___Incontinent	___Help to trans.	___Indep.
___Help	___Help to toilet	___Indep. amb.	___Super.
	___Spec. prob.	___Equip. needed	___Help

2. COMMUNICATION:

A. SPEECH	B. HEARING	C. VISION	D. WRITING
___Normal	___Normal	___Norm./correct.	___Normal
___Deficit	___Aided	___Dist. deficit	___Deficit
___Variable	___Deficit	___Reads	___Left-handed
___Lang. dif.	___Under Rx	___Reading def.	

3. PATTERNS AND HABITS:

A. NUTRITION	B. SLEEP	C. TOBACCO	D. ALCOHOL/ DRUGS
___Good	___Good	___Non-user	
___Limited	___Poor	___Lt./mod. use	___Non-user
___Spec. diet	___Interrupted	___Hvy. use	___Lt./mod. alco.
___Overweight	___Naps	___Adv. to stop	___Alcohol prob.
___Underweight			___Reg. drugs
			___Drug prob.

4. LEARNING ABILITY:

A. COGNITION	B. MEMORY	C. MOTIVATION	D. STRESS LEVEL
___Normal	___Good	___Present	
___Diminished	___Short	___Developing	___High now
___Variable	___Variable	___Poor	___Norm. high
___Poor concen.	___Aids help		___Norm. low
___Disorient.	___Poor		___Managed

5. SOCIAL/FINANCIAL SITUATIONS:

A. FAMILY/ FRIENDS	B. LIVING SITUATION	C. FINANCES	D. INSURANCE
___Active	___Ret. to former	___Ret. to employ	___Medicare/-aid
___Supportve	___Changing	___Leave avail.	___H.M.O./Pvt.
___Limited	___Shared	___Supported	___Dr./Clin.
___No support	___Alone	___Pension or aid	___Home care
		___Uncertain	___No insur.

6. CONTINUING CARE:

A. MEDICAL FOLLOW-UP	B. NURSING CARE	C. COMM. SERV.	D. EQUIPMENT
___Reg. MD	___None	___Social work	___Indoor mobil.
___Spec. MD	___Family	___Ment. Hlth./ Couns.	___Outdoor mobil.
___Clinic	___Skilled	___Supp. group	___Ventilation
___Other: _____	___Home care	___Therapies	___Communication

Needs Identification Completed by _____on _____

FORM 4. *NEEDS IDENTIFICATION—DEFINITIONS AND DESCRIPTIONS*

1. SELF-CARE

A. ACTIVITIES OF DAILY LIVING:	(Indep.)	Able to feed, dress, and bathe self independently.
	(Super.)	Needs to be supervised during eating, dressing, or bathing activities. *Specify level of supervision needed.*
	(Help)	Needs help with eating, dressing, or bathing. *Specify kinds of help needed.*
B. BLADDER/ BOWELS:	(Continent)	Has full bladder and bowel control.
	(Incontinent)	Does not have full bladder and/or bowel control. *Specify under what conditions incontinence occurs and how usually managed. Note approximate daily urine output and frequency of bowel movements.*
	(Help to toilet)	Needs help in using special equipment (e.g., commode, urinal) or in getting to toilet. *Specify kind of help needed and frequency.*
	(Spec. prob.)	There are special problems associated with bladder or bowel function (e.g. catheter, ostomy). *Specify nature of problem and how it is usually managed.*
C. MOBILITY:	(Indep. trans.)	Able to transfer from bed to chair and back independently. *Note present schedule for being up in chair and anticipated progress.*
	(Help to trans.)	Needs help in transferring from bed to chair and back. *Specify kind and frequency of help needed.*
	(Indep. amb.)	Able to ambulate independently. *Note present schedule for ambulation, including time or distance limitations.*
	(Equip. needed)	Special equipment or assistance needed (e.g., walker, wheelchair, cane, braces). *Specify kind of equipment or assistive devices needed and anticipated length of time required.*
D. INSTRUM. A.D.Ls:	(Indep.)	Able to prepare own meals, wash and iron clothes. *Note any exceptions to above and other abilities such as shopping, driving, etc.*
	(Super.)	Needs supervision while preparing meals, washing, or ironing. *Specify reason for and level of needed supervision.*
	(Help)	Needs help with meal preparation and clothes upkeep. *Note kind and frequency of help needed.*

2. COMMUNICATION

A. SPEECH:	(Normal)	Able to express self understandably in English. *Note any hesitation to express needs, desires, or emotions.*

FORM 4 *Continued*

	(Deficit)	Has a speech impediment or aphasia. *Specify nature and severity of difficulty.*
	(Variable)	Ability to communicate verbally is variable. *Note conditions that affect variability (e.g., stress, time of day, etc.)*
	(Lang. dif.)	Speaks with accent or hard to understand. *Specify degree of language difficulty and what language is preferred by patient. Note how difficulty is managed or overcome.*
B. HEARING:	(Normal)	Able to hear normal speech.
	(Aided)	Uses a hearing aid. *Note kind, frequency of use, and whether help is needed.*
	(Deficit)	Hearing is limited. *Specify kind and severity of deficit. Note how deficit is managed or overcome.*
	(Under Rx)	Under care for deficit or resulting handicap. *Specify nature of care, frequency, and name of caregiver.*
C. VISION:	(Norm./correct.)	Normal or fully corrected vision. *Note whether glasses or contacts are used.*
	(Dist. deficit)	Patient has limited distance vision. *Specify severity of deficit and limitations it imposes on patient.*
	(Reads)	Normal or corrected close (reading) vision. *Note whether glasses or contacts are used and whether enlarged print is necessary.*
	(Reading def.)	Unable to read due to physical or educational handicap. *Specify nature and severity of deficit.*
D. WRITING:	(Normal)	Able to write legible English. *Note whether writing is an especially important form of communication to the patient.*
	(Deficit)	Has physical or educational handicap that limits writing ability. *Specify nature and severity of limitation.*
	(Left-handed)	Prefers left hand over right for writing and other tasks.

3. PATTERNS AND HABITS

A. NUTRITION:	(Good)	Generally well nourished. *Note usual meal and snack pattern and any supplements usually taken.*
	(Limited)	Nutrition limited due to food preferences or poor appetite. *Specify food preferences and ways in which these are managed. Note reason for present poor appetite and/or appetite history.*
	(Spec. diet)	Receiving special diet. *Note reason for diet and expected duration.*

Form continued on following page

FORM 4 *Continued*

	(Overweight)	Significantly overweight for height and bone structure. *Note any recommendations that have been made regarding weight control.*
	(Underweight)	Significantly underweight for height and bone structure. *Note any known reasons for weight loss, duration of problem, and recommendations given.*
B. SLEEP:	(Good)	Sleeps well each night and feels rested. *Note usual bed and arising times and times of naps during day.*
	(Poor)	Sleeps poorly and seldom feels rested. *Note probable causes of poor sleep.*
	(Interrupted)	Sleep is normally interrupted. *Note reason for interruption and frequency (toilet, medication, dreams, etc.)*
	(Naps)	Takes naps during the day. *Note usual frequency and length of naps and whether they affect nighttime sleep.*
C. TOBACCO:	(Non-user)	Does not now or never has used tobacco. *Note whether patient ever has used tobacco and in what form.*
	(Lt./mod. use)	Smokes up to one pack of cigarettes per day or uses other forms of tobacco. *Note what form of tobacco is used, usual consumption pattern, and duration of habit.*
	(Hvy. use)	Heavy user of tobacco on a regular basis. *Note what form of tobacco is used, usual consumption pattern, and duration of habit.*
	(Adv. to stop)	Trying to stop smoking or has been advised to stop. *Note present attitudes and goals and past history of trying to stop.*
D. ALCOHOL/ DRUGS:	(Non-user)	Does not consume alcohol or use potentially addictive drugs. *Note whether patient has ever used alcohol or drugs and to what extent.*
	(Lt./mod. alco.)	Regularly consumes light to moderate amount of alcoholic beverages. *Note kind and pattern of daily consumption.*
	(Alcohol prob.)	Alcohol use has been or now is a problem for patient or family. *Note severity of problem and what advice has been given.*
	(Reg. drugs)	Regularly takes tranquilizers, sedatives, narcotics, or other drugs. *Specify kind of drugs used and pattern of use.*
	(Drug prob.)	Drug use has been or now is a problem for patient or family. *Note severity of problem and what advice has been given.*

4. LEARNING ABILITY

A. COGNITION:	(Normal)	Ability to think and reason normal.

FORM 4 *Continued*

	(Diminished)	Ability to think and reason clearly diminished. *Note probable cause and evidence used to make this judgment.*
	(Variable)	Alertness and ability to reason varies. *Note any observable pattern to variation and probable causes.*
	(Poor concen.)	Able to reason normally but has short attention span or poor ability to concentrate. *Note probable cause and evidence used to make this judgment.*
	(Disorient.)	Mentally confused or disoriented as to time, person, or place. *Note any variations in disorientation.*
B. MEMORY:	(Good)	Both short- and long-term memory seem to be within normal limits.
	(Short)	Able to recall facts or ideas for only a short period of time. *Note nature of memory difficulty and whether problem existed prior to acute episode.*
	(Variable)	Memory good at times, poor at others. *Note possible causes of variability, such as medication. Note any categories of information that seem to be retained more reliably.*
	(Aids help)	Memory is improved by use of aids such as timers, written reminders, etc. *Specify kinds of memory aids that have been tried and which are most effective.*
	(Poor)	Unable to recall facts or ideas long enough to use them effectively. *Note any known causes for poor memory and length of time problem has existed.*
C. MOTIVATION:	(Present)	Wants to learn about health and continuing care. *Note phrases listed or others that describe patient's dominant attitudes: asks questions, interested in explanations, applies knowledge.*
	(Developing)	Developing awareness of need to learn or change behaviors. *Note areas in which awareness is developing and evidence of increased motivation.*
	(Poor)	Uninterested in learning about present care and rehabilitation. *Note phrases listed or others that describe patient's dominant attitudes: passive toward care, unaware of potential, hostile toward teacher or teaching. Note any known factors that may contribute to patient's lack of interest in learning.*
D. STRESS LEVEL:	(High now)	Stress level presently high enough to interfere with learning or decision making. *Specify cause of high stress level and evidence of its effect.*

Form continued on following page

FORM 4 *Continued*

(Norm. high) Describes self as having a normally high stress level.
Note usual causes of high stress and effect on patient's life.

(Norm. low) Describes self as having a normally low stress level.
Note patient's perception of present stress level and how it is affecting him.

(Managed) Able to use stress management techniques to keep level under control.
Specify management techniques used and their effectiveness for patient.

5. SOCIAL/FINANCIAL SITUATIONS:

A. FAMILY/ FRIENDS: (Active) Family members or friends are actively involved with patient's care and future plans.
Identify those most involved by name and relationship.

(Supportive) Family members or friends support patient in efforts to get well and care for his or her health.
Identify those most supportive by name, and note in what ways support is given.

(Limited) Involvement of family or friends in patient care or planning limited.
Note apparent reason for limited involvement by name and relationship.

(No support) Family members or friends are not available or not involved with care or plans.
Note apparent reason for lack of support or involvement.

B. LIVING SITUATION: (Ret. to former) Return to former living situation following discharge is anticipated.
Note anticipated adequacy of this living arrangement.

(Changing) Discharge to a different living situation anticipated.
Note progress of decision making about altered living situation.
Note patient's response to anticipated change.

(Shared) Housing is or will be shared with others.
Identify persons in household.

(Alone) Anticipates living alone.
Note whether patient has lived alone in the past.

C. FINANCES: (Ret. to employ) Expects to return to full- or part-time employment.
Note name of employer, nature of job, and approximate length of time before return.

(Leave avail.) Has work leave benefits that will allow patient to recuperate from acute episode.
Note whether leave is paid or unpaid and how supportive employer is to continuing care.

FORM 4 *Continued*

	(Supported)	Is fully supported or has independent source of income. *Note any relevant details about level of support.*
	(Pens. or aid)	Receives Social Security, retirement pension, welfare, or other financial aid. *Note whether income is adequate for expected needs.*
	(Uncertain)	Source of a regular income now uncertain. *Note reasons for uncertainty and whether help is needed in applying for aid.*
D. INSURANCE:	(Medicare/-aid)	Eligible for continuing care benefits from Medicare and/or Medicaid. *Note present status of benefits.*
	(H.M.O./Pvt.)	Member of a Health Maintenance Organization or has private insurance with extended benefits. *Note present status of benefits.*
	(Dr./Clin.)	Visits to doctor's office or clinic for medical follow-up partly or fully covered. *Note level of coverage.*
	(Home care)	Home care assistance partly or fully covered. *Note level of coverage and whether adequate for needs.*
	(No insur.)	Has no insurance coverage for continuing care. *Note whether financial counseling and/or assistance is needed and by whom.*
6. CONTINUING CARE		
A. MEDICAL FOLLOW-UP:	(Reg. MD)	Will be returning to the care of own physician for follow-up care. *Note name of doctor and level of involvement in hospital care.*
	(Spec. MD)	Will receive follow-up care from a specialist physician. *Note name of doctor and plan for follow-up.*
	(Clinic)	Will receive follow-up care from an out-patient facility or clinic. *Note name of clinic and plan for follow-up.*
	(Other)	*Specify plan for medical follow-up, including name of doctor and/or facility.*
B. NURSING CARE:	(None)	No need for nursing care anticipated. *Note any treatments or procedures that will be done by the patient.*
	(Family)	Nursing care needs will be met by family members. *Note extent of nursing care anticipated and plan for family instruction.*
	(Skilled)	Need for skilled nursing care is anticipated. *Note how this need is expected to be met.*
	(Home care)	Need for home care is anticipated. *Specify what kind of care will be needed and for approximately what period of time.*

Form continued on following page

FORM 4 *Continued*

C. COMMUNITY   (Social work)   Needs social work consultation or
SERVICES: assistance.
Note how this need is expected to be met
and whether a referral has been made.

(Ment. Hlth./   Needs assistance from a mental health or
Couns.)   counseling professional.
Note how this need is expected to be met
and whether a referral has been made.

(Supp. group)   Support from a community group is
expected to be helpful to patient.
Note how this need is expected to be met
and whether a referral has been made.

(Therapies)   Needs physical, occupational, respiratory,
or speech therapy.
Note how this need is expected to be met
and whether a referral has been made.

D. EQUIPMENT: (Indoor mobil.)   Needs assistive equipment to improve
mobility or safety indoors.
Specify kinds of equipment or aids and
source(s) of supply.

(Outdoor   Needs assistive equipment to improve
mobil.)   mobility or safety outdoors.
Specify kinds of equipment or aids and
source(s) of supply.

(Ventilation)   Needs assistive equipment to improve or
monitor breathing.
Specify kinds of equipment or aids and
source(s) of supply.

(Communication)   Needs assistive equipment to aid
communication.
Specify kinds of equipment or aids and
source(s) of supply.

MAKING A TEACHING PLAN

When a patient needs help with learning in several areas or it is anticipated that care immediately after discharge will be complex, it is worthwhile to complete a Teaching Plan. Such a plan clarifies goals and priorities so that teaching can proceed more efficiently and it serves to coordinate the efforts of several teachers. A teaching plan is especially important when skills need to be learned or when learning involves major behavior changes. An ordered, carefully planned approach will ensure that learning will result from teaching.

Form 5 is designed to help caregivers identify areas of learning needs and construct learning objectives quickly. These objectives then become the framework for patient and family teaching. The subjects on this form parallel those indicated in the third section of the Discharge Plan Summary.

Remember that the only useful learning objectives are REALISTIC ones. They should be attainable in the time available, and the desired behavior should be observable by the teacher(s).

Elements of this form are described below.

Identification of Learners. Those people who are to be included in some or all teaching sessions are listed across the top of the form. The nurse may want to write the telephone numbers of visitor-learners, as well as their names, to simplify coordination. Where notations are made about a learner other than the patient, they may be referred to by number. For example, the motivation of the patient may be "developing," but for learner "#2," it may be already "present."

Subject of Teaching. Eight common subjects for discharge teaching have been listed on the form. The nurse may indicate that teaching in this subject area is not needed. If it is needed, the next three lines provide a record of teaching progress from planning through evaluation. Updating the teaching plan by checking the description that currently applies to teaching in each subject area will alert other caregivers to what has been done. They can then actively cooperate with the learning process by stimulating further patient interest in the subject and reinforcing learning. Following the completion of teaching, learning may be evaluated through tests, verbal questions, demonstrations, or other methods. Verifying that an objective has been successfully reached is positive feedback for both teacher and learner.

Motivation. Attention to a person's motivation to learn particular subjects is extremely important for effective and efficient teaching. If motivation to learn is poor, the nurse will want to work on this before attempting to teach content in an area. Changes in motivation can be recorded with a check or an arrow. When several learners are involved, those with more motivation may be able to help the others understand the importance of the subject.

Prior Knowledge or Experience. A short phrase is usually enough to record the basis on which new learning can be built. Finding out what a learner already knows about a subject takes only moments, but it allows the teacher to start with relevant material, thereby improving both motivation and learning ability. It is best not to make any assumptions about what the learner knows; a person may have taken a medication for ten years but not know what it is for or why it is important!

Learning Objective. The construction of learning objectives is a simple but often unfamiliar activity to those who are not full-time teachers. An objective or learning goal starts with the phrase *"The learner will be able to..."* This is followed by a verb indicating the **level of complexity** at which learning must take place. To "adapt" learning to different situations is, for example, much more complex than simply "remembering" it. We have suggested a number of possible verbs that may be used.

Next, a learning objective defines the **subject** of concern and what kind of **behavior** is expected as a result of learning. Remember that the stated behavior must be observable in the time available, and therefore objectives for learning in acute care settings will necessarily be short-term and limited. The ultimate goal in teaching a person about available community services might be, for example, that he or she appropriately utilize these services after discharge. A realistic learning objective while the person is in the hospital, however, might be that he or she be able to describe the services of the Senior Citizen's Center and give three examples of how to use them.

Finally, writing down a **time** for learning to be completed gives both learners and teachers a target toward which to work.

Notes. Noting what teaching approaches have been used (for example, "demonstrated safe use of crutches"), the response learners have had to them, the priority given certain subjects, and plans for learning evaluation are all important pieces of information to share with other caregivers. Current notes kept in a known location are essential when several teachers are involved or learning needs are complex.

FORM 5. *DISCHARGE TEACHING PLAN FOR:* _____

OTHER THAN PATIENT, THOSE TO BE INVOLVED AS LEARNERS
INCLUDE: *(Note name and relationship to patient.)*
   #1:   #2:   #3:

1. MEDICAL/FOLLOW-UP:
    Teaching: __not needed   Motivation: __present   Prior knowledge/
          __planned   __developing experience: _____
          __in progress   __poor
          __learning   _____
           evaluated

Learner will be able to: _____ By _____
                       (level)   (specific subject)   (behavior)   (date)
       (e.g., remember, understand, apply information, make decisions about)

2. MEDICATIONS:
    Teaching: __not needed   Motivation: __present   Prior knowledge/
          __planned   __developing experience: _____
          __in progress   __poor
          __learning   _____
           evaluated

Learner will be able to: _____ By _____
                       (level)   (specific subject)   (behavior)   (date)
       (e.g., remember, understand, apply information, respond, evaluate)

3. TREATMENTS/PROCEDURES:
    Teaching: __not needed   Motivation: __present   Prior knowledge/
          __planned   __developing experience: _____
          __in progress   __poor
          __learning   _____
           evaluated

Learner will be able to: _____ By _____
                       (level)   (specific subject)   (behavior)   (date)
       (e.g., remember, understand, apply information, perform, adapt, evaluate)

4. ACTIVITIES/EXERCISES:
    Teaching: __not needed   Motivation: __present   Prior knowledge/
          __planned   __developing experience: _____
          __in progress   __poor
          __learning   _____
           evaluated

Learner will be able to: _____ By _____
                       (level)   (specific subject)   (behavior)   (date)
       (e.g., remember, recognize, understand, apply information, perform, adapt)

5. NUTRITION/DIET:
    Teaching: __not needed   Motivation: __present   Prior knowledge/
          __planned   __developing experience: _____
          __in progress   __poor
          __learning   _____
           evaluated

Learner will be able to: _____ By _____
                     (level)   (specific subject)   (behavior)   (date)
       (e.g., remember, recognize, understand, apply information, prepare, adapt)
                                      Form continued on following page

FORM 5 *Continued*

6. COMPLICATION MANAGEMENT:

Teaching: __not needed Motivation: __present Prior knowledge/
   __planned   __developing experience: _____
   __in progress   __poor
   __learning   _____
   evaluated

Learner will be able to: _____ By _____
        (level) (specific subject) (behavior)   (date)
     (e.g., remember, recognize, understand, evaluate, perform, adapt)

7. HEALTH MAINTENANCE/PROMOTION:

Teaching: __not needed Motivation: __present Prior knowledge/
   __planned   __developing experience: _____
   __in progress   __poor
   __learning   _____
   evaluated

Learner will be able to: _____ By _____
        (level) (specific subject) (behavior)   (date)
    (e.g., remember, understand, apply information, perform, realistically plan)

8. COMMUNITY SERVICES/RESOURCES:

Teaching: __not needed Motivation: __present Prior knowledge/
   __planned   __developing experience: _____
   __in progress   __poor
   __learning   _____
   evaluated

Learner will be able to: _____ By _____
        (level) (specific subject) (behavior)   (date)
     (e.g., remember, understand, apply information, plan, utilize)

9. OTHER LEARNING OBJECTIVES:

Learner will be able to _____ by _____

Learner will be able to _____ by _____

Teaching Plan initiated by _____ on _____

NOTES ON TEACHING (what was taught, methods/materials used, response, etc.)

B/2

How to Build a Plan for Rehabilitation

Patients for whom rehabilitation has been identified as a realistic goal of continuing care have lost some normal bodily function as a result of an acute episode, but have a reasonable chance of regaining it or learning to compensate for its loss. Discharge planning for these patients is a special challenge for caregivers for a number of reasons. One aspect of that challenge is that even while the patient is experiencing grief over a lost function he or she must be helped to focus on realistic goals for the future. (See Section 3.1 for a discussion of the stages of a crisis response.) Encouraging the development of motivation to work toward recovery and independence demands that caregivers are fully aware of the patient's emotional state and the details of his or her socio-cultural world, as well as physical abilities and limitations. The sooner comprehensive information is available, the more effective is the discharge planning process.

Another major aspect of the challenge facing the nurse is the coordination of effort among the many people involved in the rehabilitation patient's care. Any gap in communication or inconsistency of messages given to the patient will interrupt the development of a sense of trust and erode motivation. It is therefore especially important that the intervention of caregivers be fully documented and that communication channels be opened early with community caregivers.

The motivation of the patient and continuity of care offered by hospital and community caregivers make the difference in whether rehabilitation goals are reached.

Whether the rehabilitation process is expected to be long- or short-term, discharge planning will be intensive. The approaches to gathering information, summarizing goals, and organizing teaching presented in this section will help the nurse improve communication with the patient and family, and among caregivers. Four separate but coordinated forms are suggested as the basis for this communication. They are:

263

- the Discharge Plan Summary,
- a Detailed Needs Identification and associated Definitions and Descriptions, and
- a Discharge Teaching Plan.

Together they make it possible to record comprehensive information relevant to the discharge planning process with ease and clarity so that it is easily shared by caregivers who can, as a result, better coordinate their efforts.

A written **Discharge Plan** is a method used for communication and coordination of effort among caregivers. It is also appropriately used to involve patients and their family members in the discharge planning process by including them in the gathering of data and the clarification of objectives and priorities. Form 6 represents a *summary* of information collected from several sources and combined to give an overview of professional intervention. It is designed to reflect the progression of needs identification, patient and family teaching, and decision making about plans for continuing care. It should be begun as early in the patient's care as possible and updated regularly so that caregivers have a clear picture of the state of the discharge planning process. Especially important is information about where more detailed information can be located in the patient's medical record. This item alone can save caregivers a great deal of time and frustration.

In addition to the summary, guidance is given for completing a **Detailed Needs Identification** using the associated **Definitions and Descriptions** (Forms 7 and 8). The comprehensive information that they contain may be considered essential when the rehabilitation process is expected to be lengthy, when several caregivers or agencies will be involved in the community care, or when a major bodily function has been entirely lost due to an acute episode.

The success of rehabilitation depends upon the learning of behaviors that promote recovery of function. High-quality patient and family teaching begun early in care not only help the patient learn information and skills needed later, but also helps develop positive attitudes toward overcoming the disability and returning to independence. Such attitudes are the beginning of the motivation that the patient will so badly need to persevere through the discomforts, frustrations, and setbacks of rehabilitation.

The **Teaching Plan** format (Form 9) that we suggest here will help the nurse organize learning experiences for patient and family and coordinate the teaching input of several caregivers. Together, these approaches represented by the four forms ensure that caregivers have a comprehensive "picture" of the patient and his or her continuing care needs and a clear view of caregiving objectives.

FORM 6. *DISCHARGE PLAN SUMMARY FOR:* _____

PATIENT IDENTIFICATION NO.: _____ UNIT/ROOM: _____

GENERAL GOAL: Rehabilitation during which patient will compensate for disability
or recover function of _____ .

A. SPECIAL SERVICES DURING ACUTE CARE:
Note with + those that will/may need to be continued AFTER discharge.

__None	__Respiratory therapy	__Patient/family
__Intensive care	__Physical therapy	counseling
__Isolation	__Occupational therapy	__Mental health/
__Surgery	__Speech therapy	psychiatric
__Blood transfusion	__Social services	__Discharge planning
__Other: _____		team
		__Rehabilitation team

B. IDENTIFICATION OF RISKS/DEFICITS   Patient's age is _____
*Note with * those risks present BEFORE admission.*
Note with ↑ areas in which IMPROVED FUNCTION is expected.

__No special risks	__Mobility/Strength
identified	__Toileting
__Activities of daily	__Mental state
living	__Motivation
__Senses	__Social situation
__Communication	__Economic situation

C. TEACHING NEEDED FOR PATIENT OR FAMILY IN SUBJECTS OF:
__No separate teaching plan
Note names and phone numbers of family or others involved in teaching.

__Med./Rehab. follow-up	__Activities/Exercises	__Health Promotion
__in progress	__in progress	__in progress
__completed	__completed	__completed
__Medications	__Nutrition/diet	__Community services
__in progress	__in progress	__in progress
__completed	__completed	__completed
__Treatments/Procedures	__Complication manag.	__Other: _____
__in progress	__in progress	__in progress
__completed	__completed	__completed

D. POST-HOSPITAL SERVICES: __None needed.
Medical follow-up by:

_____

Home Care: __Needed   __Decision in progress

Referral made to _____on _____by _____
Rehab. services: __Needed   __Decision in progress

Referral made to _____on _____by _____
Social Services: __Needed   __Decision in progress

Referral made to _____on _____by _____
Form continued on following page

FORM 6 *Continued*

Mental Health: ___Needed ___Decision in progress

Referral made to _____on _____by _____

Special Equip: ___Needed ___Decision in progress

Referral made to _____on _____by _____

Note details of services needed, options considered, and agencies/caregivers involved. Continue on back of sheet if needed.

E. SPECIFIC OBJECTIVES OF CONTINUING CARE: *Detail plans and goals for up to three months after discharge.*

ANTICIPATED DISCHARGE TO _____ ON OR ABOUT _____
WITH CARE COORDINATED BY _____

F. COORDINATION OF INFORMATION: *Note exactly where information can be located (e.g., "Nursing Care Plan" or "Form 111")*
___Initial **assessment** of discharge risks can be found: _____
___Further details of continuing care **needs and plans** can be found: _____
___Details of **teaching** planned and/or completed can be found: _____
___Copies of **referrals** or detailed plans can be found: _____

PLAN INITIATED BY _____ ON _____ .
UPDATED: _____

INTRODUCTION TO DETAILED NEEDS
IDENTIFICATION

When a person loses normal body functions or mobility due to accident, stroke, neurological problem, or spinal injury, all aspects of his or her life are interrupted. The first step in helping patients toward a realistic program of rehabilitation is to understand as much as possible about them and the "world" to which they will be returning. Gathering and recording such comprehensive information serves several purposes: it provides a resource for personal understanding for all caregivers, it involves the patient and family in interaction whose goal is future oriented, and it establishes trust by confirming the nurse's interest in the patient as a whole person.

The Detailed Needs Identification is one approach to information gathering and the projection of probable needs. The reader will notice that spaces are left on Form 7 for making individualized comments about specific patient needs. More than one choice may be appropriate to some items. The subject areas that are included parallel those listed in the second section of the Discharge Planning Summary. The Needs Identification focuses on realistic *anticipation* of what can and should be done to help the patient successfully begin and continue a rehabilitation program.

A suggested format for recording information is shown on Form 7. Form 8 defines each option shown on Form 7 and describes specific information that may be important to the patient's continuing care. Many aspects of the patient's strengths and resources are included. For rehabilitation patients, it is especially useful to note which abilities or functions are expected to change or are in a current state of change. These may be marked with " ↑ " rather than the usual check mark.

For nurses who are unfamiliar with discharge planning, these definitions and descriptions provide a basis for understanding the kinds and quality of information that have important implications for the patient's future well-being. Nurses are encouraged to read through the descriptive material and then use it in conjunction with the first few discharge plans they complete. They will soon find that they have become alert to significant information and will only need to refer to the details occasionally to refresh their memory.

It should be noted that the scope of information included on this form and in the descriptions is extremely complete and represents an ideal. When working with real patient situations and commonly experienced time limitations, the nurse will find that some items are inappropriate or too time-consuming to pursue. Should the nurse choose to skip an item, it is helpful to note whether it is "N.A." (Not Applicable) or "Unk." (Unknown).

In addition to providing details of patient needs for caregivers in the acute care setting so that they might better help patient and family plan rehabilitation, a form such as this can be invaluable to community professionals who need to begin providing sensitive care and encouragement immediately after discharge. Gaps that occur at this time of transition may undermine the patient's motivation. Of course, sharing such information must be with the full consent of the patient, and all aspects of professional confidentiality must be observed.

FORM 7. *DETAILED NEEDS IDENTIFICATION FOR* _____ *I.D.* ___

INSTRUCTIONS: Check all appropriate options for each item. Mark with ↑ the abilities that are expected to improve with rehab.

1. ACTIVITIES OF DAILY LIVING:

A. EATING	B. DRESSING	C. BATHING	D. ORAL CARE
__Indep.	__Indep.	__Indep.	__Indep.
__Super.	__Super.	__Super.	__Super.
__Help	__Help	__Help	__Help
__Total care	__Total Care	__Total care	__Total care

2. SENSES:

A. VISION	B. HEARING	C. TOUCH	D. TASTE/SMELL
__Full dist.	__Normal	__Normal	__Normal
__Full close	__Aided	__Hot/cold only	__Deficit
__Deficit	__Deficit	__Other deficit	
__Under Rx	__Under Rx		

3. COMMUNICATION:

A. SPEECH	B. READING	C. WRITING
__Normal	__Normal	__Normal
__Deficit	__Deficit	__Deficit
__Variable	__Non-Eng.	__Left-handed
__Lang. dif.		

4. MOBILITY/STRENGTH:

A. TRANSFER	B. AMBULATION	C. GROOMING	D. INSTRU. ADLs *(meal prep., care of clothes)*
__Indep.	__Indep.	__Indep.	
__Equip.	__Equip.	__Super.	__Indep.
__Help	__Help	__Help	__Help
__Confined to bed	__Non-amb.	__Total care	__Depen.

5. HABITS AND PATTERNS:

A. APPETITE	B. SLEEP	C. BLADDER	D. BOWELS
__Good	__Good	__Continent	__Continent
__Limited	__Poor	__Help	__Regular
__Spec. diet	__Interrupted	__Incont.	__Help
	__Pre-bed rit.	__Frequen.	__Lax./Soft.
	__Naps	__Fluid def.	__Incont.

E. SMOKING/ALCOHOL/DRUG USE:

__Tobacco
__Stop tobac.
__Alcohol   _____
__Alco. prob.   _____
__Stop alco.   _____
__Drugs
__Stop drugs

Form continued on following page

FORM 7 *Continued*

6. MENTAL STATE:

A. COGNITION	B. AWARENESS	C. RESP. TO CARE	D. MEMORY
__Normal	__Alert	__Pos.	__Good
__Diminished	__Aware of Dx.	__Neg.	__Short
__Variable	__Realistic	__Guard.	__Variable
__Poor concen.	__Unreal.	__Upset	__Aids help
__Disorient.	__Unaware		__Poor

7. MOTIVATION:

A. FOR SELF-CARE	B. LEARNING	C. PERSONAL-ITY	D. DECISION MAKING
__Active	__Interested	__Present orien.	__Involved
__Self respon.	__Disabled	__Future orien.	__Near ready
__Unreal.	__Uninterested	__Time consc.	__Unready
__Demoralized		__Easygoing	__Optimistic
			__Pessimistic

8. SOCIAL SITUATION:

A. FAMILY INVOLVEMENT	B. COMMUNITY PARTICIP.	C. LIVING SITUATION	D. SPECIAL GROUP
__Active	__Soc. groups	__Ret. to former	__Minority
__Realistic	__Rel. groups	__Changing	__Handicap
__Supportive	__Support	__Shared	__Adjust. prob.
__Limited	__Involved friends	__Alone	
__Not avail.	__Few friends	__Resid. care	
__No support	__No support	__Needs modifi.	

9. ECONOMIC SITUATION:

A. FINANCES	B. REHAB. INS. BENEFIT
__Ret. to employ.	__Medicare/-aid
__Leave avail.	__H.M.O.
__Supported	__Pvt. insur.
__S.S./Retir.	__Dr./clin. visits
__Receive aid	__Home care
__Uncertain	__No insur.

10. CONTINUING CARE:

A. REHAB. PROGRAM	B. NURSING CARE	C. COMM. SERV.	D. EQUIPMENT
__Reg. MD	__None	__Social work	__Indoor mobil.
__Spec. MD	__Family	__Counseling	__Outdoor mobil.
__In-pt. unit	__Skilled	__Mental Hlth.	__Ventilation
__Clinic	__Home care	__Supp. group	__Communication
__Other: ____		__Therapies	__Other: ____

Needs Identification completed by ____ on _____. Updated: ____

FORM 8. *DETAILED NEEDS IDENTIFICATION—DEFINITIONS AND DESCRIPTIONS*

Instructions: Check all appropriate descriptions on Detailed Needs Identification Form and follow each with short notes.

1. ACTIVITIES OF DAILY LIVING (ADL)

A. EATING:	(Indep.)	Feeds self.
	(Super.)	Needs to be supervised while eating. *Specify level of supervision needed.*
	(Help)	Needs help with certain foods or drink. *Specify kinds of help needed.*
	(Total care)	Needs to be fed. *Note food preferences.*
B. DRESSING:	(Indep.)	Selects appropriate clothing and dresses self.
	(Super.)	Needs supervision while dressing. *Specify whether clothing must be selected or level of supervision.*
	(Help)	Needs help with certain clothing or fasteners. *Specify kinds of help needed. Note right- or left-handedness.*
	(Total care)	Needs to be dressed. *Note clothing preferences.*
C. BATHING:	(Indep.)	Bathes self. *Note whether patient regularly takes tub, shower, or sponge baths.*
	(Super.)	Needs supervision while bathing. *Specify reason for and level of supervision needed.*
	(Help)	Needs help preparing for bath or while bathing. *Specify kinds of help needed.*
	(Total care)	Needs to be bathed. *Note frequency and preferred time of baths.*
D. ORAL CARE:	(Indep.)	Able to brush and floss teeth without help. *Note whether person has dentures or whether special oral care procedures are used.*
	(Super.)	Needs supervision during oral care procedures. *Specify reason for and level of supervision needed.*
	(Help)	Needs help with oral care. *Specify kind of help needed.*
	(Total care)	Unable to perform own oral care. *Note kinds of care to be given and frequency. Note preferences for oral care equipment and products.*

2. SENSES

A. VISION:	(Full dist.)	Normal or fully corrected distance vision. *Note whether glasses or contacts are used.*
	(Full close)	Normal or corrected close (reading) vision. *Note whether glasses or contacts are used.*
	(Deficit)	Patient has limited vision. *Specify kind and severity of deficit.*

Form continued on following page

FORM 8 *Continued*

	(Under Rx)	Under care for deficit or resulting handicap. *Specify nature of care, frequency, and name of caregiver.*
B. HEARING:	(Normal)	Able to hear normal speech.
	(Aided)	Uses a hearing aid. *Note kind, frequency of use, and whether help is needed.*
	(Deficit)	Hearing is limited. *Specify kind and severity of deficit. Note how deficit is managed or overcome.*
	(Under Rx)	Under care for deficit or resulting handicap. *Specify nature of care, frequency, and name of caregiver.*
C. TOUCH:	(Normal)	Has normal touch sensations.
	(Hot/Cold only)	Able to sense only hot and cold. *Specify areas of the body affected and the degree to which change is anticipated.*
	(Other deficit)	Sense of touch is limited. *Specify nature of deficit and part of body involved. Note how deficit is managed or overcome.*
D. TASTE/ SMELL:	(Normal)	Normal taste and smell sensations.
	(Deficit)	Taste or smell sensations are limited. *Specify nature and severity of deficit. Note how deficit is managed or overcome.*

3. COMMUNICATION

A. SPEECH:	(Normal)	Able to express self understandably in English. *Note any hesitation to express needs, desires, or emotions.*
	(Deficit)	Has a speech impediment or aphasia. *Specify nature and severity of difficulty.*
	(Variable)	Ability to communicate verbally is variable. *Note conditions that affect variability (e.g. stress, time of day, etc.)*
	(Lang. dif.)	Speaks with accent or hard to understand. *Specify degree of language difficulty and what language is preferred by patient. Note how difficulty is managed or overcome.*
B. READING:	(Normal)	Able to read English in newspaper-sized print. *Note apparent strength of interest in reading and preferred subjects.*
	(Deficit)	Has physical or educational handicap that limits reading ability. *Specify nature and severity of limitation.*
	(Non-Eng.)	Reads in language other than English. *Note language preference and apparent strength of interest in reading.*
C. WRITING:	(Normal)	Able to write legible English. *Note whether writing is an especially important form of communication to the patient.*

FORM 8 *Continued*

(Deficit) Has physical or educational handicap that limits writing ability.
Specify nature and severity of limitation.
(Left-handed) Prefers left hand over right for writing and other tasks.

4. MOBILITY/STRENGTH
A. TRANSFER: (Indep.) Able to transfer from bed to chair or chair to chair without help.
(Equip.) Uses special equipment to aid transfer.
Specify kind of equipment used (rail, walker, special chairs, etc.).
(Help) Needs help to transfer.
Specify kind of help needed and weight-bearing limitations of patient.
(Confined to bed) Unable to be out of bed at all.
Note reason for confinement and whether temporary or long-term.

B. AMBULA-TION: (Indep.) Able to ambulate by self and climb stairs.
Note any time or distance restrictions.
(Equip.) Uses special equipment to aid ambulation.
Specify kind of equipment used (walker, crutches, cane, braces, elastic stockings).
Note if patient uses wheelchair all or part time.
(Help) Needs help with ambulation.
Specify kind and amount of help needed and weight-bearing limitations.
Note usual schedule and destination of ambulation.
(Non-amb.) Not ambulatory.

C. GROOMING: (Indep.) Able to comb and shampoo hair, shave, or apply makeup without help.
(Super.) Needs supervision during grooming activities.
Specify reason for and level of supervision needed.
(Help) Needs help with grooming activities.
Specify activity and kind of help needed.
Note right- or left-handedness.
(Total care) Unable to groom self.
Note preferences and frequency of activities.

D. INSTRUMEN-TAL ACTIVI-TIES: (Indep.) Able to prepare own meals, wash and iron clothes.
Note any exceptions to above and other abilities such as shopping, driving, etc.
(Help) Needs help with meal preparation and clothes upkeep.
Note kind and frequency of help needed.
(Depen.) Mostly unable to prepare meals or maintain clothes.
Note any exceptions to dependency.

5. HABITS AND PATTERNS
A. APPETITE: (Good) Good appetite for patient's size and level of activity.
Note frequency of meals and snacks and time of main meal.

Form continued on following page

FORM 8 *Continued*

	(Limited)	Nutrition limited due to food preferences or poor appetite. *Specify food preferences and ways in which these are managed. Note reason for present poor appetite and/or appetite history.*
	(Spec. diet)	Receiving special diet. *Note reason for diet and expected duration.*
B. SLEEP:	(Good)	Sleeps well each night and feels rested. *Note usual bed and arising times and times of naps during day.*
	(Poor)	Sleeps poorly and seldom feels rested. *Note probable causes of poor sleep.*
	(Interrupted)	Sleep is normally interrupted. *Note reason for interruption and frequency (toilet, medication, dreams, etc.)*
	(Pre-bed rit.)	Ability to sleep is improved by certain routines or rituals. *Specify snacks, medications, pre-bed activities, and preferred clothing.*
	(Naps)	Takes naps during the day. *Note usual frequency and length of naps and whether they affect nighttime sleep.*
C. BLADDER:	(Continent)	Has full bladder control. *Note approximate daily output.*
	(Help)	Needs help in using equipment or getting to toilet. *Specify kind of help needed and frequency. Note any special equipment required such as high toilet seat, urinal, bedpan, or catheter.*
	(Incont.)	Patient is incontinent of urine. *Specify under what conditions incontinence occurs and how usually managed. Note whether bladder training program is part of rehabilitation.*
	(Frequen.)	Patient urinates frequently enough to disturb daytime activities or sleep. *Note approximate frequency of urination and probable cause.*
	(Fluid def.)	Needs assistance in getting appropriate level of fluid intake. *Specify nature of fluid deficit and how it is usually managed.*
D. BOWELS:	(Continent)	Has bowel control and regular bowel habits.
	(Regular)	Has regular pattern of bowel movements. *Note frequency of bowel movements and usual time of day.*
	(Help)	Needs help in getting to the toilet or using special equipment. *Specify kind of help or equipment needed (toilet seat, commode, bedpan).*
	(Lax./Soft.)	Uses laxatives, stool softeners, special foods, or procedures to improve regularity. *Note when and how frequently special foods or medications, laxatives, enemas, etc., are used.*

FORM 8 *Continued*

	(Incont.)	Patient is incontinent. *Specify under what conditions incontinence occurs and how usually managed.* *Note whether bowel training program is part of rehabilitation.*
E. SMOKING/ ALCOHOL DRUG USE:	(Tobacco)	Smokes regularly or uses tobacco in other forms. *Note what form of tobacco is used and usual frequency.*
	(Stop tobac.)	Trying to stop smoking or has been advised to stop. *Note present attitudes and goals and past history of trying to stop.*
	(Alcohol)	Regularly consumes alcoholic beverages. *Note approximate usual daily intake of alcohol and preferences.*
	(Alco. prob.)	Alcohol use has been a problem for patient or family in the past. *Note severity of problem and how it has been managed.*
	(Stop alco.)	Trying to limit or stop alcohol use. *Note present attitudes and goals.*
	(Drugs)	Regularly takes tranquilizers, sedatives, narcotics, or other drugs. *Note whether patient considers self to have a current or potential drug habit.* *Note any past history of problem drug use and whether drugs used are prescription or otherwise.*
	(Stop drugs)	Trying to limit or stop drug use. *Note present attitudes and goals.*

6. MENTAL STATE

A. COGNITION:	(Normal)	Ability to think and reason normally.
	(Diminished)	Ability to think and reason clearly is diminished. *Note probable cause and evidence used to make this judgment.*
	(Variable)	Alertness and ability to reason varies. *Note any observable pattern to variation and probable causes.*
	(Poor concen.)	Able to reason normally but has short attention span or poor ability to concentrate. *Note probable cause and evidence used to make this judgment.*
	(Disorient.)	Mentally confused or disoriented as to time, person, or place. *Note any variations in disorientation.*
B. AWARENESS:	(Alert)	Alert to present situation and able to report symptoms and needs.
	(Aware of Dx.)	Aware of diagnosis and its consequences for future health. *Note words listed or others that describe patient's attitude toward diagnosis:* *optimistic, pessimistic, depressed, uninterested, angry, passive, anxious.*

Form continued on following page

FORM 8 Continued

	(Realistic)	Mostly uses reality-based thinking when discussing continuing care.
	(Unreal.)	Expresses unrealistic goals, plans, or fears related to continuing care. *Specify nature of unrealistic thinking and note how others have responded to this.*
	(Unaware)	Not able to understand diagnosis or consequences. *Note reason for inability and whether family members or friends are aware.*
C. RESP. TO CARE:	(Pos.)	Has mostly positive attitudes toward care and caregivers. *Note words listed or others that describe patient's dominant attitudes: friendly, cooperative, alert, active in care, forms relationships easily.*
	(Neg.)	Has mostly negative attitudes toward care and caregivers. *Note words listed or others that describe patient's dominant attitudes: angry, uncooperative, critical, distrustful, withdrawn.*
	(Guard.)	Uses mostly guarded, defensive, or passive responses to care or caregivers. *Note whether there are variations in response and under what circumstances.*
	(Upset)	Seems upset by care and caregivers. *Note words listed or others that describe patient's dominant attitudes: disoriented, easily confused, nervous, embarrassed, demanding, depressed. Note any known factors that may contribute to patient's attitudes.*
D. MEMORY:	(Good)	Both short- and long-term memory seem to be within normal limits.
	(Short)	Able to recall facts or ideas for only a short period of time. *Note nature of memory difficulty and whether problem existed prior to acute episode.*
	(Variable)	Memory good at times, poor at others. *Note possible causes of variability, such as medication. Note any categories of information that seem to retained more reliably.*
	(Aids help)	Memory is improved by use of aids such as timers, written reminders, etc. *Specify kinds of memory aids that have been tried and which are most effective.*
	(Poor)	Unable to recall facts or ideas long enough to use them effectively. *Note any known causes for poor memory and length of time problem has existed.*

FORM 8 *Continued*

7. MOTIVATION

A. FOR SELF-CARE: (Active) Actively taking steps toward understanding potential and planning rehabilitation.
Note any specific evidence of positive/active motivation.

(Self-respon.) Demonstrates desire to be self-responsible and work toward improved abilities.
Note specific evidence of self-responsibility.

(Unreal.) Has unrealistic expectations of self or others related to future.
Note specific evidence of unrealistic thinking.

(Demoralized) Seems demoralized, depressed, or helpless in present circumstances.
Note evidence of demoralization or lack of motivation for self-care.

B. LEARNING: (Interested) Wants to learn about present care and rehabilitation.
Note phrases listed or others that describe patient's dominant attitudes:
asks questions, interested in explanations, applies knowledge.
Note teaching approaches that have been successful.

(Disabled) Unable to learn effectively.
Note reason for disability, such as mental impairment, confusion, poor memory, etc.

(Uninterested) Uninterested in learning about present care and rehabilitation.
Note phrases listed or others that describe patient's dominant attitudes:
passive toward care, unaware of potential, hostile toward teacher or teaching.
Note any known factors that may contribute to patient's lack of interest in learning.

C. PERSONALITY: (Present orien.) Describes self as practical, realistic, and concerned about "here and now."
Note how characteristic may affect teaching or rehab. program.

(Future orien.) Describes self as concerned with the overall picture and future potential.
Note how characteristic may affect teaching or rehab. program.

(Time consc.) Describes self as feeling some pressure until tasks are done and decisions made.
Note how characteristic may affect teaching or rehab. program.

(Easygoing) Describes self as easygoing and uncomfortable with deadlines and rules.
Note how characteristic may affect teaching or rehab. program.

D. DECISION MAKING: (Involved) Actively involved in plans for rehabilitation.
Note a word or phrase that describes patient's involvement such as:
discussing options, making plans, organizing help.

Form continued on following page

FORM 8 *Continued*

(Near ready)   Seems ready to begin decision making and planning rehabilitation.
Note evidence of readiness such as asking questions or talking about future needs.

(Unready)   Seems as yet unable to plan for future.
Note any known factors that may contribute to lack of readiness.

(Optimistic)   Has positive attitude toward ability to achieve rehabilitation goals.

(Pessimistic)   Has negative or unrealistic attitude toward achieving rehabilitation goals.

8. SOCIAL SITUATION
  A. FAMILY IN-VOLVEMENT: (Active)   Family members or close friends are actively involved with patient's care and future plans.
Identify those most involved by name and relationship.

(Realistic)   Family members or close friends seem to have realistic expectations for patient's progress.
Note evidence of realistic thinking and role that they anticipate for themselves.

(Supportive)   Family members support patient in rehab. efforts and participate in learning opportunities.
Identify those most supportive by name, and note in what ways support is given.

(Limited)   Involvement of family or friends in patient care or planning limited.
Note apparent reason for limited involvement by name and relationship.

(Not avail.)   Family not available due to geography or alienation.
Note reason for unavailability of family or friends.

(No support)   Family members or close friends visit but do not encourage rehabilitation efforts or planning.
Note apparent reason for lack of encouragement and support.

  B. COMMUNITY PARTICIP.:   (Soc. groups)   Has actively participated in community social groups or organizations.
Specify groups and note level of anticipated future involvement.

(Rel. groups)   Has actively participated in religious groups or activities.
Specify groups and note level of anticipated future involvement.

(Support)   Evidence of support and encouragement from community social or religious groups.
Note kind of support given and response of patient to it.

(Involved friends)   Friends visit regularly and seem actively involved with patient's well-being.
Note identity of any particularly involved.

FORM 8 *Continued*

	(Few friends)	Seems to have a limited social support network or speaks of self as having few friends. *Note apparent reason for limited friendships, such as personality, frequent moves, etc.*
	(No support)	Little or no evidence of support or encouragement from groups or friends. *Note apparent reasons for lack of a supportive social group and the patient's response to this.*
C. LIVING SITU-ATION:	(Ret. to former)	Return to former living situation following discharge is anticipated. *Note anticipated adequacy of this living arrangement.*
	(Changing)	Discharge to a different living situation anticipated. *Note progress of decision-making about altered living situation.* *Note patient's response to anticipated change.*
	(Shared)	Housing is or will be shared with others. *Identify persons in household.*
	(Alone)	Anticipates living alone. *Note whether patient has lived alone in the past.*
	(Resid. care)	Anticipates discharge to skilled nursing, rehab., or other residential care facility. *Note whether patient has lived in residential care in the past, and if so, for how long.*
	(Needs modifi.)	Needs structural modifications made to house/apartment. *Specify kinds of modifications that need to be made and available sources of help.*
D. SPECIAL GROUP:	(Minority)	Belongs to minority cultural or ethnic group that influences patient's language, diet, life-style, or values. *Specify group and anticipated impact on future care.*
	(Handicap)	Has a physical or mental handicap that will continue to limit activities or interaction. *Specify nature of handicap and limitations imposed by it.*
	(Adjust. prob.)	Needs special help in adjusting to care in the community. *Note kind of help needed and by whom.*

9. ECONOMIC SITUATION

A. FINANCES:	(Ret. to employ)	Expects to return to full- or part-time employment. *Note name of employer and nature of job.*
	(Leave avail.)	Has work leave benefits that will allow patient to recuperate from acute episode. *Note whether leave is paid or unpaid and how supportive employer is to rehab. program.*

Form continued on following page

FORM 8 *Continued*

(Supported)	Is fully supported or has independent source of income. *Note any relevant details about level of support.*
(S.S./Retir.)	Receives Social Security or retirement benefits. *Note whether income is adequate for expected needs.*
(Receive aid)	Receives disability, welfare, or other financial aid. *Note source and adequacy of income.*
(Uncertain)	Source of a regular income now uncertain. *Note reasons for uncertainty and whether help is needed in applying for aid.*

B. REHAB. IN-SURANCE BENEFITS

(Medicare/-aid)	Eligible for continuing care/rehab. benefits from Medicare and/or Medicaid. *Note present status of benefits.*
(H.M.O.)	Member of a Health Maintenance Organization with rehabilitation benefits. *Note present status of benefits.*
(Pvt. insur.)	Eligible for private insurance benefits for rehabilitation. *Note present status of benefits.*
(Dr./Clin.)	Visits to doctor's office or clinic for medical and rehab. follow-up partly or fully covered. *Note level of coverage.*
(Home care)	Home care assistance partly or fully covered. *Note level of coverage and whether adequate for needs.*
(No insurance)	Has no insurance coverage for continuing care/ rehabilitation. *Note whether financial counseling and/or assistance is needed and by whom.*

10. CONTINUING CARE

A. REHAB. PRO-GRAM:

(Reg. MD)	Will be returning to the care of own physician for follow-up care and rehab. supervision. *Note name of doctor and anticipated level of involvement in rehab. program.*
(Spec. MD)	Will receive follow-up care and/or rehab. supervision from a specialist physician. *Note name of doctor and plan for follow-up.*
(In-pt. unit)	Will initially receive rehab. services in an in-patient unit. *Note anticipated length of stay in unit and major rehab. goals to be reached.*
(Clinic)	Will receive follow-up care and/or rehab. supervision from an out-patient facility or clinic. *Note name of clinic and plan for follow-up.*
(Other)	Specify plan for medical and rehab. follow-up, including name of doctor and/or facility.

FORM 8 *Continued*

B. NURSING CARE:	(None)	No need for nursing care anticipated. *Note any treatments or procedures that will be done by the patient.*
	(Family)	Nursing care needs will be met by family members. *Note extent of nursing care anticipated and plan for family instruction.*
	(Skilled)	Need for skilled nursing care is anticipated. *Note how this need is expected to be met.*
	(Home care)	Need for home care is anticipated. *Specify what kind of care will be needed and for approximately what period of time.*
C. COMMUNITY SERVICES:	(Social work)	Needs social work consultation or assistance. *Note how this need is expected to be met and whether a referral has been made.*
	(Counseling)	Needs counseling assistance with personal problem solving. *Note how this need is expected to be met and whether a referral has been made.*
	(Mental Hlth.)	Needs consultation or assistance from a mental health professional. *Note how this need is expected to be met and whether a referral has been made.*
	(Supp. group)	Support from a community group is expected to be helpful to patient. *Note how this need is expected to be met and whether a referral has been made.*
	(Therapies)	Needs physical, occupational, respiratory, or speech therapy. *Note how this need is expected to be met and whether a referral has been made.*
D. EQUIPMENT:	(Indoor mobil.)	Needs assistive equipment to improve mobility or safety indoors. *Specify kinds of equipment or aids and source(s) of supply.*
	(Outdoor mobil.)	Needs assistive equipment to improve mobility or safety outdoors. *Specify kinds of equipment or aids and source(s) of supply.*
	(Ventilation)	Needs assistive equipment to improve or monitor breathing. *Specify kinds of equipment or aids and source(s) of supply.*
	(Communication)	Needs assistive equipment to aid communication. *Specify kinds of equipment or aids and source(s) of supply.*
	(Other)	Specify other kinds of equipment or aids needed and source(s) of supply.

MAKING A TEACHING PLAN

The early initiation of a Teaching Plan for the rehabilitation patient is especially important because of the complexity of learning goals and the need to coordinate the efforts of several teachers. While all aspects of learning needs may not be clear right away, the fact that a basic plan has been started and teaching begun in some areas will stimulate modification of the plan as needs emerge and promote continuing evaluation of patient progress toward rehabilitation goals. The Discharge Teaching Plan (Form 9) is designed to help caregivers identify areas of learning needs and construct learning objectives quickly. These objectives then become the framework for patient and family teaching. The subjects on this form parallel those indicated in the third section of the Discharge Plan Summary.

Remember that the only useful learning objectives are REALISTIC ones. They should be attainable in the time available, and the desired behavior should be observable by the teacher(s).

Elements of this form are described below.

Identification of Learners. Those people who are to be included in some or all teaching sessions are listed across the top of the form. The nurse may want to write the telephone numbers of visitor-learners, as well as their names, to simplify coordination. Where notations are made about a learner other than the patient, they may be referred to by number. For example, the motivation of the patient may be "developing," but for learner "#2" it may be already "present."

Subject of Teaching. Eight common subjects for discharge teaching have been listed on the form. The nurse may indicate that teaching in this subject area is not needed. If it is needed, the next three lines provide a record of teaching progress from planning thorough evaluation. Updating the teaching plan by checking the description that currently applies to teaching in each subject area will alert other caregivers to what has been done. They can then actively cooperate with what has been done. They can then actively cooperate with the learning process by stimulating further patient interest in the subject and reinforcing learning. Following the completion of teaching, learning may be evaluated through tests, verbal questions, demonstrations, or other methods. Verifying that an objective has been successfully reached is positive feedback for both teacher and learner.

Motivation. For the rehabilitation patient, motivation is both the beginning and the end point for learning. Motivation to learn is essential for effective progress in acquiring new knowledge, attitudes, and skills. Motivation to implement the rehabilitation program is the major goal of teaching. If motivation to learn is poor, the nurse will want to work on this before attempting to teach content in an area. Changes in motivation can be recorded with a check or an arrow. When several learners are involved, those with more motivation may be able to help the others understand the importance of the subject. Due to the fact that the rehabilitation patient may well still be in a state of crisis when teaching needs to begin, positive reinforcement of attempts to learn and progress as it is made are especially important to the patient's level of motivation.

Prior Knowledge or Experience. A short phrase is usually enough to record the basis on which new learning can be built. Finding out what a learner already knows about a subject takes only moments, but it allows the teacher to start with relevant material, thereby improving both motivation and learning ability. It is best not to make any assumptions about what the learner knows; a person may have eaten fresh fruits and vegetables for years but not know why they are particularly nutritious!

Learning Objective. The construction of learning objectives is a simple but often unfamiliar activity to those who are not full-time teachers. An objective or learning goal starts with the phrase *"The learner will be able to . . . "* This is followed by a verb indicating the **level of complexity** at which learning must take place. To "adapt" learning to different situations is, for example, much more complex than simply "remembering" it. We have suggested a number of possible verbs that may be used.

Next, a learning objective defines the specific **subject** of concern and what kind of **behavior** is expected as a result of learning. Remember that the stated behavior must be observable in the time available, and therefore objectives for learning in acute care settings will necessarily be short-term and limited. The ultimate goal in teaching a person how to do a number of strengthening exercises might be, for example, that he or she regularly perform these at home. A realistic learning objective while in hospital, however, might be that the person demonstrate the exercises and describe why they are important to rehabilitation. Finally, writing down a **time** for learning to be completed gives both learners and teachers a target toward which to work.

Notes. Noting what teaching approaches have been used (for example, "videotape on safe transfer procedures shown") and the response learners have had to them, the priority given certain subjects, and plans for learning evaluation are all important pieces of information to share with other caregivers. Current notes kept in a known location are essential when several teachers are involved or learning needs are complex.

FORM 9. *DISCHARGE TEACHING PLAN FOR:* _____

OTHER THAN PATIENT, THOSE TO BE INVOLVED AS LEARNERS
INCLUDE: *(Note name and relationship to patient.)*
#1:   #2:   #3:

1. MEDICAL/REHAB. FOLLOW-UP:
   Teaching: ___not needed   Motivation: ___present   Prior knowledge/
   ___planned   ___developing experience: _____
   ___in progress   ___poor
   ___learning   _____
   evaluated

   Learner will be able to: _____ By _____
                            (level)   (specific subject)   (behavior)   (date)
          (e.g., remember, understand, apply information, make decisions about)

2. MEDICATIONS:
   Teaching: ___not needed   Motivation: ___present   Prior knowledge/
   ___planned   ___developing experience: _____
   ___in progress   ___poor
   ___learning   _____
   evaluated

   Learner will be able to: _____ By _____
                            (level)   (specific subject)   (behavior)   (date)
          (e.g., remember, understand, apply information, respond, evaluate)

3. TREATMENTS/PROCEDURES:
   Teaching: ___not needed   Motivation: ___present   Prior knowledge/
   ___planned   ___developing experience: _____
   ___in progress   ___poor
   ___learning   _____
   evaluated

   Learner will be able to: _____ By _____
                            (level)   (specific subject)   (behavior)   (date)
          (e.g., remember, understand, apply information, perform, adapt, evaluate)

4. ACTIVITIES/EXERCISES:
   Teaching: ___not needed   Motivation: ___present   Prior knowledge/
   ___planned   ___developing experience: _____
   ___in progress   ___poor
   ___learning   _____
   evaluated

   Learner will be able to: _____ By _____
                            (level)   (specific subject)   (behavior)   (date)
          (e.g., remember, recognize, understand, apply information, perform, adapt)

5. NUTRITION/DIET:
   Teaching: ___not needed   Motivation: ___present   Prior knowledge/
   ___planned   ___developing experience: _____
   ___in progress   ___poor
   ___learning   _____
   evaluated

   Learner will be able to: _____ By _____
                            (level)   (specific subject)   (behavior)   (date)
          (e.g., remember, recognize, understand, apply information, prepare, adapt)

FORM 9 *Continued*

6. COMPLICATION MANAGEMENT:
   Teaching: __not needed   Motivation: __present   Prior knowledge/
   __planned   __developing experience: _____
   __in progress   __poor
   __learning   _____
   evaluated

   Learner will be able to: _____ By _____
                           (level)   (specific subject)   (behavior)   (date)
   (e.g., remember, recognize, understand, evaluate, perform, adapt)

7. HEALTH MAINTENANCE/PROMOTION:
   Teaching: __not needed   Motivation: __present   Prior knowledge/
   __planned   __developing experience: _____
   __in progress   __poor
   __learning   _____
   evaluated

   Learner will be able to: _____ By _____
                           (level)   (specific subject)   (behavior)   (date)
   (e.g., remember, understand, apply information, perform, realistically plan)

8. COMMUNITY SERVICES/RESOURCES:
   Teaching: __not needed   Motivation: __present   Prior knowledge/
   __planned   __developing experience: _____
   __in progress   __poor
   __learning   _____
   evaluated

   Learner will be able to: _____ By _____
                           (level)   (specific subject)   (behavior)   (date)
   (e.g., remember, understand, apply information, plan, utilize)

9. OTHER LEARNING OBJECTIVES:
   Learner will be able to _____ by _____

   Learner will be able to _____ by _____

Teaching Plan initiated by _____on _____

NOTES ON TEACHING (what was taught, methods/materials used, response, etc.)

B/3

How to Build a Plan for Management of Chronic Disease

Most people with chronic diseases are able to remain at home during most or all of the course of their illness. Their ability to do so is dependent on their receiving continuing care from health professionals and support from family and friends. These patients need intensive help from the nurse to build a discharge plan that will help them maintain independence while meeting their ongoing health care needs. Whether a person suffers from diabetes, multiple sclerosis, arthritis, or many other chronic or progressive diseases, their basic needs for maintaining supported self-reliance are similar.

In this section an approach is outlined that includes the use of four separate but coordinated forms. They are:

- the Discharge Plan Summary,
- a Detailed Needs Identification and associated Definitions and Descriptions, and
- a Discharge Teaching Plan.

Together they make it possible to record comprehensive information relevant to the discharge planning process with ease and clarity so that it is easily shared by caregivers who can, as a result, better coordinate their efforts.

A written **Discharge Plan** is a method used for communication and coordination of effort among caregivers. It is also appropriately used to involve patients and their family members in the discharge planning process by including them in the gathering of data and the clarification of objectives and priorities. Form 10 represents a *summary* of information collected from several sources and combined to give an overview of professional intervention. It is designed to reflect the progression of need identification, patient and family teaching, and

286

decision making about plans for continuing care. It should be begun as early in the patient's care as possible and updated regularly so that caregivers have a clear picture of the state of the discharge planning process. Especially important is information about where more detailed information can be located in the patient's medical record. This item alone can save caregivers a great deal of time and frustration.

In addition to the summary, guidance is given for completing a **Detailed Needs Identification** using the associated **Definitions and Descriptions** (Forms 11 and 12). The comprehensive information that they contain is especially useful when care is complex, when the patient has several diagnoses, or when the need for professional care at home is anticipated.

Patients who will be managing a chronic condition are particularly in need of high-quality teaching. We show the nurse how to make a **Teaching Plan** to help organize learning experiences for patient and family and coordinate efforts when several teachers are involved. Together, these approaches ensure that caregivers have a comprehensive "picture" of the patient and his or her continuing care needs.

FORM 10. *DISCHARGE PLAN SUMMARY FOR:* _____

PATIENT IDENTIFICATION NO.: _____ UNIT/ROOM: _____

GENERAL GOAL: Management of chronic disease while maintaining/improving other aspects of patient's health.

A. SPECIAL SERVICES DURING ACUTE CARE:
Note with + those that will/may need to be continued AFTER discharge.

___None   ___Radiation therapy   ___Patient/family
___Intensive care   ___Respiratory therapy   counseling
___Isolation   ___Physical therapy   ___Social services
___Surgery   ___Occupational therapy   ___Mental health/
___Blood transfusion ___Speech therapy   psychiatric
___Other: _____   ___Discharge planning
                                                     team
                                                 ___Rehabilitation team

B. IDENTIFICATION OF RISKS/DEFICITS   Patient's age is _____
*Note with * those risks present BEFORE admission.*
Note limitations expected to continue AFTER discharge.

___No special risks   ___Toileting
   identified   ___Mental state
___Activities of daily   ___Motivation
   living   ___Social situation
___Senses   ___Economic situation
___Communication
___Mobility

C. TEACHING NEEDED FOR PATIENT OR FAMILY IN SUBJECTS OF:
___No separate teaching plan
Note names and phone numbers of family or others involved in teaching.

___Medical follow-up   ___Activities   ___Health Promotion
   ___in progress   ___in progress   ___in progress
   ___completed   ___completed   ___completed

___Medications   ___Nutrition/diet   Community services
   ___in progress   ___in progress   ___in progress
   ___completed   ___completed   ___completed

___Treatments/procedures ___Complication manag.   ___Other: _____
   ___in progress   ___in progress   ___in progress
   ___completed   ___completed   ___completed

FORM 10 *Continued*

D. POST-HOSPITAL SERVICES: ___None needed.
Medical follow-up by: _____

   Home Care: ___Needed   ___Decision in progress

Referral made to _____on _____by _____

   Extended Care: ___Needed   ___Decision in progress

Referral made to _____on _____by _____

   Social Services: ___Needed   ___Decision in progress

Referral made to _____on _____by _____

   Mental Health: ___Needed   ___Decision in progress

Referral made to _____on _____by _____

   Special Equip: ___Needed   ___Decision in progress

Referral made to _____on _____by _____

Note details of services needed, options considered, and agencies/caregivers involved. Continue on back of sheet if needed.

E. SPECIFIC OBJECTIVES OF CONTINUING CARE: *Detail plans and goals for up to three months after discharge.*

ANTICIPATED DISCHARGE TO _____
ON OR ABOUT _____UNDER CARE OF DOCTOR_____

F. COORDINATION OF INFORMATION: *Note exactly where information can be located (e.g., "Nursing Care Plan" or "Form 111")*
___Initial **assessment** of discharge risks can be found: _____
___Further details of continuing care **needs and plans** can be found: _____
___Details of **teaching** planned and/or completed can be found: _____
___Copies of **referrals** or detailed plans can be found: _____

PLAN INITIATED BY: _____ON: _____. UPDATED: _____

INTRODUCTION TO DETAILED NEEDS
IDENTIFICATION

When patients have multiple diagnoses or several areas of risk have been identified, it is especially important to successful discharge planning that the full range of their needs be determined. The Detailed Needs Identification form is one approach to gathering and recording complete information. The reader will notice that spaces are left on Form 11 for making individualized comments about specific patient needs. More than one choice may be appropriate to some items. The subject areas that are included parallel those listed in the second section of the Discharge Planning Summary. The Needs Identification focuses on realistic *anticipation* of what can and should be done to help the patient successfully manage his or her disease after discharge.

A suggested format for recording information is shown on Form 11. Form 12 defines each option shown on Form 11 and describes specific information that may be important to the patient's continuing care. Many aspects of the patient's strengths and resources are included. Typically, a chronic disease affects many areas of one's life.

Those providing care, support, and supervision for disease management are able to respond more quickly and accurately to problems and to guide patients more effectively when they have access to information about how patients manage their life as well as their disease.

For nurses who are unfamiliar with discharge planning, these definitions and descriptions provide a basis for understanding the kinds and quality of information that have important implications for the patient's future well-being. Nurses are encouraged to read through the descriptive material and then use it in conjunction with the first few discharge plans they complete.

When working with real patient situations and commonly experienced time limitations, the nurse will find that some items are inappropriate or too time-consuming to pursue. Should the nurse choose to skip an item, it is helpful to note whether it is "N.A." (Not Applicable) or "Unk." (Unknown).

In addition to providing details of patient needs for caregivers in the acute care setting so that they might better help both patient and family plan continuing care, a form such as this is also helpful to community professionals who are involved in the plan's implementation. Of course, sharing such information must be with the full consent of the patient, and all aspects of professional confidentiality must be observed.

FORM 11. *DETAILED NEEDS IDENTIFICATION FOR* _____
I.D. _____

INSTRUCTIONS: *Check all appropriate options for each item. Note individual aspects of need and how care will be affected.*

1. ACTIVITIES OF DAILY LIVING:

A. EATING	B. DRESSING	C. BATHING	D. ORAL CARE
___Indep.	___Indep.	___Indep.	___Indep.
___Super.	___Super.	___Super.	___Super.
___Help	___Help	___Help	___Help
___Total care	___Total care	___Total care	___Total care

2. SENSES:

A. VISION	B. HEARING	C. TOUCH	D. TASTE/SMELL
___Full dist.	___Normal	___Normal	___Normal
___Full close	___Aided	___Deficit	___Deficit
___Deficit	___Deficit		
___Under Rx	___Under Rx		

3. COMMUNICATION:

A. SPEECH	B. READING	C. WRITING
___Normal	___Normal	___Normal
___Deficit	___Deficit	___Deficit
___Lang. dif.	___Non-Eng.	

4. MOBILITY:

A. TRANSFER	B. AMBULATION	C. GROOMING	D. INSTRU. ADLs *(meal prep., care of clothes)*
___Indep.	___Indep.	___Indep.	
___Equip.	___Equip.	___Super.	___Indep.
___Help	___Help	___Help	___Help
___Confined to bed	___Non-amb.	___Total care	___Depen.

5. HABITS AND PATTERNS:

A. APPETITE	B. SLEEP	C. BLADDER	D. BOWELS
___Good	___Good	___Continent	___Continent
___Limited	___Poor	___Help	___Regular
___Spec. diet	___Interrupted	___Incont.	___Help
	___Pre-bed rit.	___Frequen.	___Lax./Soft.
	___Naps	___Fluid def.	___Incont.

E. SMOKING/ALCOHOL/DRUG USE

___Tobacco	___Stop alco.
___Stop tobac.	___Drugs
___Alcohol	___Stop drugs
___Alco. prob.	

Form continued on following page

FORM 11 *Continued*

6. MENTAL STATE:

A. COGNITION	B. AWARENESS	C. RESP. TO CARE	D. MEMORY
___Normal	___Alert	___Pos.	___Good
___Diminished	___Aware of Dx.	___Neg.	___Short
___Variable	___Realistic	___Guard.	___Variable
___Poor concen.	___Unreal.	___Upset	___Poor
___Disorient.	___Unaware		

7. MOTIVATION:

A. FOR SELF-CARE	B. LEARNING	C. PERSONAL-ITY	D. DECISION MAKING
___Active	___Interested	___Present orien.	___Involved
___Self-respon.	___Disabled	___Future orien.	___Near ready
___Unreal.	___Uninterest.	___Time consc.	___Unready
___Demoralized		___Easygoing	___Optimistic
			___Pessimistic

8. SOCIAL SITUATION:

A. FAMILY IN-VOLVEMENT	B. COMMUNITY PARTICIP.	C. LIVING SITU-ATION	D. SPECIAL GROUP
___Active	___Soc. groups	___Ret. to former	___Minority
___Realistic	___Rel. groups	___Changing	___Handicap
___Supportive	___Support	___Shared	___Adjust. prob.
___Limited	___Involved friends	___Alone	
___Not avail.	___Few friends	___Resid. care	
___No support	___No support	___Needs modifi.	

9. ECONOMIC SITUATION:

A. FINANCES	B. CONT. INS. BENEFITS
___Ret. to employ.	
___Leave avail.	___Medicare/-aid
___Supported	___H.M.O.
___S.S./retir.	___Pvt. insur.
___Receive aid	___Dr. visit
___Uncertain	___Home care
	___No insur.

10. CONTINUING CARE:

A. MEDICAL FOLLOW-UP	B. NURSING CARE	C. COMM. SERV.	D. EQUIPMENT
___Reg. MD	___None	___Social work	___Indoor mobil.
___Spec. MD	___Family	___Counseling	___Outdoor mobil.
___Clinic	___Skilled	___Mental Hlth.	___Ventilation
___Other: _____	___Home care	___Supp. group	___Communication
		___Therapies	___Other: _____

Needs Identification completed by _____ on _____. Updated: _____

FORM 12. *DETAILED NEEDS IDENTIFICATION—DEFINITIONS AND DESCRIPTIONS*

Instructions: Check all appropriate descriptions on Detailed Needs Identification Form and follow each with short notes.

1. ACTIVITIES OF DAILY LIVING (ADL)
   A. EATING:
	(Indep.)	Feeds self.
	(Super.)	Needs to be supervised while eating.
		Specify level of supervision needed.
	(Help)	Needs help with certain foods or drink.
		Specify kinds of help needed.
	(Total care)	Needs to be fed.
		Note food preferences.

   B. DRESSING:
	(Indep.)	Selects appropriate clothing and dresses self.
	(Super.)	Needs supervision while dressing.
		Specify whether clothing must be selected or level of supervision.
	(Help)	Needs help with certain clothing or fasteners.
		Specify kinds of help needed.
		Note right- or left-handedness.
	(Total care)	Needs to be dressed.
		Note clothing preferences.

   C. BATHING:
	(Indep.)	Bathes self.
		Note whether patient regularly takes tub, shower, or sponge baths.
	(Super.)	Needs supervision while bathing.
		Specify reason for and level of supervision needed.
	(Help)	Needs help preparing for bath or while bathing.
		Specify kinds of help needed.
	(Total care)	Needs to be bathed.
		Note frequency and preferred time of baths.

   D. ORAL CARE:
	(Indep.)	Able to brush and floss teeth without help.
		Note whether person has dentures or whether special oral care procedures are used.
	(Super.)	Needs supervision during oral care procedures.
		Specify reason for and level of supervision needed.
	(Help)	Needs help with oral care.
		Specify kind of help needed.
	(Total care)	Unable to perform own oral care.
		Note kinds of care to be given and frequency.
		Note preferences for oral care equipment and products.

2. SENSES
   A. VISION:
	(Full dist.)	Normal or fully corrected distance vision.
		Note whether glasses or contacts are used.
	(Full close)	Normal or corrected close (reading) vision.
		Note whether glasses or contacts are used.
	(Deficit)	Patient has limited vision.
		Specify kind and severity of deficit.
	(Under Rx)	Under care for deficit or resulting handicap.
		Specify nature of care, frequency, and name of caregiver.

Form continued on following page

FORM 12 *Continued*

B. HEARING:	(Normal)	Able to hear normal speech.
	(Aided)	Uses a hearing aid.
		Note kind, frequency of use, and whether help is needed.
	(Deficit)	Hearing is limited.
		Specify kind and severity of deficit.
		Note how deficit is managed or overcome.
	(Under Rx)	Under care for deficit or resulting handicap.
		Specify nature of care, frequency, and name of caregiver.
C. TOUCH:	(Normal)	Has normal touch sensations.
	(Deficit)	Sense of touch is limited.
		Specify nature of deficit and part of body involved. Note how deficit is managed or overcome.
D. TASTE/ SMELL:	(Normal)	Normal taste and smell sensations.
	(Deficit)	Taste or smell sensations are limited.
		Specify nature and severity of deficit. Note how deficit is managed or overcome.

3. COMMUNICATION

A. SPEECH:	(Normal)	Able to express self understandably in English. Note any hesitation to express needs, desires, or emotions.
	(Deficit)	Has a speech impediment or aphasia.
		Specify nature and severity of difficulty.
	(Lang. dif.)	Speaks with accent or hard to understand.
		Specify degree of language difficulty and what language is preferred by patient.
		Note how difficulty is managed or overcome.
B. READING:	(Normal)	Able to read English in newspaper-sized print.
		Note apparent strength of interest in reading and preferred subjects.
	(Deficit)	Has physical or educational handicap that limits reading ability.
		Specify nature and severity of limitation.
	(Non-Eng.)	Reads in language other than English.
		Note language preference and apparent strength of interest in reading.
C. WRITING:	(Normal)	Able to write legible English.
		Note whether writing is an especially important form of communication to the patient.
	(Deficit)	Has physical or educational handicap that limits writing ability.
		Specify nature and severity of limitation.

4. MOBILITY

A. TRANSFER:	(Indep.)	Able to transfer from bed to chair or chair to chair without help.
	(Equip.)	Uses special equipment to aid transfer.
		Specify kind of equipment used (rail, walker, special chairs, etc.).
	(Help)	Needs help to transfer.
		Specify kind of help needed and weight-bearing limitations of patient.

FORM 12 *Continued*

	(Confined to bed)	Unable to be out of bed at all. *Note reason for confinement and whether temporary or long-term.*
B. AMBULA-TION:	(Indep.)	Able to ambulate by self and climb stairs. *Note any time or distance restrictions.*
	(Equip.)	Uses special equipment to aid ambulation. *Specify kind of equipment used (walker, crutches, cane, braces, elastic stockings). Note if patient uses wheelchair all or part time.*
	(Help)	Needs help with ambulation. *Specify kind and amount of help needed and weight-bearing limitations. Note usual schedule and destination of ambulation.*
	(Non-amb.)	Not ambulatory.
C. GROOMING:	(Indep.)	Able to comb and shampoo hair, shave, or apply makeup without help.
	(Super.)	Needs supervision during grooming activities. *Specify reason for and level of supervision needed.*
	(Help)	Needs help with grooming activities. *Specify activity and kind of help needed. Note right- or left-handedness.*
	(Total care)	Unable to groom self. *Note preferences and frequency of activities.*
D. INSTRU-MENTAL ADLs:	(Indep.)	Able to prepare own meals, wash and iron clothes. *Note any exceptions to above and other abilities such as shopping, driving, etc.*
	(Help)	Needs help with meal preparation and clothes upkeep. *Note kind and frequency of help needed.*
	(Depen.)	Mostly unable to prepare meals or maintain clothes. *Note any exceptions to dependency.*

5. HABITS AND PATTERNS

A. APPETITE:	(Good)	Good appetite for patient's size and level of activity. *Note frequency of meals and snacks and time of main meal.*
	(Limited)	Nutrition limited due to food preferences or poor appetite. *Specify food preferences and ways in which these are managed. Note reason for present poor appetite and/or appetite history.*
	(Spec. diet)	Receiving special diet. *Note reason for diet and expected duration.*
B. SLEEP:	(Good)	Sleeps well each night and feels rested. *Note usual bed and arising times and times of naps during day.*
	(Poor)	Sleeps poorly and seldom feels rested. *Note probable causes of poor sleep.*
	(Interrupted)	Sleep is normally interrupted. *Note reason for interruption and frequency (toilet, medication, dreams, etc.)*

Form continued on following page

FORM 12 *Continued*

	(Pre-bed rit.)	Ability to sleep is improved by certain routines or rituals. *Specify snacks, medications, pre-bed activities, and preferred clothing.*
	(Naps)	Takes naps during the day. *Note usual frequency and length of naps and whether they affect nighttime sleep.*
C. BLADDER:	(Continent)	Has full bladder control. *Note approximate daily output.*
	(Help)	Needs help in using equipment or getting to toilet. *Specify kind of help needed and frequency. Note any special equipment required such as high toilet seat, urinal, bedpan, or catheter.*
	(Incont.)	Patient is incontinent of urine. *Specify under what conditions incontinence occurs and how usually managed.*
	(Frequen.)	Patient urinates frequently enough to disturb daytime activities or sleep. *Note approximate frequency of urination and probable cause.*
	(Fluid def.)	Needs assistance in getting appropriate level of fluid intake. *Specify nature of fluid deficit and how it is usually managed.*
D. BOWELS:	(Continent)	Has bowel control and regular bowel habits.
	(Regular)	Has regular pattern of bowel movements. *Note frequency of bowel movements and usual time of day.*
	(Help)	Needs help in getting to the toilet or using special equipment. *Specify kind of help or equipment needed (toilet seat, commode, bedpan).*
	(Lax./Soft.)	Uses laxatives, stool softeners, special foods, or procedures to improve regularity. *Note when and how frequently special foods or medications, laxatives, enemas, etc., are used.*
	(Incont.)	Patient is incontinent. *Specify under what conditions incontinence occurs and how usually managed.*
E. SMOKING/ ALCOHOL DRUG USE:	(Tobacco)	Smokes regularly or uses tobacco in other forms. *Note what form of tobacco is used and usual frequency.*
	(Stop tobac.)	Trying to stop smoking or has been advised to stop. *Note present attitudes and goals and past history of trying to stop.*
	(Alcohol)	Regularly consumes alcoholic beverages. *Note approximate usual daily intake of alcohol and preferences.*
	(Alco. prob.)	Alcohol use has been a problem for patient or family in the past. *Note severity of problem and how it has been managed.*
	(Stop Alco.)	Trying to limit or stop alcohol use. *Note present attitudes and goals.*

FORM 12 *Continued*

	(Drugs)	Regularly takes tranquilizers, sedatives, narcotics, or other drugs. *Note whether patient considers self to have a current or potential drug habit. Note any past history of problem drug use and whether drugs used are prescription or otherwise.*
	(Stop drugs)	Trying to limit or stop drug use. *Note present attitudes and goals.*

6. MENTAL STATE

A. COGNITION:	(Normal)	Ability to think and reason normal.
	(Diminished)	Ability to think and reason clearly diminished. *Note probable cause and evidence used to make this judgment.*
	(Variable)	Alertness and ability to reason varies. *Note any observable pattern to variation and probable causes.*
	(Poor concen.)	Able to reason normally but has short attention span or poor ability to concentrate. *Note probable cause and evidence used to make this judgment.*
	(Disorient.)	Mentally confused or disoriented as to time, person, or place. *Note any variations in disorientation.*
B. AWARENESS:	(Alert)	Alert to present situation and able to report symptoms and needs.
	(Aware of Dx.)	Aware of diagnosis and its consequences for future health. *Note words listed or others that describe patient's attitude toward diagnosis: optimistic, pessimistic, depressed, uninterested, angry, passive, anxious.*
	(Realistic)	Mostly uses reality-based thinking when discussing continuing care.
	(Unreal.)	Expresses unrealistic goals, plans, or fears related to continuing care. *Specify nature of unrealistic thinking and note how others have responded to this.*
	(Unaware)	Not able to understand diagnosis or consequences. *Note reason for inability and whether family members or friends are aware.*
C. RESP. TO CARE:	(Pos.)	Has mostly positive attitudes toward care and caregivers. *Note words listed or others that describe patient's dominant attitudes:* friendly, cooperative, alert, active in care, forms relationships easily.
	(Neg.)	Has mostly negative attitudes toward care and caregivers. *Note words listed or others that describe patient's dominant attitudes:* angry, uncooperative, critical, distrustful, withdrawn.

Form continued on following page

FORM 12 *Continued*

	(Guard.)	Uses mostly guarded, defensive, or passive responses to care or caregivers. *Note whether there are variations in response and under what circumstances.*
	(Upset)	Seems upset by care and caregivers. *Note words listed or others that describe patient's dominant attitudes: disoriented, easily confused, nervous, embarrassed, demanding, depressed. Note any known factors that may contribute to patient's attitudes.*
D. MEMORY:	(Good)	Both short- and long-term memory seem to be within normal limits.
	(Short)	Able to recall facts or ideas for only a short period of time. *Note nature of memory difficulty and whether problem existed prior to acute episode.*
	(Variable)	Memory good at times, poor at others. *Note possible causes of variability such as medication. Note any categories of information that seem to be retained more reliably.*
	(Poor)	Unable to recall facts or ideas long enough to use them effectively. *Note any known causes for poor memory and length of time problem has existed.*
7. MOTIVATION A. FOR SELF- CARE:	(Active)	Actively taking steps toward understanding diagnosis and planning for future. *Note any specific evidence of positive/active motivation.*
	(Self-respon.)	Demonstrates self-responsibility and motivation to attempt self-management. *Note specific evidence of self-responsibility.*
	(Unreal.)	Has unrealistic expectations of self or others related to future care. *Note specific evidence of unrealistic thinking.*
	(Demoralized)	Seems demoralized, depressed, or helpless in present circumstances. *Note evidence of demoralization or lack of motivation for self-care.*
B. LEARNING:	(Interested)	Wants to learn about illness and future care. *Note phrases listed or others that describe patient's dominant attitudes: asks questions, interested in explanations, attentive to procedures. Note teaching approaches that have been successful.*
	(Disabled)	Unable to learn effectively. *Note reason for inability such as unconsciousness, mental impairment, confusion, or inability to concentrate.*

FORM 12 *Continued*

	(Uninterested)	Uninterested in learning about illness and future care. *Note phrases listed or others that describe patient's dominant attitudes: passive toward care, unaware of needs, hostile toward teaching. Note any known factors that may contribute to patient's disinterest in learning.*
C. PERSON-ALITY:	(Present orien.)	Describes self as practical, realistic, and concerned about "here and now." *Note how characteristic may affect teaching or care plans.*
	(Future orien.)	Describes self as concerned with the overall picture and future potential. *Note how characteristic may affect teaching or care plans.*
	(Time consc.)	Describes self as feeling some pressure until tasks done and decisions made. *Note how characteristic may affect teaching or care plans.*
	(Easygoing)	Describes self as easygoing and uncomfortable with deadlines and rules. *Note how characteristic may affect teaching or care plans.*
D. DECISION MAKING:	(Involved)	Actively involved in plans for chronic disease management. *Note a word or phrase that describes patient's involvement such as: discussing options, making plans, organizing help.*
	(Near ready)	Seems ready to begin decision making and planning about future care. *Note evidence of readiness such as asking questions or talking about previous experiences.*
	(Unready)	Seems as yet unable to plan for future. *Note any known factors that may contribute to lack of readiness.*
	(Optimistic)	Has positive attitude toward ability to manage disease.
	(Pessimistic)	Has negative or unrealistic attitude toward ability to manage disease.

8. SOCIAL SITUATION

A. FAMILY INVOLVE-MENT:	(Active)	Family members or close friends are actively involved with patient's care. *Identify those most involved by name and relationship.*
	(Realistic)	Family members or close friends seem to have realistic expectations for patient's progress. *Note evidence of realistic thinking and role that they anticipate for themselves.*
	(Supportive)	Family members support patient in self-care and participate in learning opportunities. *Identify those most supportive by name and note in what ways support is given.*

Form continued on following page

FORM 12 Continued

	(Limited)	Involvement of family or friends in patient care limited. *Note apparent reason for limited involvement by name and relationship.*
	(Not avail.)	Family not available due to geography or alienation. *Note reason for unavailability of family or friends.*
	(No support)	Family or close friends visit but give patient no encouragement or support. *Note apparent reasons for lack of encouragement or support.*
B. COMMUNITY PARTICIP.:	(Soc. groups)	Participates in community social groups or organizations. *Specify groups and note level of involvement.*
	(Rel. groups)	Participates in religious groups or activities. *Specify groups and any implications for future care.*
	(Support)	Evidence of support and encouragement from community social or religious groups. *Note kind of support given and response of patient to it.*
	(Involved friends)	Friends visit regularly and seem actively involved with patient's well-being. *Note identity of any particularly involved.*
	(Few friends)	Seems to have a limited social support network or speaks of self as having few friends. *Note apparent reason for limited friendships such as personality, frequent moves, etc.*
	(No support)	Little or no evidence of support or encouragement from groups or friends. *Note apparent reasons for lack of a supportive social group and the patient's response to this.*
C. LIVING SITUATION:	(Ret. to former)	Return to former living situation following discharge is anticipated. *Note anticipated adequacy of this living arrangement.*
	(Changing)	Discharge to a different living situation anticipated. *Note progress of decision making about altered living situation. Note patient's response to anticipated change.*
	(Shared)	Housing is or will be shared with others. *Identify persons in household.*
	(Alone)	Anticipates living alone. *Note whether patient has lived alone in the past.*
	(Resid. care)	Anticipates discharge to skilled nursing or other residential care facility. *Note whether patient has lived in residential care in the past, and if so, for how long.*
	(Needs modifi.)	Needs structural modifications made to house/apartment. *Specify kinds of modifications that need to be made and available sources of help.*

FORM 12 *Continued*

D. SPECIAL GROUP:	(Minority)	Belongs to minority cultural or ethnic group that influences patient's language, diet, lifestyle, or values. *Specify group and anticipated impact on future care.*
	(Handicap)	Has a physical or mental handicap that limits activities or interaction. *Specify nature of handicap and limitations imposed by it.*
	(Adjust. prob.)	Needs special help in adjusting to care in the community. *Note kind of help needed and by whom.*

9. ECONOMIC SITUATION

A. FINANCES:	(Ret. to employ)	Expects to return to full- or part-time employment. *Note name of employer and nature of job.*
	(Leave avail.)	Has work leave benefits that will allow patient to recuperate from acute episode. *Note whether leave is paid or unpaid and how supportive employer is to disease management.*
	(Supported)	Is fully supported or has independent source of income. *Note any relevant details about level of support.*
	(S.S./Retir.)	Receives Social Security or retirement benefits. *Note whether income is adequate for expected needs.*
	(Receive aid)	Receives disability, welfare, or other financial aid. *Note source and adequacy of income.*
	(Uncertain)	Source of a regular income now uncertain. *Note reasons for uncertainty and whether help is needed in applying for aid.*
B. CONTINUING INSURANCE BENEFITS:	(Medicare/-aid)	Eligible for continuing care benefits from Medicare and/or Medicaid. *Note present status of benefits.*
	(H.M.O.)	Member of a Health Maintenance Organization with continuing care benefits. *Note present status of benefits.*
	(Pvt. insur.)	Eligible for private insurance benefits for continuing care. *Note present status of benefits.*
	(Dr. visit)	Medical follow-up visits to doctor's offices or clinic partly or fully covered. *Note level of coverage.*
	(Home care)	Home care assistance partly or fully covered. *Note level of coverage and whether adequate for needs.*
	(No insurance)	Has no insurance coverage for continuing care. *Note whether financial counseling and/or assistance is needed and by whom.*

10. CONTINUING CARE

A. MEDICAL FOLLOW-UP:	(Reg. MD)	Will be returning to the care of own physician for follow-up care. *Note name of doctor and level of involvement in hospital care.*

Form continued on following page

FORM 12 *Continued*

	(Spec. MD)	Will receive follow-up care from a specialist physician. *Note name of doctor and any anticipated difficulty with patient access.*
	(Clinic)	Will receive follow-up care from an out-patient facility or clinic. *Note name of clinic and whether patient has received care there previously.*
	(Other)	*Specify plan for medical follow-up, including name of doctor and/or facility.*
B. NURSING CARE:	(None)	No need for nursing care anticipated. *Note any treatments or procedures that will be done by the patient.*
	(Family)	Nursing care needs will be met by family members. *Note extent of nursing care anticipated and plan for family instruction.*
	(Skilled)	Need for skilled nursing care is anticipated. *Note how this need is expected to be met.*
	(Home care)	Need for home care is anticipated. *Specify what kind of care will be needed and for approximately what period of time.*
C. COMMUNITY SERVICES:	(Social work)	Needs social work consultation or assistance. *Note how this need is expected to be met and whether a referral has been made.*
	(Counseling)	Needs counseling assistance with personal problem solving. *Note how this need is expected to be met and whether a referral has been made.*
	(Mental Hlth.)	Needs consultation or assistance from a mental health professional. *Note how this need is expected to be met and whether a referral has been made.*
	(Supp. group)	Support from a community group is expected to be helpful to patient. *Note how this need is expected to be met and whether a referral has been made.*
	(Therapies)	Needs physical, occupational, respiratory, or speech therapy. *Note how this need is expected to be met and whether a referral has been made.*
D. EQUIPMENT:	(Indoor mobil.)	Needs assistive equipment to improve mobility or safety indoors. *Specify kinds of equipment or aids and source(s) of supply.*
	(Outdoor mobil.)	Needs assistive equipment to improve mobility or safety outdoors. *Specify kinds of equipment or aids and source(s) of supply.*
	(Ventilation)	Needs assistive equipment to improve or monitor breathing. *Specify kinds of equipment or aids and source(s) of supply.*
	(Communication)	Needs assistive equipment to aid communication. *Specify kinds of equipment or aids and source(s) of supply.*
	(Other)	*Specify other kinds of equipment or aids needed and source(s) of supply.*

MAKING A TEACHING PLAN

A Teaching Plan completed early in a patient's care allows caregivers to coordinate their teaching efforts and continuously evaluate patient progress toward discharge objectives. The Discharge Teaching Plan (Form 13) is designed to help caregivers identify areas of learning needs and construct learning objectives quickly. These objectives then become the framework for patient and family teaching. The subjects on this form parallel those indicated in the third section of the Discharge Plan Summary.

Remember that the only useful learning objectives are REALISTIC ones. They should be attainable in the time available, and the desired behavior should be observable by the teacher(s).

Elements of this form are described below.

Identification of Learners. Those people who are to be included in some or all teaching sessions are listed across the top of the form. The nurse may want to write the telephone numbers of visitor-learners, as well as their names, to simplify coordination. Where notations are made about a learner other than the patient, they may be referred to by number. For example, the motivation of the patient may be "developing," but for learner "#2" it may be already "present."

Subject of Teaching. Eight common subjects for discharge teaching have been listed on the form. The nurse may indicate that teaching in this subject area is not needed. If it is needed, the next three lines provide a record of teaching progress from planning through evaluation. Updating the teaching plan by checking the description that currently applies to teaching in each subject area will alert other caregivers to what has been done. They can then actively cooperate with the learning process by stimulating further patient interest in the subject and reinforcing learning. Following the completion of teaching, learning may be evaluated through tests, verbal questions, demonstrations, or other methods. Verifying that an objective has been successfully reached is positive feedback for both teacher and learner.

Motivation. Attention to a person's motivation to learn particular subjects is extremely important for effective and efficient teaching. If motivation is poor, the nurse will want to work on this before attempting to teach content in an area. Changes in motivation can be recorded with a check or an arrow. When several learners are involved, those with more motivation may be able to help the others understand the importance of the subject.

Prior Knowledge or Experience. A short phrase is usually enough to record the basis on which new learning can be built. Finding out what a learner already knows about a subject takes only moments, but it allows the teacher to start with relevant material, thereby improving both motivation and learning ability. It is best not to make any assumptions about what the learner knows; a person may have experienced mild symptoms of a disease process for years without recognizing their importance or the role they play in disease management.

Learning Objective. The construction of learning objectives is a simple but often unfamiliar activity to those who are not full-time teachers. An objective or learning goal starts with the phrase *"The learner will be able to . . . "* This is followed by a verb indicating the **level of complexity** at which learning must take place. To "adapt" learning to different situations is, for example, much more complex than simply "remembering" it. We have suggested a number of possible words that may be used.

Next, a learning objective defines the **specific subject** of concern and states what kind of **behavior** is expected as a result of learning. Remember that the stated behavior must be observable in the time available, and therefore objectives for learning in acute care settings will necessarily be short-term and limited. The ultimate goal in teaching a person about diet modification, for example, might be a reduction in cholesterol level. A realistic learning objective while the person is in the hospital, however, might be the appropriate choice of foods from the daily menu. Finally, writing down a **time** for learning to be completed gives both learners and teachers a target toward which to work.

Notes. Noting what teaching approaches have been used, (for example, "videotape on heart disease shown") and the response learners have had to them, the priority given certain subjects, and plans for learning evaluation are all important pieces of information to share with other caregivers. Current notes kept in a known location are essential when several teachers are involved or learning needs are complex.

FORM 13. *DISCHARGE TEACHING PLAN FOR:* _____

OTHER THAN PATIENT, THOSE TO BE INVOLVED AS LEARNERS
INCLUDE: *(Note name and relationship to patient.)*
    #1:   #2:   #3:

1. DIAGNOSIS/MEDICAL FOLLOW-UP:
    Teaching: ___not needed   Motivation: ___present   Prior knowledge/
          ___planned   ___developing experience: _____
          ___in progress   ___poor
          ___learning   _____
          evaluated

Learner will be able to: _____ By _____
                          (level)   (specific subject)   (behavior)   (date)
          (e.g., remember, understand, apply information, make decisions about)

2. MEDICATIONS:
    Teaching: ___not needed   Motivation: ___present   Prior knowledge/
          ___planned   ___developing experience: _____
          ___in progress   ___poor
          ___learning   _____
          evaluated

Learner will be able to: _____ By _____
                          (level)   (specific subject)   (behavior)   (date)
          (e.g., remember, understand, apply information, respond, evaluate)

3. TREATMENTS/PROCEDURES:
    Teaching: ___not needed   Motivation: ___present   Prior knowledge/
          ___planned   ___developing experience: _____
          ___in progress   ___poor
          ___learning   _____
          evaluated

Learner will be able to: _____ By _____
                          (level)   (specific subject)   (behavior)   (date)
          (e.g., remember, understand, apply information, perform, adapt, evaluate)

4. ACTIVITIES:
    Teaching: ___not needed   Motivation: ___present   Prior knowledge/
          ___planned   ___developing experience: _____
          ___in progress   ___poor
          ___learning   _____
          evaluated

Learner will be able to: _____ By _____
                          (level)   (specific subject)   (behavior)   (date)
          (e.g., remember, recognize, understand, apply information, perform, adapt)

5. NUTRITION/DIET:
    Teaching: ___not needed   Motivation: ___present   Prior knowledge/
          ___planned   ___developing experience: _____
          ___in progress   ___poor
          ___learning   _____
          evaluated
Learner will be able to: _____ By _____
                          (level)   (specific subject)   (behavior)   (date)
          (e.g., remember, recognize, understand, apply information, prepare, adapt)
                                          Form continued on following page

FORM 13 *Continued*

6. COMPLICATION MANAGEMENT:
    Teaching: __not needed   Motivation: __present   Prior knowledge/
    __planned   __developing   experience: _____
    __in progress   __poor
    __learning   _____
    evaluated

Learner will be able to: _____ By _____
                          (level)   (specific subject)   (behavior)   (date)
          (e.g., remember, recognize, understand, evaluate, perform, adapt)

7. HEALTH MAINTENANCE/PROMOTION:
    Teaching: __not needed   Motivation: __present   Prior knowledge/
    __planned   __developing   experience: _____
    __in progress   __poor
    __learning   _____
    evaluated

Learner will be able to: _____ By _____
                          (level)   (specific subject)   (behavior)   (date)
          (e.g., remember, understand, apply information, perform, realistically plan)

8. COMMUNITY SERVICES/RESOURCES:
    Teaching: __not needed   Motivation: __present   Prior knowledge/
    __planned   __developing   experience: _____
    __in progress   __poor
    __learning   _____
    evaluated

Learner will be able to: _____ By _____
                          (level)   (specific subject)   (behavior)   (date)
          (e.g., remember, understand, apply information, plan, utilize)

9. OTHER LEARNING OBJECTIVES:
    Learner will be able to _____ by _____

    Learner will be able to _____ by _____

Teaching Plan initiated by _____ on _____

NOTES ON TEACHING (what was taught, methods/materials used, response, etc.)

B/4

How to Build a Plan for Residential Care

The vast majority of people who are unable to maintain independent living with or without the help of family and friends have disabling chronic conditions. For them, some form of residential care where meals and housekeeping are provided are the best option. The frail aged, even those without an overriding medical condition, also often need this kind of protected environment.

Residential care facilities are divided into categories based on the kind and amount of care they offer. "Intermediate" facilities, including "Board and Care Homes," provide some supervision for those who are basically able to manage the activities of daily living. They are an appropriate choice for some frail elderly, mentally ill, or developmentally handicapped individuals. "Skilled Nursing Facilities" (SNFs) provide full nursing services emphasizing restorative and rehabilitative care. They are a realistic destination for patients leaving acute care who need nursing care in excess of what can be provided at home. "Nursing Homes" may offer skilled nursing to some patients, but usually the majority of their residents need long-term custodial care with varying degrees of help with activities of daily living.

In building a plan for patients to be discharged to a residential facility, there are three major concerns. One is the emotional aspects of the decision-making process that precedes placement. It is appropriate for the nurse to encourage family members and the patient to talk through their hopes and fears and their feelings of guilt, abandonment, or relief that are the prelude to rational and realistic decisions. A second concern is the financial aspects of a decision in favor of residential care. Insurance benefits even for rehabilitative or skilled nursing care are limited. It is important that the patient and family have good information about costs as they make their decisions. Finally, the nurse is concerned with giving the recipient residential facility good quality information concerning the patient's needs so that the transition can go smoothly and the level of care offered is appropriate.

In order to help the nurse focus on these concerns and begin need identification and teaching activities early in the patient's acute care, four separate but coordinated forms are outlined in this section. They are:

- the Discharge Plan Summary,
- a Detailed Needs Identification and associated Definitions and Descriptions, and
- a Discharge Teaching Plan.

Together they make it possible to record comprehensive information relevant to the discharge planning process with ease and clarity so that it is easily shared by caregivers who can, as a result, better coordinate their efforts.

A written **Discharge Plan** is a method used for communication and coordination of effort among caregivers. It is also appropriately used to involve patients and their family members in the discharge planning process by including them in the gathering of data and the clarification of objectives and priorities. Form 14 represents a *summary* of information collected from several sources and combined to give an overview of professional intervention. It is designed to reflect the progression of need identification, patient and family teaching, and decision-making about plans for continuing care. It should be begun as early in the patient's care as possible and updated regularly so that caregivers have a clear picture of the state of the discharge planning process. Especially important is information about where in the patient's medical record more detailed information can be located. This item alone can save caregivers a great deal of time and frustration.

In addition to the summary, guidance is given for completing a **Detailed Needs Identification** using the associated **Definitions and Descriptions** (Forms 15 and 16). The comprehensive information they contain helps caregivers understand many dimensions of the patient's needs, allowing them to give more sensitive support for the decision-making process.

It is often unclear early in patients' acute care whether their discharge destination will be their own home, the home of a relative, or a residential facility, although it may be quite clear that they will need intensive help wherever they go. One of the first steps in helping patients and their families decide among their options is to help them learn realistically what kind of care is involved. They also need help with learning about the financial aspects of various options and how to appropriately use the help offered by health care professionals. Family members may need special help anticipating their continuing social and emotional relationship with the patient and learning how to investigate facilities. We show the nurse how to make a **Teaching Plan** that will help organize learning experiences for patient and family and coordinate efforts when several teachers are involved. Together, these approaches ensure that caregivers have a comprehensive "picture" of the patient and his or her continuing care needs.

FORM 14. *DISCHARGE PLAN SUMMARY FOR:* _____

PATIENT IDENTIFICATION NO.: _____ UNIT/ROOM: _____

GENERAL GOAL: Management of the medical and physical care needs in a residential setting that promotes health and independence.

A. SPECIAL SERVICES DURING ACUTE CARE:
Note with + those that will/may need to be continued AFTER discharge.

__None	__Radiation therapy	__Discharge planning
__Intensive care	__Respiratory therapy	team
__Isolation	__Physical therapy	__Patient/family
__Surgery	__Speech therapy	counseling
__Blood transfusion	__Mental health/	__Social services
__Other: _____	psychiatric	__Financial assistance

B. IDENTIFICATION OF RISKS/DEFICITS: Patient's age is _____
Note limitations expected to continue AFTER discharge.
*Note with * those risks present BEFORE admission.*

__No special risks	__Bladder/bowels
identified	__Skin condition
__Activities of daily	__Mental state
living	__Social situation
__Senses	__Economic situation
__Communication	
__Mobility	

C. TEACHING NEEDED FOR PATIENT OR FAMILY IN SUBJECTS OF:
__No separate teaching plan
Note names and phone numbers of family or others involved in teaching.

__Medical needs	__Complication manag.	__Emot./Soc. aspects of
__in progress	__in progress	transition
__completed	__completed	__in progress
__Post-hosp. nursing	__Options for contin.	__completed
needs	care	__Community resources
__in progress	__in progress	__in progress
__completed	__completed	__completed
__Nutritional needs	__Financial aspects of	__Other: _____
__in progress	care	__in progress
__completed	__in progress	__completed
	__completed	

FORM 14 *Continued*

D. POST-HOSPITAL SERVICES: __None needed.
Medical follow-up by:

_____

   Extend./Resid. Care: __Needed   __Decision in progress

Referral made to _____on _____by _____
   Special Equipment: __Needed   __Decision in progress

Referral made to _____on _____by _____
   Ment. Hlth./Couns.:   __Needed   __Decision in progress

Referral made to _____on _____by _____
   Social Services: __Needed   __Decision in progress

Referral made to _____on _____by _____
   Financial assist.:   __Needed   __Decision in progress

Referral made to _____on _____by _____

Note details of services needed, options considered, and agencies/caregivers involved. Continue on back of sheet if needed.

E. SPECIFIC OBJECTIVES OF CONTINUING CARE: *Detail plans and goals for up to three months after discharge.*

ANTICIPATED DISCHARGE TO _____
ON OR ABOUT _____UNDER CARE OF DOCTOR _____

F.   COORDINATION OF INFORMATION: *Note exactly where information can be located (e.g., "Nursing Care Plan" or "Form 111")*
__Initial **assessment** of discharge risks can be found: _____
__Further details of continuing care **needs and plans** can be found: _____
__Details of **teaching** planned and/or completed can be found: _____
__Copies of **referrals** or detailed plans can be found: _____

PLAN INITIATED BY _____ON _____. UPDATED: _____

INTRODUCTION TO DETAILED NEEDS
IDENTIFICATION

The acute care of the patient who will probably or certainly need the resources of residential care typically involves caregivers from several disciplines. Specialist physicians, a social worker, members of the discharge planning team, and perhaps a clergyman or pyschologist as well as nursing staff all may have intense input to the decision-making and planning stages of the discharge planning process. As they work with the patient and the family, it is essential that they not lose their focus on the patient and his or her specific and individual needs. Early identification and recording of those needs help everyone better coordinate the help they offer.

The Detailed Needs Identification form is one approach to gathering and recording complete information. The reader will notice that spaces are left on Form 15 for making individualized comments about specific patient needs. More than one choice may be appropriate to some items. The subject areas that are included parallel those listed in the second section of the Discharge Planning Summary. It is especially helpful to colleagues if the nurse notes with an arrow (↑ or ↓) those items that are changing rapidly or are likely to change for better or worse in the near future. The Needs Identification focuses on realistic *anticipation* of what can and should be done to help both patient and family decide on and arrange the appropriate level of care following discharge.

A suggested format for recording information is shown on Form 15. Form 16 defines each option shown on Form 15 and describes specific information that may be important to the patient's continuing care. Many aspects of the patient's strengths and resources are included. For nurses who are unfamiliar with discharge planning, these definitions and descriptions provide a basis for understanding the kinds and quality of information that have important implications for the patient's future well-being. Nurses are encouraged to read through the descriptive material and then use it in conjunction with the first few discharge plans they complete. When working with real patient situations and commonly experienced time limitations, the nurse will find that some items are inappropriate or too time-consuming to pursue. Should the nurse choose to skip an item, it is helpful to note whether it is "N.A." (Not Applicable) or "Unk." (Unknown).

In addition to providing details of patient needs for caregivers in the acute care setting so that they might better help the patient and family plan continuing care, a form such as this is extremely valuable to caregivers in the residential facility who will be working with the patient. Of course, sharing such information must be with the full consent of the patient, and all aspects of professional confidentiality must be observed.

FORM 15. *DETAILED NEEDS IDENTIFICATION FOR* _____
I.D. _____

*INSTRUCTIONS: Check all appropriate options for each item. Note with an arrow
(↑ or ↓) items now changing or expected to change.*

1. ACTIVITIES OF DAILY LIVING:

A. EATING	B. DRESSING	C. BATHING	D. ORAL CARE
___Indep.	___Indep.	___Indep.	___Indep.
___Super.	___Super.	___Super.	___Super.
___Help	___Help	___Help	___Help
___Total care	___Total care	___Total care	___Total care

2. SENSES:

A. VISION	B. HEARING	C. TOUCH	D. TASTE/SMELL
___Full dist.	___Normal	___Normal	___Normal
___Full close	___Aided	___Deficit	___Deficit
___Deficit	___Deficit		
___Under Rx	___Under Rx		

3. COMMUNICATION:

A. SPEECH	B. READING	C. WRITING	D. RESP. TO CARE
___Normal	___Normal	___Normal	___Pos.
___Deficit	___Deficit	___Deficit	___Guard.
___Lang. dif.	___Non-Eng.	___Left-handed	___Upset
			___Neg./hostile

4. MOBILITY:

A. TRANSFER	B. AMBULA-TION	C. GROOMING	D. LEISURE ACTIV.
___Indep.		___Indep.	___Conversation
___Equip.	___Indep.	___Super.	___Music
___Help	___Equip.	___Help	___Crafts
___Confined to bed	___Help	___Total care	___Other: _____
	___Non-amb.		

5. ELIMINATION/SKIN:

A. BLADDER	B. BOWELS	C. SKIN CONDITION
___Continent	___Continent	___Good
___Help	___Regular	___Fragile
___Incont.	___Help	___Spec. care/extrem.
___Frequen.	___Lax./Soft.	___Spec. care/pressure
___Fluid def.	___Incont.	___Open areas/Rx.

Form continued on following page

FORM 15 *Continued*

6. MENTAL STATE:

A. COGNITION	B. AWARE OF	C. MEMORY	D. DECISION
—Normal/alert	CARE NEEDS	—Good	MAKING
—Diminished	—Aware of prog.	—Short	—Involved
—Variable	—Prior resid. care	—Variable	—Near ready
—Poor concen.	—Realistic	—Poor	—Unready
—Disorient.	—Unrealistic		—Optimistic
	—Unaware		—Pessimistic

7. PATTERNS AND HABITS:

A. NUTRITION	B. SLEEP	C. TOBACCO	D. ALCOHOL/
—Good	—Good	—Non-user	DRUGS
—Limited	—Poor	—Lt./mod. use	—Non-user
—Spec. diet	—Interrupted	—Hvy. use	—Lt./mod. alco.
—Overweight	—Naps	—Adv. to stop	—Alcohol prob.
—Underweight			—Reg. drugs
			—Drug prob.

8. SOCIAL SITUATION:

A. FAMILY	B. COMMUNITY	C. RESPONSE	D. SPECIAL
INVOLVEMENT	SUPPORT	TO VISITORS	GROUP
—Active	—Soc. groups	—Positive	—Minority
—Realistic	—Rel. groups	—Guarded	—Handicap
—Supportive	—Involved friends	—Upset	—Poor skills
—Limited	—Few friends	—Neg./hostile	—Adjust. prob.
—Not avail.	—No support	—Little or none	
—No support			

9. CONTINUING CARE:

A. NURSING	B. EQUIPMENT	C. FINANCIAL	D. COVER. FOR
CARE	—Indoor mobil.	SITUATION	CARE
—None	—Outdoor mobil.	—Supported	—Medicare/-aid
—Minimal	—Ventilation	—Pension or aid	—Pvt. insur.
—Skilled	—Communication	—Savings	—No insur.
—Rehab.	—Other: _____	—Other sources	—Indep. funds
—Custodial		—Uncertain	—Fam. funds

Needs Identification completed by _____ on _____. Updated: _____

FORM 16. *DETAILED NEEDS IDENTIFICATION—DEFINITIONS AND DESCRIPTIONS*

Instructions: Check all appropriate descriptions on Detailed Needs Identification Form adding notes for clarification as needed.

1. ACTIVITIES OF DAILY LIVING (ADL)

A. EATING:
- (Indep.) — Feeds self.
- (Super.) — Needs to be supervised while eating. *Specify level of supervision needed.*
- (Help) — Needs help with certain foods or drink. *Specify kinds of help needed.*
- (Total care) — Needs to be fed. *Note food preferences.*

B. DRESSING:
- (Indep.) — Selects appropriate clothing and dresses self.
- (Super.) — Needs supervision while dressing. *Specify whether clothing must be selected or level of supervision.*
- (Help) — Needs help with certain clothing or fasteners. *Specify kinds of help needed. Note right- or left-handedness.*
- (Total care) — Needs to be dressed. *Note clothing preferences.*

C. BATHING:
- (Indep.) — Bathes self. *Note whether patient regularly takes tub, shower, or sponge baths.*
- (Super.) — Needs supervision while bathing. *Specify reason for and level of supervision needed.*
- (Help) — Needs help preparing for bath or while bathing. *Specify kinds of help needed.*
- (Total care) — Needs to be bathed. *Note frequency and preferred time of baths.*

D. ORAL CARE:
- (Indep.) — Able to brush and floss teeth without help. *Note whether person has dentures or whether special oral care procedures are used.*
- (Super.) — Needs supervision during oral care procedures. *Specify reason for and level of supervision needed.*
- (Help) — Needs help with oral care. *Specify kind of help needed.*
- (Total care) — Unable to perform own oral care. *Note kinds of care to be given and frequency. Note preferences for oral care equipment and products.*

2. SENSES

A. VISION:
- (Full dist.) — Normal or fully corrected distance vision. *Note whether glasses or contacts are used.*
- (Full close) — Normal or corrected close (reading) vision. *Note whether glasses or contacts are used.*
- (Deficit) — Patient has limited vision. *Specify kind and severity of deficit.*
- (Under Rx) — Under care for deficit or resulting handicap. *Specify nature of care, frequency, and name of caregiver.*

Form continued on following page

FORM 16 *Continued*

B. HEARING:	(Normal)	Able to hear normal speech.
	(Aided)	Uses a hearing aid.
		Note kind, frequency of use, and whether help is needed.
	(Deficit)	Hearing is limited.
		Specify kind and severity of deficit. Note how deficit is managed or overcome.
	(Under Rx)	Under care for deficit or resulting handicap.
		Specify nature of care, frequency, and name of caregiver.
C. TOUCH:	(Normal)	Has normal touch sensations.
	(Deficit)	Sense of touch is limited.
		Specify nature of deficit and part of body involved. Note how deficit is managed or overcome.
D. TASTE/ SMELL:	(Normal)	Normal taste and smell sensations.
	(Deficit)	Taste or smell sensations are limited.
		Specify nature and severity of deficit. Note how deficit is managed or overcome.

3. COMMUNICATION

A. SPEECH:	(Normal)	Able to express self understandably in English.
		Note any hesitation to express needs, desires, or emotions.
	(Deficit)	Has a speech impediment or aphasia.
		Specify nature and severity of difficulty.
	(Lang. dif.)	Speaks with accent or hard to understand.
		Specify degree of language difficulty and what language is preferred by patient.
		Note how difficulty is managed or overcome.
B. READING:	(Normal)	Able to read English in newspaper-sized print.
		Note apparent strength of interest in reading and preferred subjects.
	(Deficit)	Has physical or educational handicap that limits reading ability.
		Specify nature and severity of limitation.
	(Non-Eng.)	Reads in language other than English.
		Note language preference and apparent strength of interest in reading.
C. WRITING:	(Normal)	Able to write legible English.
		Note whether writing is an especially important form of communication to the patient.
	(Deficit)	Has physical or educational handicap that limits writing ability.
		Specify nature and severity of limitation.
	(Left-handed)	Prefers using left hand for writing and other tasks.
D. RESP. TO CARE:	(Pos.)	Has mostly positive attitudes toward care and caregivers.
		Note words listed or others that describe patient's dominant attitudes:
		friendly, cooperative, alert, active in care, forms relationships easily.
	(Guard.)	Uses mostly guarded, defensive, or passive responses to care or caregivers.
		Note whether there are variations in response and under what circumstances.

FORM 16 *Continued*

	(Upset)	Seems upset by care and caregivers. *Note words listed or others that describe patient's dominant attitudes: disoriented, easily confused, nervous, embarrassed, demanding, depressed. Note any known factors that may contribute to patient's attitudes.*
	(Neg./hostile)	Has mostly negative attitudes toward care and caregivers. *Note words listed or others that describe patient's dominant attitudes: angry, uncooperative, critical, distrustful, withdrawn.*

4. MOBILITY

A. TRANSFER:	(Indep.)	Able to transfer from bed to chair or chair to chair without help.
	(Equip.)	Uses special equipment to aid transfer. *Specify kind of equipment used (rail, walker, special chairs, etc.).*
	(Help)	Needs help to transfer. *Specify kind of help needed and weight-bearing limitations of patient.*
	(Confined to bed)	Unable to be out of bed at all. *Note reason for confinement and whether temporary or long-term.*
B. AMBULA-TION:	(Indep.)	Able to ambulate by self and climb stairs. *Note any time or distance restrictions.*
	(Equip.)	Uses special equipment to aid ambulation. *Specify kind of equipment used (walker, crutches, cane, braces, elastic stockings). Note if patient uses wheelchair all or part time.*
	(Help)	Needs help with ambulation. *Specify kind and amount of help needed and weight-bearing limitations. Note usual schedule and destination of ambulation.*
	(Non-amb.)	Not ambulatory.
C. GROOMING:	(Indep.)	Able to comb and shampoo hair, shave, or apply makeup without help.
	(Super.)	Needs supervision during grooming activities. *Specify reason for and level of supervision needed.*
	(Help)	Needs help with grooming activities. *Specify activity and kind of help needed. Note right- or left-handedness.*
	(Total care)	Unable to groom self. *Note preferences and frequency of activities.*
D. LEISURE ACTIVITIES:	(Conversation)	Enjoys participating in conversation with family, friends, or acquaintances. *Note any especially favored topics and limitations on ability to hold conversation.*
	(Music)	Enjoys listening to, playing an instrument, or dancing to music. *Note degree of activity or involvement in musical events.*

Form continued on following page

FORM 16 Continued

	(Crafts)	Enjoys participating in handcrafts or other creative activities. *Note kinds of crafts favored and estimate of fine-muscle control.*
	(Other)	*Specify other leisure activities enjoyed by patient.*

5. ELIMINATION/SKIN

A. BLADDER:	(Continent)	Has full bladder control. Note approximate daily output.
	(Help)	Needs help in using equipment or getting to toilet. *Specify kind of help needed and frequency. Note any special equipment required such as high toilet seat, urinal, bedpan, or catheter.*
	(Incont.)	Patient is incontinent of urine. *Specify under what conditions incontinence occurs and how usually managed.*
	(Frequen.)	Patient urinates frequently enough to disturb daytime activities or sleep. *Note approximate frequency of urination and probable cause.*
	(Fluid def.)	Needs assistance in getting appropriate level of fluid intake. *Specify nature of fluid deficit and how it is usually managed.*
B. BOWELS:	(Continent)	Has bowel control and regular bowel habits.
	(Regular)	Has regular pattern of bowel movements. *Note frequency of bowel movements and usual time of day.*
	(Help)	Needs help in getting to the toilet or using special equipment. *Specify kind of help or equipment needed (toilet seat, commode, bedpan).*
	(Lax./Soft.)	Uses laxatives, stool softeners, special foods, or procedures to improve regularity. *Note when and how frequently special foods or medications, laxatives, enemas, etc., are used.*
	(Incont.)	Patient is incontinent. *Specify under what conditions incontinence occurs and how usually managed.*
C. SKIN COND.:	(Good)	Skin is in good condition with normal color. *Note any exceptions to otherwise good condition.*
	(Fragile)	Skin in basically good condition but is easily damaged or is sensitive. *Specify in what ways skin condition is damaged.*
	(Sp. care/ext.)	Skin on arms, legs, hands, or feet requires special care to maintain good condition. *Specify any areas of skin breakdown and treatments or procedures presently used.*
	(Sp. care/pres.)	Skin on coccyx, heels, elbows, shoulders, or head requires special care to prevent breakdown. *Specify any areas of skin breakdown and treatments or procedures presently used.*

FORM 16 *Continued*

(Open areas/Rx) There are presently open areas (decubitus, abrasions, incisions) under treatment. *Specify area involved, current treatment or procedures, and anticipated healing time.*

6. MENTAL STATE
A. COGNITION: (Normal) — Ability to think and reason normal.
(Diminished) — Ability to think and reason clearly is diminished. *Note probable cause and evidence used to make this judgment.*
(Variable) — Alertness and ability to reason varies. *Note any observable pattern to variation and probable causes.*
(Poor concen.) — Able to reason normally but has short attention span or poor ability to concentrate. *Note probable cause and evidence used to make this judgment.*
(Disorient.) — Mentally confused or disoriented as to time, person, or place. *Note any variations in disorientation.*

B. AWARE OF CARE NEEDS: (Aware of prog.) — Aware of prognosis and its consequences for future health care. *Note words listed or others that describe patient's attitude toward diagnosis/prognosis: optimistic, pessimistic, depressed, uninterested, angry, passive, anxious.*
(Prior resid.) — Previously in residential care. *Specify name of facility and level of care provided. Note whether patient expects to return there.*
(Realistic) — Mostly uses reality-based thinking when discussing continuing care.
(Unreal.) — Expresses unrealistic goals, plans, or fears related to continuing care. *Specify nature of unrealistic thinking and note how others have responded to this.*
(Unaware) — Not able to understand prognosis or consequences. *Note reason for inability and whether family members or friends are aware.*

C. MEMORY: (Good) — Both short- and long-term memory seem to be within normal limits.
(Short) — Able to recall facts or ideas for only a short period of time. *Note nature of memory difficulty and whether problem existed prior to acute episode.*
(Variable) — Memory good at times, poor at others. *Note possible causes of variability, such as medication. Note any categories of information that seem to retained more reliably.*
(Poor) — Unable to recall facts or ideas long enough to use them effectively. *Note any known causes for poor memory and length of time problem has existed.*

Form continued on following page

FORM 16 *Continued*

D. DECISION
MAKING:

(Involved)   Actively involved in plans for continuing care.
Note a word or phrase that describes patient's involvement such as:
discussing options, making plans, organizing help.

(Near ready)   Seems ready to begin decision-making and planning about future care.
Note evidence of readiness such as asking questions or talking about previous experiences.

(Unready)   Seems as yet unable to plan for future.
Note any known factors that may contribute to lack of readiness.

(Optimistic)   Has positive attitude toward residential care.

(Pessimistic)   Has negative or unrealistic attitude toward residential care.

7. PATTERNS AND HABITS

A. NUTRITION:

(Good)   Generally well nourished.
Note usual meal and snack pattern and any supplements usually taken.

(Limited)   Nutrition limited due to food preferences or poor appetite.
Specify food preferences and ways in which these are managed.
Note reason for present poor appetite and/or appetite history.

(Spec. diet)   Receiving special diet.
Note reason for diet and expected duration.

(Overweight)   Significantly overweight for height and bone structure.
Note any recommendations that have been made regarding weight control.

(Underweight)   Significantly underweight for height and bone structure.
Note any known reasons for weight loss, duration of problem, and recommendations given.

B. SLEEP:

(Good)   Sleeps well each night and feels rested.
Note usual bed and arising times and times of naps during day.

(Poor)   Sleeps poorly and seldom feels rested.
Note probable causes of poor sleep.

(Interrupted)   Sleep is normally interrupted.
Note reason for interruption and frequency (toilet, medication, dreams, etc.)

(Naps)   Takes naps during the day.
Note usual frequency and length of naps and whether they affect nighttime sleep.

C. TOBACCO:

(Non-user)   Does not now or never has used tobacco.
Note whether patient ever has used tobacco and in what form.

(Lt./mod. use)   Smokes up to one pack of cigarettes per day or uses other forms of tobacco.
Note what form of tobacco is used, usual consumption pattern, and duration of habit.

FORM 16 *Continued*

	(Hvy. use)	Heavy user of tobacco on a regular basis. *Note what form of tobacco is used, usual consumption pattern, and duration of habit.*
	(Adv. to stop)	Trying to stop smoking or has been advised to stop. *Note present attitudes and goals and past history of trying to stop.*
D. ALCOHOL/ DRUGS:	(Non-user)	Does not consume alcohol or use potentially addictive drugs. *Note whether patient has ever used alcohol or drugs and to what extent.*
	(Lt./mod. alco.)	Regularly consumes light to moderate amount of alcoholic beverages. *Note kind and pattern of daily consumption.*
	(Alco. prob.)	Alcohol use has been or now is a problem for patient or family. *Note severity of problem and what advice has been given about stopping.*
	(Reg. drugs)	Regularly takes tranquilizers, sedatives, narcotics, or other drugs. *Specify kind of drugs used and pattern of use.*
	(Drug prob.)	Drug use has been or now is a problem for patient or family. *Note severity of problem and what advice has been given.*

8. SOCIAL SITUATION

A. FAMILY INVOLVE-MENT:	(Active)	Family members or close friends are actively involved with patient's care and decisions. *Identify those most involved by name and relationship.*
	(Realistic)	Family members or close friends seem to have realistic expectations for patient's progress. *Note evidence of realistic thinking and role that they anticipate for themselves.*
	(Supportive)	Family members offer emotional support to patient through attention and loving concern. *Identify those most supportive by name and specify ways in which support is demonstrated.*
	(Limited)	Involvement of family or friends in patient care limited. *Note apparent reason for limited involvement by name and relationship.*
	(Not avail.)	Family not available due to geography or alienation. *Note reason for unavailability of family or friends.*
	(No support)	Family or close friends visit but give patient no encouragement or support. *Note apparent reasons for lack of encouragement or support.*
B. COMMUNITY SUPPORT:	(Soc. groups)	Has been active in community social groups or organizations. *Specify groups and note level of involvement.*

Form continued on following page

FORM 16 *Continued*

	(Rel. groups)	Has been active in religious groups or activities. *Specify groups and any implications for future care.*
	(Involved friends)	Friends visit regularly and seem actively involved with patient's well-being. *Note identity of any particularly involved.*
	(Few friends)	Seems to have a limited social support network or speaks of self as having few friends. *Note apparent reason for limited friendships such as personality, frequent moves, etc.*
	(No support)	No evidence of community involvement with patient or support.
C. RESPONSE TO VISITORS:	(Positive)	Mostly pleased to have visitors and interacts positively with them. *Note any exceptions that have been observed.*
	(Guarded)	Uses mostly guarded, defensive, or passive responses with visitors. *Note whether there are variations in response and under what circumstances.*
	(Upset)	Seems upset with visitors. *Note words listed or others that describe patient's dominant attitudes: disoriented, easily confused, nervous, embarrassed, demanding, depressed. Note any known factors that may contribute to patient's attitudes.*
	(Neg./hostile)	Has mostly negative attitudes toward visitors. *Note words listed or others that describe patient's dominant attitudes: angry, uncooperative, critical, distrustful, withdrawn.*
	(Little or none)	Gives little or no response to visitors. *Note probable reasons for lack of response, e.g., does not recognize, disoriented, etc.*
D. SPECIAL GROUP:	(Minority)	Belongs to minority cultural or ethnic group that influences patient's language, diet, life-style, or values. *Specify group and anticipated impact on future care.*
	(Handicap)	Has a physical or mental handicap that limits activities or interaction. *Specify nature of handicap and limitations imposed by it.*
	(Poor skills)	Has poor social skills that act to limit relationships with others. *Note whether personality, mental state, social isolation, or other factors have contributed.*
	(Adjust. prob.)	It is anticipated that special help will be needed in adjusting to residential care. *Note kind of help needed and by whom.*
9. CONTINUING CARE A. NURSING CARE:	(None)	No need for nursing care anticipated. *Note any treatments or procedures that will be done by the patient.*
	(Minimal)	Nursing care needs are minimal and/or are expected to continue for only a short time. *Specify kind of care needed and how long need is anticipated to continue.*

FORM 16 *Continued*

(Skilled) — Need for skilled nursing care is anticipated. *Specify kind of care needed and how long need is anticipated to continue.*

(Rehab.) — Need for rehabilitation care (e.g., physical therapy) in addition to nursing care is anticipated. *Specify what kind of care will be needed and the goal of rehabilitation care.*

(Custodial) — Need for long-term custodial care (e.g., assistance with ADLs) is anticipated. *Specify level of care needed.*

B. EQUIPMENT: (Indoor mobil.) — Needs assistive equipment to improve mobility or safety indoors. *Specify kinds of equipment or aids.*

(Outdoor mobil.) — Needs assistive equipment to improve mobility or safety outdoors. *Specify kinds of equipment or aids.*

(Ventilation) — Needs assistive equipment to improve or monitor breathing. *Specify kinds of equipment or aids.*

(Communi-cation) — Needs assistive equipment to aid communication. *Specify kinds of equipment or aids.*

(Other) — *Specify other kinds of equipment or aids needed.*

C. FINANCIAL SITUATION: (Supported) — Has full financial support. *Specify source of support and note any relevant details about level of support.*

(Pension or aid) — Receives Social Security, retirement pension, disability, welfare, or other financial aid. *Specify source of pension or aid and note whether income is adequate for expected needs.*

(Savings) — Patient and/or spouse have savings that will be considered when arranging residential care. *Note whether patient expects to use savings to finance care.*

(Other sources) — Has other sources of income such as investments. *Note any relevant details about these sources and whether they will influence residential care.*

(Uncertain) — Source of support or income now uncertain. *Note reasons for uncertainty and whether help is needed in applying for aid.*

D. COVERAGE FOR CARE: (Medicare/-aid) — Eligible for continuing care benefits from Medicare and/or Medicaid. *Note present status and extent of benefits.*

(Pvt. insur.) — Eligible for private insurance benefits for residential care. *Note present status and extent of benefits.*

(No insurance) — Has no insurance coverage for residential care. *Note whether financial counseling and/or assistance is needed and by whom.*

(Indep. funds) — Has access to independent means of financing residential care. *Note whether funds are likely to be adequate for needs.*

(Fam. funds) — Members of family will contribute to residential care costs. *Note who is acting as financial coordinator.*

MAKING A TEACHING PLAN

When it is anticipated that long-term or residential care will be needed to meet post-hospital patient needs, the focus of the patient and family teaching program is to help them through a problem solving process. By learning how to identify and understand needs for care and by developing realistic goals for the patient, they are able to actively participate in deciding among available options. A plan for residential care has both an emotional side for patient and family and a practical side involving choices about finances and the quality of care. There is a great deal of information that needs to be heard and understood in an emotional environment that sometimes limits learning ability. The following Discharge Teaching Plan (Form 17) is designed to help caregivers identify areas of learning needs and construct learning objectives quickly. These objectives then become the framework for patient and family teaching. The subjects on this form parallel those indicated in the third section of the Discharge Plan Summary.

Remember that the only useful learning objectives are REALISTIC ones. They should be attainable in the time available, and the desired behavior should be observable by the teacher(s).

Elements of Form 17 are described below.

Identification of Learners. Those people who are to be included in some or all teaching sessions are listed across the top of the form. The nurse may want to write the telephone numbers of visitor-learners, as well as their names, to simplify coordination. Where notations are made about a learner other than the patient, they may be referred to by number. For example, the motivation of the patient may be "developing," but for learner "#2" it may be already "present".

Subject of Teaching. Eight common subjects for discharge teaching have been listed on the form. The nurse may indicate that teaching in this subject area is not needed. If it is needed, the next three lines provide a record of teaching progress from planning through evaluation. Updating the teaching plan by checking the description that currently applies to teaching in each subject area will alert other caregivers to what has been done. They can then actively cooperate with the learning process by stimulating further patient interest in the subject and reinforcing learning. Following the completion of teaching, learning may be evaluated through tests, verbal questions, demonstrations, or other methods. Verifying that an objective has been successfully reached is positive feedback for both teacher and learner.

Motivation. Attention to a person's motivation to learn particular subjects is extremely important to effective and efficient teaching. If motivation is poor, the nurse will want to work on this before attempting to teach content in an area. Changes in motivation can be recorded with a check or an arrow. When several learners are involved, those with more motivation may be able to help the others understand the importance of the subject.

Prior Knowledge or Experience. A short phrase is usually enough to record the basis on which new learning can be built. Finding out what a learner already knows about a subject takes only moments, but it allows the teacher to start with relevant material, thereby improving both motivation and learning ability. It is best not to make any assumptions about what the learner knows; a person may have visited friends at a particular residential facility but know very little about what professional services are offered there.

Learning Objective. The construction of learning objectives is a simple but often unfamiliar activity to those who are not full-time teachers. An objective or learning goal starts with the phrase *"The learner will be able to . . . "* This is followed by a verb indicating the **level of complexity** at which learning must take place. To "adapt" learning to different situations is, for example, much more complex than simply "remembering" it. We have suggested a number of possible words that may be used.

Next, a learning objective defines the **specific subject** of concern and states what kind of **behavior** is expected as a result of learning. Remember that the stated behavior must be observable in the time available, and therefore objectives for learning in acute care settings will necessarily be short-term and limited. The ultimate goal in teaching a person about investigating residential facilities, for example, might be for that person to weigh all available information logically and reach the best possible decision about continuing care. A realistic learning objective while in the hospital, however, might be for the person to list important criteria and and cooperate with a family member who can visit the available options. Finally, writing down a **time** for learning to be completed gives both learners and teachers a target toward which to work.

Notes. Noting what teaching approaches have been used, (for example, "videotape on custodial care shown") and the response learners have had to them, the priority given certain subjects, and plans for learning evaluation are all important pieces of information to share with other caregivers. Current notes kept in a known location are essential when several teachers are involved or learning needs are complex.

FORM 17. *DISCHARGE TEACHING PLAN FOR:* _____

OTHER THAN PATIENT, THOSE TO BE INVOLVED AS LEARNERS
INCLUDE: *(Note name and relationship to patient.)*
#1:   #2:   #3:

1. MEDICAL NEEDS:
   Teaching: __not needed   Motivation: __present   Prior knowledge/
             __planned   __developing experience: _____
             __in progress   __poor
             __learning   _____
             evaluated

   Learner will be able to: _____ By _____
                            (level)   (specific subject)   (behavior)   (date)
   (e.g., remember, understand, apply information, make decisions about)

2. POST-HOSPITAL NURSING NEEDS:
   Teaching: __not needed   Motivation: __present   Prior knowledge/
             __planned   __developing experience: _____
             __in progress   __poor
             __learning   _____
             evaluated

   Learner will be able to: _____ By _____
                            (level)   (specific subject)   (behavior)   (date)
   (e.g., remember, understand, apply information, respond, evaluate,
                                                make decisions about)

3. NUTRITIONAL NEEDS:
   Teaching: __not needed   Motivation: __present   Prior knowledge/
             __planned   __developing experience: _____
             __in progress   __poor
             __learning   _____
             evaluated

   Learner will be able to: _____ By _____
                            (level)   (specific subject)   (behavior)   (date)
   (e.g., remember, understand, apply information, respond, evaluate)

4. PROGNOSIS/COMPLICATION MANAGEMENT:
   Teaching: __not needed   Motivation: __present   Prior knowledge/
             __planned   __developing experience: _____
             __in progress   __poor
             __learning   _____
             evaluated

   Learner will be able to: _____ By _____
                            (level)   (specific subject)   (behavior)   (date)
   (e.g., remember, understand, apply information, make decisions about, adapt)

5. OPTIONS FOR CONTINUING CARE:
   Teaching: __not needed   Motivation: __present   Prior knowledge/
             __planned   __developing experience: _____
             __in progress   __poor
             __learning   _____
             evaluated
   Learner will be able to: _____ By _____
                            (level)   (specific subject)   (behavior)   (date)
   (e.g., remember, understand, apply information, evaluate, make decisions about)

FORM 17 *Continued*

6. FINANCIAL ASPECTS OF CARE:
   Teaching: __not needed   Motivation: __present   Prior knowledge/
   __planned   __developing experience: _____
   __in progress   __poor
   __learning   _____
   evaluated

   Learner will be able to: _____ By _____
                            (level)   (specific subject)   (behavior)   (date)
                    (e.g., understand, evaluate, adapt, make decisions about)

7. EMOTIONAL/SOCIAL ASPECTS OF TRANSITION:
   Teaching: __not needed   Motivation: __present   Prior knowledge/
   __planned   __developing experience: _____
   __in progress   __poor
   __learning   _____
   evaluated

   Learner will be able to: _____ By _____
                            (level)   (specific subject)   (behavior)   (date)
              (e.g., remember, understand, evaluate, apply information, realistically plan)

8. COMMUNITY RESOURCES:
   Teaching: __not needed   Motivation: __present   Prior knowledge/
   __planned   __developing experience: _____
   __in progress   __poor
   __learning   _____
   evaluated

   Learner will be able to: _____ By _____
                            (level)   (specific subject)   (behavior)   (date)
                  (e.g., remember, understand, apply information, plan, utilize)

9. OTHER LEARNING OBJECTIVES:
   Learner will be able to _____ by _____

   Learner will be able to _____ by _____

Teaching Plan initiated by _____on _____

NOTES ON TEACHING (what was taught, methods/materials used, response, etc.)

B/5

How to Build a Plan for Terminal Care

It is always emotionally difficult for caregivers to acknowledge that the disease process is likely to overwhelm their best efforts, but of course, we have learned that denial of a terminal condition is no favor to the patient or family. A major contribution can be made by the nurse who helps the patient face the realities of impending death and plan with family and friends for the kinds of support wanted and needed.

There are a number of options that may be available to these patients. They may be able to remain at home or at the home of a relative for the terminal period. There they might receive the services of a home care agency or a home-based hospice service. Some communities have residential hospice care, while in others, a nursing home or hospital are the only options for residential care.

The challenge of building a plan for terminal care is to help patients retain as much control over planning and their own care management as possible. Although they may make choices that seem wrong or irrational to caregivers, it is the caregivers' responsibility to allow them that independence and, within economic and legal limits, to implement their plans.

The nurse's involvement in planning revolves around three principal activities: identification of needs, patient and family teaching, and emotional support during decision-making. Four separate but coordinated forms are presented in this section that will help the nurse plan these activities early in the patient's acute care. They are:

- the Discharge Plan Summary,
- a Detailed Needs Identification and associated Definitions and Descriptions, and
- a Discharge Teaching Plan.

Together they make it possible to record comprehensive information relevant to the discharge planning process with ease and clarity so that it is easily shared by caregivers who can, as a result, better coordinate their efforts.

A written **Discharge Plan** is a method used for communication and coordination of effort among caregivers. It is also appropriately used to involve patients and their family members in the discharge planning process by including them in the gathering of data and the clarification of objectives and priorities. Form 18 represents a *summary* of information collected from several sources and combined to give an overview of professional intervention. It is designed to reflect the progression of need identification, patient and family teaching, and decision-making about plans for continuing care. It should be begun as early in the patient's care as possible and updated regularly so that caregivers have a clear picture of the state of the discharge planning process. Especially important is information about where in the patient's medical record more detailed information can be located. This item alone can save caregivers a great deal of time and frustration.

In addition to the summary, guidance is given for completing a **Detailed Needs Identification** using the associated **Definitions and Descriptions** (Forms 19 and 20). The comprehensive information they contain helps caregivers understand many dimensions of the patient's needs allowing them to give more sensitive support for the decision-making process.

It is often unclear early in a patient's acute care whether their discharge destination will be their own home, the home of a relative, or a residential facility, although it may be quite clear that they will need intensive help wherever they go. One of the first steps in helping patients and their families decide among their options is to help them learn realistically what to expect in terms of length and quality of life and manner of death. They also need help with learning about the financial aspects of various options and how to appropriately use the help offered by health care professionals. It is important that teaching begin early so that both patient and family have time to deal with the emotional as well as practical issues. We have suggested a **Teaching Plan** (Form 21) that will help nurses organize appropriate teaching and coordinate these with the efforts of their medical and nursing colleagues. Together, these approaches ensure that caregivers have a comprehensive "picture" of the patient and his or her continuing care needs.

FORM 18. *DISCHARGE PLAN SUMMARY FOR:* _____

PATIENT IDENTIFICATION NO.: _____UNIT/ROOM: _____

GENERAL GOAL: Management of the terminal phase of illness and as pain-free and dignified death as possible.

A. SPECIAL SERVICES DURING ACUTE CARE:
Note with + those that will/may need to be continued AFTER discharge.

____None
____Intensive care
____Isolation
____Surgery
____Blood transfusion

____Radiation therapy
____Respiratory therapy
____Physical therapy
____Occupational therapy
____Speech therapy
____Mental health/
psychiatric

____Discharge planning
team
____Patient/family
counseling
____Social services
____Financial assistance
____Other: _____

B. IDENTIFICATION OF RISKS/DEFICITS: Patient's age is _____
Note limitations expected to continue AFTER discharge.
*Note with * those risks present BEFORE admission.*

____No special risks
identified
____Activities of daily
living
____Senses
____Communication
____Mobility

____Bladder/bowels
____Skin condition
____Mental state
____Social situation
____Financial situation

C. TEACHING NEEDED FOR PATIENT OR FAMILY IN SUBJECTS OF:
____No separate teaching plan
Note names and phone numbers of family or others involved in teaching.

____Medical needs
____in progress
____completed
____Treatments/procedures
____in progress
____completed
____Nutritional needs
____in progress
____completed

____Pain management
____in progress
____completed
____Prognosis/crisis manag.
____in progress
____completed
____Financial/legal planning
____in progress
____completed

____Emot./soc. aspects of
care
____in progress
____completed
____Community services
____in progress
____completed
____Other: _____
____in progress
____completed

FORM 18 *Continued*

D. POST-HOSPITAL SERVICES: ___None needed.
Medical follow-up by:

_____

| **Home/Resid. care:** | ___Needed | ___Decision in progress |

Referral made to _____on _____by _____
Special Equipment: ___Needed   ___Decision in progress

Referral made to _____on _____by _____
Ment. Hlth./Couns.   ___Needed   ___Decision in progress

Referral made to _____on _____by _____
Social Services: ___Needed   ___Decision in progress

Referral made to _____on _____by _____
Financial assist.:   ___Needed   ___Decision in progress

Referral made to _____on _____by _____

Note details of services needed, options considered, and agencies/caregivers involved. Continue on back of sheet if needed.

E. SPECIFIC OBJECTIVES OF CONTINUING CARE: *Detail plans and goals of care.*

ANTICIPATED DISCHARGE TO _____
ON OR ABOUT _____UNDER CARE OF DOCTOR _____

F. COORDINATION OF INFORMATION: *Note exactly where information can be located (e.g., "Nursing Care Plan" or "Form 111")*
___Initial **assessment** of discharge risks can be found: _____
___Further details of continuing care **needs and plans** can be found: _____
___Details of **teaching** planned and/or completed can be found: _____
___Copies of **referrals** or detailed plans can be found: _____

PLAN INITIATED BY: _____ON: _____. UPDATED: _____

INTRODUCTION TO DETAILED NEEDS
IDENTIFICATION

Planning the discharge of a terminally ill person typically involves caregivers from several disciplines. Specialist physicians, a social worker, members of the discharge planning team, and perhaps a clergyman or pyschologist as well as nursing staff all may have intense input to the decision-making and planning stages of the discharge planning process. As they work with both patient and family, it is essential that they not lose their focus on the patient and his or her specific and individual needs and preferences. Early identification and recording of those needs help provide baseline information against which changes in condition can be measured and prognosis more realistically assessed.

The Detailed Needs Identification form is one approach to gathering and recording complete information. The reader will notice that spaces are left on Form 19 for making individualized comments about specific patient needs. More than one choice may be appropriate to some items. The subject areas that are included parallel those listed in the second section of the Discharge Planning Summary. It is especially helpful to colleagues if the nurse notes with an arrow (↑ or ↓) those items that are changing rapidly or are likely to change for better or worse in the near future. The Needs Identification focuses on realistic **anticipation** of what can and should be done to help patient and family decide on and arrange the appropriate level of care following discharge.

A suggested format for recording information is shown on Form 19. Form 20 defines each option shown on Form 19 and describes specific information that may be important to the patient's continuing care. Many aspects of the patient's strengths and resources are included. For nurses who are unfamiliar with discharge planning, these definitions and descriptions provide a basis for understanding the kinds and quality of information that have important implications for the patient's future well-being. Nurses are encouraged to read through the descriptive material and then use it in conjunction with the first few discharge plans they complete. When working with real patient situations and commonly experienced time limitations, the nurse will find that some items are inappropriate or too time-consuming to pursue. Should the nurse choose to skip an item, it is helpful to note whether it is "N.A." (Not Applicable) or "Unk." (Unknown).

In addition to providing details of patient needs for caregivers in the acute care setting so that they might better help both patient and family plan for continuing care, a form such as this is extremely valuable to caregivers in the community who will provide care and support. Of course, sharing such information must be with the full consent of the patient, and all aspects of professional confidentiality must be observed.

FORM 19. *DETAILED NEEDS IDENTIFICATION FOR* _____ *I.D.* _____

INSTRUCTIONS: Check all appropriate options for each item. Note with an arrow (↑ or ↓) items now changing or expected to change.

1. ACTIVITIES OF DAILY LIVING:

A. EATING	B. DRESSING	C. BATHING	D. ORAL CARE
___Indep.	___Indep.	___Indep.	___Indep.
___Super.	___Super.	___Super.	___Super.
___Help	___Help	___Help	___Help
___Total care	___Total care	___Total care	___Total care

2. SENSES:

A. VISION	B. HEARING	C. TOUCH	D. TASTE/SMELL
___Full dist.	___Normal	___Normal	___Normal
___Full close	___Aided	___Deficit	___Deficit
___Deficit	___Deficit		
___Under Rx	___Under Rx		

3. COMMUNICATION:

A. SPEECH	B. READING	C. WRITING	D. RESP. TO CARE
___Normal	___Normal	___Normal	___Pos.
___Deficit	___Deficit	___Deficit	___Guard.
___Lang. dif.	___Non-Eng.	___Left-handed	___Upset
			___Neg./hostile

4. MOBILITY:

A. TRANSFER	B. AMB.	C. GROOMING	D. ACTIVITIES
___Indep.	___Indep.	___Indep.	___Conversation
___Equip.	___Equip.	___Super.	___Music
___Help	___Help	___Help	___Crafts
___Confined to bed	___Non-amb.	___Total care	___Other:_____

5. ELIMINATION/SKIN:

A. BLADDER	B. BOWELS	C. SKIN CONDITION
___Continent	___Continent	___Good
___Help	___Regular	___Fragile
___Incont.	___Help	___Spec. care/extrem.
___Frequen.	___Lax. Soft.	___Spec. care/pres.
___Fluid def.	___Incont.	___Open areas/Rx.

6. MENTAL STATE:

A. COGNITION	B. AWARENESS	C. MEMORY	D. DECISION MAKING
___Normal/alert	___Aware of prog.	___Good	___Involved
___Diminished	___Decided prefer.	___Short	___Near ready
___Variable	___Realistic	___Variable	___Unready
___Poor concen.	___Unrealistic	___Poor	___Optimistic
___Disorient.	___Unaware		___Pessimistic

Form continued on following page

FORM 19 *Continued*

7. PATTERNS AND HABITS:

A. NUTRITION	B. SLEEP	C. TOBACCO	D. ALCOHOL/ DRUGS
__Good	__Good	__Non-user	__Non-user
__Limited	__Poor	__Lt./mod. use	__Lt./mod. alco.
__Spec. diet	__Interrupted	__Hvy. use	__Alcohol prob.
__Overweight	__Naps	__Adv. to stop	__Reg. drugs
__Underweight			__Drug prob.

8. SOCIAL SITUATION:

A. FAMILY INVOLVEMENT	B. COMMUNITY SUPPORT	C. LIVING SITUATION	D. FINANCIAL SITUATION
__Active	__Soc. groups	__Ret. to former	__Medicare/-aid
__Realistic	__Rel. groups	__Changing	__H.M.O./pvt.
__Supportive	__Gr. support	__Shared	__No insurance
__Limited	__Involved friends	__Resid. care	__Indep. funds
__Not avail.	__Few friends	__Needs modifi.	__Fam. funds
__No support	__No support		

9. CONTINUING CARE:

A. MEDICAL SUPER.	B. NURSING CARE	C. EQUIPMENT	D. PAIN MANAGEMENT
__Reg. MD	__None	__Hosp. bed	__Oral meds
__Spec. MD	__Minimal	__Mobility aids	__I.M. meds
__Clinic	__Skilled	__Ventilation	__I.V. meds
__Other: _____	__Custodial	__Treatment sup.	__Slf-reg. pump
		__Other: ___	__Other: _____

Needs Identification completed by _____ on _____ . Updated: _____

FORM 20. *DETAILED NEEDS IDENTIFICATION—DEFINITIONS AND DESCRIPTIONS*

Instructions: Check all appropriate descriptions on Detailed Needs Identification Form, adding notes for clarification as needed.

1. ACTIVITIES OF DAILY LIVING (ADL)

A. EATING:	(Indep.)	Feeds self.
	(Super.)	Needs to be supervised while eating. *Specify level of supervision needed.*
	(Help)	Needs help with certain foods or drink. *Specify kinds of help needed.*
	(Total care)	Needs to be fed. *Note food preferences.*
B. DRESSING:	(Indep.)	Selects appropriate clothing and dresses self.
	(Super.)	Needs supervision while dressing. *Specify whether clothing must be selected or level of supervision.*
	(Help)	Needs help with certain clothing or fasteners. *Specify kinds of help needed. Note right- or left-handedness.*
	(Total care)	Needs to be dressed. *Note clothing preferences.*
C. BATHING:	(Indep.)	Bathes self. *Note whether patient regularly takes tub, shower, or sponge baths.*
	(Super.)	Needs supervision while bathing. *Specify reason for and level of supervision needed.*
	(Help)	Needs help preparing for bath or while bathing. *Specify kinds of help needed.*
	(Total care)	Needs to be bathed. *Note frequency and preferred time of baths.*
D. ORAL CARE:	(Indep.)	Able to brush and floss teeth without help. *Note whether person has dentures or whether special oral care procedures are used.*
	(Super.)	Needs supervision during oral care procedures. *Specify reason for and level of supervision needed.*
	(Help)	Needs help with oral care. *Specify kind of help needed.*
	(Total care)	Unable to perform own oral care. *Note kinds of care to be given and frequency. Note preferences for oral care equipment and products.*

2. SENSES

A. VISION:	(Full dist.)	Normal or fully corrected distance vision. *Note whether glasses or contacts are used.*
	(Full close)	Normal or corrected close (reading) vision. *Note whether glasses or contacts are used.*
	(Deficit)	Patient has limited vision. *Specify kind and severity of deficit.*
	(Under Rx)	Under care for deficit or resulting handicap. *Specify nature of care, frequency, and name of caregiver.*

Form continued on following page

FORM 20 *Continued*

B. HEARING:	(Normal)	Able to hear normal speech.
	(Aided)	Uses a hearing aid.
		Note kind, frequency of use, and whether help is needed.
	(Deficit)	Hearing is limited.
		Specify kind and severity of deficit. Note how deficit is managed or overcome.
	(Under Rx)	Under care for deficit or resulting handicap.
		Specify nature of care, frequency, and name of caregiver.
C. TOUCH:	(Normal)	Has normal touch sensations.
	(Deficit)	Sense of touch is limited.
		Specify nature of deficit and part of body involved. Note how deficit is managed or overcome.
D. TASTE/ SMELL:	(Normal)	Normal taste and smell sensations.
	(Deficit)	Taste or smell sensations are limited.
		Specify nature and severity of deficit. Note how deficit is managed or overcome.

3. COMMUNICATION

A. SPEECH:	(Normal)	Able to express self understandably in English.
		Note any hesitation to express needs, desires, or emotions.
	(Deficit)	Has a speech impediment or aphasia.
		Specify nature and severity of difficulty.
	(Lang. dif.)	Speaks with accent or hard to understand.
		Specify degree of language difficulty and what language is preferred by patient.
		Note how difficulty is managed or overcome.
B. READING:	(Normal)	Able to read English in newspaper-sized print.
		Note apparent strength of interest in reading and preferred subjects.
	(Deficit)	Has physical or educational handicap that limits reading ability.
		Specify nature and severity of limitation.
	(Non-Eng.)	Reads in language other than English.
		Note language preference and apparent strength of interest in reading.
C. WRITING:	(Normal)	Able to write legible English.
		Note whether writing is an especially important form of communication to the patient.
	(Deficit)	Has physical or educational handicap that limits writing ability.
		Specify nature and severity of limitation.
	(Left-handed)	Prefers using left hand for writing and other tasks.
D. RESP. TO CARE:	(Pos.)	Has mostly positive attitudes toward care and caregivers.
		Note words listed or others that describe patient's dominant attitudes:
		friendly, cooperative, alert, active in care, forms relationships easily.
	(Guard.)	Uses mostly guarded, defensive, or passive responses to care or caregivers.
		Note whether there are variations in response and under what circumstances.

FORM 20 *Continued*

	(Upset)	Seems upset by care and caregivers. *Note words listed or others that describe patient's dominant attitudes: disoriented, easily confused, nervous, embarrassed, demanding, depressed. Note any known factors that may contribute to patient's attitudes.*
	(Neg./hostile)	Has mostly negative attitudes toward care and caregivers. *Note words listed or others that describe patient's dominant attitudes: angry, uncooperative, critical, distrustful, withdrawn.*

4. MOBILITY

A. TRANSFER:	(Indep.)	Able to transfer from bed to chair or chair to chair without help.
	(Equip.)	Uses special equipment to aid transfer. *Specify kind of equipment used (rail, walker, special chairs, etc.).*
	(Help)	Needs help to transfer. *Specify kind of help needed and weight-bearing limitations of patient.*
	(Confined to bed)	Unable to be out of bed at all. *Note reason for confinement and whether temporary or long-term.*
B. AMBULA-TION:	(Indep.)	Able to ambulate by self and climb stairs. *Note any time or distance restrictions.*
	(Equip.)	Uses special equipment to aid ambulation. *Specify kind of equipment used (walker, crutches, cane, braces, elastic stockings). Note if patient uses wheelchair all or part time.*
	(Help)	Needs help with ambulation. *Specify kind and amount of help needed and weight-bearing limitations. Note usual schedule and destination of ambulation.*
	(Non-amb.)	Not ambulatory.
C. GROOMING:	(Indep.)	Able to comb and shampoo hair, shave, or apply makeup without help.
	(Super.)	Needs supervision during grooming activities. *Specify reason for and level of supervision needed.*
	(Help)	Needs help with grooming activities. *Specify activity and kind of help needed. Note right- or left-handedness.*
	(Total care)	Unable to groom self. *Note preferences and frequency of activities.*
D. ACTIVITIES:	(Conversation)	Enjoys participating in conversation with family, friends, or acquaintances. *Note any especially favored topics and limitations on ability to hold conversation.*
	(Music)	Enjoys listening to, playing an instrument, or dancing to music. *Note degree of activity or involvement in musical events.*

Form continued on following page

FORM 20 *Continued*

	(Crafts)	Enjoys participating in handcrafts or other creative activities. *Note kinds of crafts favored and estimate of fine-muscle control.*
	(Other)	*Specify other activities enjoyed by patient.*

5. ELIMINATION/SKIN

A. BLADDER:	(Continent)	Has full bladder control. *Note approximate daily output.*
	(Help)	Needs help in using equipment or getting to toilet. *Specify kind of help needed and frequency. Note any special equipment required such as high toilet seat, urinal, bedpan, or catheter.*
	(Incont.)	Patient is incontinent of urine. *Specify under what conditions incontinence occurs and how usually managed.*
	(Frequen.)	Patient urinates frequently enough to disturb daytime activities or sleep. *Note approximate frequency of urination and probable cause.*
	(Fluid def.)	Needs assistance in getting appropriate level of fluid intake. *Specify nature of fluid deficit and how it is usually managed.*
B. BOWELS:	(Continent)	Has bowel control and regular bowel habits.
	(Regular)	Has regular pattern of bowel movements. *Note frequency of bowel movements and usual time of day.*
	(Help)	Needs help in getting to the toilet or using special equipment. *Specify kind of help or equipment needed (toilet seat, commode, bedpan).*
	(Lax./Soft.)	Uses laxatives, stool softeners, special foods, or procedures to improve regularity. *Note when and how frequently special foods or medications, laxatives, enemas, etc., are used.*
	(Incont.)	Patient is incontinent. *Specify under what conditions incontinence occurs and how usually managed.*
C. SKIN COND.:	(Good)	Skin is in good condition with normal color. *Note any exceptions to otherwise good condition.*
	(Fragile)	Skin in basically good condition but is easily damaged or is sensitive. *Specify in what ways skin condition is damaged.*
	(Sp. care/ext.)	Skin on arms, legs, hands, or feet requires special care to maintain good condition. *Specify any areas of skin breakdown and treatments or procedures presently used.*
	(Sp. care/pres.)	Skin on coccyx, heels, elbows, shoulders, or head requires special care to prevent breakdown. *Specify any areas of skin breakdown and treatments or procedures presently used.*

FORM 20 *Continued*

(Open areas/Rx) There are presently open areas (decubitus, abrasions, incisions) under treatment. *Specify area involved, current treatment or procedures, and anticipated healing time.*

6. MENTAL STATE

A. COGNITION:

(Normal/alert)	Ability to think and reason normal.
(Diminished)	Ability to think and reason clearly diminished. *Note probable cause and evidence used to make this judgment.*
(Variable)	Alertness and ability to reason varies. *Note any observable pattern to variation and probable causes.*
(Poor concen.)	Able to reason normally but has short attention span or poor ability to concentrate. *Note probable cause and evidence used to make this judgment.*
(Disorient.)	Mentally confused or disoriented as to time, person, or place. *Note any variations in disorientation.*

B. AWARE OF CARE NEEDS:

(Aware of prog.)	Aware of prognosis and its consequences for continuing care. *Note words listed or others that describe patient's attitude toward diagnosis/prognosis: optimistic, pessimistic, depressed, uninterested, angry, passive, anxious.*
(Decided pref.)	Has made basic decisions about care preferences—e.g., attitude toward code, pain relief, etc. *Specify patient's preferences for care and note any problems they present with family or doctor.*
(Realistic)	Mostly uses reality-based thinking when discussing terminal care. *Note any exceptions to awareness of condition or realistic expectations.*
(Unrealistic)	Expresses unrealistic goals, plans, or fears related to terminal care. *Specify nature of unrealistic thinking and note how others have responded to this.*
(Unaware)	Not able to understand prognosis or consequences. *Note reason for inability and degree of awareness of family or friends.*

C. MEMORY:

(Good)	Both short- and long-term memory seem to be within normal limits.
(Short)	Able to recall facts or ideas for only a short period of time. *Note nature of memory difficulty and whether problem existed prior to acute episode.*
(Variable)	Memory good at times, poor at others. *Note possible causes of variability such as medication.* *Note any categories of information that seem to be retained more reliably.*

Form continued on following page

FORM 20 *Continued*

	(Poor)	Unable to recall facts or ideas long enough to use them effectively. *Note any known causes for poor memory and length of time problem has existed.*
D. DECISION MAKING:	(Involved)	Actively involved in plans for continuing care. *Note a word or phrase that describes patient's involvement such as:* *discussing options, making plans, organizing help.*
	(Near ready)	Seems ready to begin decision-making and planning about continuing care. *Note evidence of readiness such as asking questions or talking about previous experiences.*
	(Unready)	Seems as yet unable to plan for continuing care. *Note any known factors that may contribute to lack of readiness, including stage of crisis/grief.*
	(Optimistic)	Has positive attitude toward terminal care.
	(Pessimistic)	Has negative or unrealistic attitude toward terminal care.

7. PATTERNS AND HABITS

A. NUTRITION:	(Good)	Generally well nourished. *Note usual meal and snack pattern and any supplements usually taken.*
	(Limited)	Nutrition limited due to food preferences or poor appetite. *Specify food preferences and ways in which these are managed.* *Note reason for present poor appetite and/or appetite history.*
	(Spec. diet)	Receiving special diet. *Note reason for diet and expected duration.*
	(Overweight)	Significantly overweight for height and bone structure. *Note any recommendations that have been made regarding weight control.*
	(Underweight)	Significantly underweight for height and bone structure. *Note any recommendations that have been made regarding weight control.*
B. SLEEP:	(Good)	Sleeps well each night and feels rested. *Note usual bed and arising times and times of naps during day.*
	(Poor)	Sleeps poorly and seldom feels rested. *Note probable causes of poor sleep.*
	(Interrupted)	Sleep is normally interrupted. *Note reason for interruption and frequency (toilet, medication, dreams, etc.)*
	(Naps)	Takes naps during the day. *Note usual frequency and length of naps and whether they affect nighttime sleep.*
C. TOBACCO:	(Non-user)	Does not now or never has used tobacco. *Note whether patient ever has used tobacco and in what form.*

FORM 20 *Continued*

	(Lt./mod. use)	Smokes up to one pack of cigarettes per day or uses other forms of tobacco. *Note what form of tobacco is used, usual consumption pattern, and duration of habit.*
	(Hvy. use)	Heavy user of tobacco on a regular basis. *Note what form of tobacco is used, usual consumption pattern, and duration of habit.*
	(Adv. to stop)	Trying to stop smoking or has been advised to stop. *Note present attitudes and goals and past history of trying to stop.*
D. ALCOHOL/ DRUGS:	(Non-user)	Does not consume alcohol or use potentially addictive drugs. *Note whether patient has ever used alcohol or drugs and to what extent.*
	(Lt./mod. alco.)	Regularly consumes light to moderate amount of alcoholic beverages. *Note kind and pattern of daily consumption.*
	(Alco. prob.)	Alcohol use has been or now is a problem for patient or family. *Note severity of problem and how it has been managed.*
	(Reg. drugs)	Regularly takes tranquilizers, sedatives, narcotics, or other drugs. *Specify kind of drugs used and pattern of use.*
	(Drug prob.)	Drug use has been or now is a problem for patient or family. *Note severity of problem and how it has been or will be managed.*

8. SOCIAL SITUATION

A. FAMILY INVOLVE-MENT:	(Active)	Family members or close friends are actively involved with patient's care and decisions. *Identify those most involved by name and relationship.*
	(Realistic)	Family members or close friends seem to have realistic expectations for patient's care. *Note evidence of realistic thinking and role that they anticipate for themselves.*
	(Supportive)	Family members offer emotional support to patient through attention and loving concern. *Identify those most supportive by name, and specify ways in which support is demonstrated.*
	(Limited)	Involvement of family or friends in patient care limited. *Note apparent reason for limited involvement by name and relationship.*
	(Not avail.)	Family not available due to geography or alienation. *Note reason for unavailability of family or friends.*
	(No support)	Family or close friends visit but give patient no encouragement or support. *Note apparent reasons for lack of encouragement or support.*

Form continued on following page

FORM 20 *Continued*

B. COMMUNITY SUPPORT:

(Soc. groups) Has been active in community social groups or organizations.
Specify groups and note level of involvement.

(Rel. groups) Has been active in religious groups or activities.
Specify groups and any implications for future care.

(Group support) Evidence of support and encouragement from community social or religious groups.
Note kind of support given and response of patient to it.

(Involved frnds) Friends visit regularly and seem actively involved with patient's care plans.
Note identity of any particularly involved.

(Few friends) Seems to have a limited social support network or speaks of self as having few friends.
Note apparent reason for limited friendships such as personality, frequent moves, etc.

(No support) No evidence of community involvement with patient or support.

C. LIVING SITUATION:

(Ret. to former) Return to former living situation following discharge is anticipated.
Note anticipated adequacy of this living arrangement.

(Changing) Discharge to a different living situation anticipated.
Note progress of decision making about altered living situation.
Note patient's response to anticipated change.

(Shared) Housing is or will be shared with others.
Identify persons in household.

(Resid. care) Anticipates discharge to skilled nursing or other residential care facility.
Note whether patient has lived in residential care in the past, and if so, for how long.

(Needs modifi.) Needs structural modifications made to house/apartment.
Specify kinds of modifications that need to be made and available sources of help.

D. FINANCIAL SITUATION:

(Medicare/-aid) Eligible for continuing care benefits from Medicare and/or Medicaid.
Note present status and extent of benefits.

(H.M.O./Pvt.) Eligible for H.M.O. or private insurance coverage for terminal care.
Note present status and extent of benefits.

(No insurance) Has no insurance coverage for terminal care.
Note whether financial counseling and/or assistance is needed and by whom.

(Indep. funds) Has access to independent means of financing needed care.
Note whether funds are likely to be adequate for needs.

(Fam. funds) Members of family will contribute financially to care costs.
Note who is acting as financial coordinator.

FORM 20 *Continued*

9. CONTINUING CARE

A. MEDICAL SUPER-VISION:	(Reg. MD)	Will be returning to the care of own physician for continuing care. *Note name of doctor and level of involvement in hospital care.*
	(Spec. MD)	Will receive continuing care from a specialist physician. *Note name of doctor and any anticipated difficulty with patient access.*
	(Clinic)	Will receive continuing care from an out-patient facility or clinic. *Note name of clinic and whether patient has received care there previously.*
	(Other)	*Specify plan for medical supervision, including name of doctor and/or facility.*
B. NURSING CARE:	(None)	No need for nursing care anticipated at this time. *Note any treatments or procedures that will be done by the patient.*
	(Minimal)	Nursing care needs are minimal and can be managed without outside help at this time. *Specify kind of care needed.*
	(Skilled)	Need for skilled nursing care is anticipated. *Specify kind of care needed and how need will be met.*
	(Custodial)	Need for custodial care (e.g., assistance with ADLs) is anticipated. *Specify level of care needed and how need will be met.*
C. EQUIPMENT:	(Hosp. bed)	Needs hospital bed to facilitate care. *Note reason for need and probable source of equipment.*
	(Mobility aids)	Needs assistive equipment to improve mobility or safety. *Specify kinds of equipment or aids and probable source.*
	(Ventilation)	Needs assistive equipment to improve or monitor breathing. *Specify kinds of equipment or aids and probable source.*
	(Treatment supplies)	Needs supplies for regular treatments (e.g., dressing changes, colostomy bags, etc.) *Specify kind and quantity of supplies needed and probable source.*
	(Other)	*Specify other kinds of equipment or aids needed.*
D. PAIN MANAGE-MENT:	(Oral meds.)	Will be discharged with oral medications to control pain. *Specify medication to be used and degree of control patient will have in use.*
	(I.M. meds.)	Will be discharged with intermuscular medications to control pain. *Specify medication to be used, who will administer it, and degree of patient control in its use.*

Form continued on following page

FORM 20 *Continued*

(I.V. meds.) Will be discharged with intravenous medications to control pain.
Specify medication to be used, who will administer it, and degree of patient control in its use.

(Self-reg. pump) Will be discharged with self-regulated subcutaneous medication pump for pain control.
Specify medication to be used and patient's attitude toward control.

(Other) *Specify medication to be used, method of administration, and degree of patient control.*

MAKING A TEACHING PLAN

Helping both patient and family learn how to meet the physical and emotional demands of terminal care requires special sensitivity on the part of the nurse. By starting early to plan teaching approaches and organizing information so that it is logically presented, the nurse can help learners develop the knowledge, attitudes, and skills they will need. Beginning teaching early will allow them time to cope with the emotional issues surrounding each topic.

One specific goal of teaching is to help patients learn what their realistic prognosis and options are. They need, in this process, to decide what they really want in terms of care and intervention. A sense of control and independence in that decision making is extremely important to their emotional adjustment and acceptance. Likewise, the family needs to learn what to realistically expect of the patient's condition and of the help and support available from others. A very important part of this teaching is to help them learn what to expect of the events leading to death. Deciding ahead how medical crises are to be managed increases the chances that the patient's wishes will be carried out.

The Discharge Teaching Plan (Form 21) is designed to help caregivers identify areas of learning needs and construct learning objectives quickly. These objectives then become the framework for patient and family teaching. The subjects on this form parallel those indicated in the third section of the Discharge Plan Summary.

Remember that the only useful learning objectives are REALISTIC ones. They should be attainable in the time available, and the desired behavior should be observable by the teacher(s).

Elements of this form are described below.

Identification of Learners. Those people who are to be included in some or all teaching sessions are listed across the top of the form. The nurse may want to write the telephone numbers of visitor-learners, as well as their names, to simplify coordination. Where notations are made about a learner other than the patient, they may be referred to by number. For example, the motivation of the patient may be "developing," but for learner "#2" it may be already "present".

Subject of Teaching. Eight common subjects for discharge teaching have been listed on the form. The nurse may indicate that teaching in this subject area is not needed. If it is needed, the next three lines provide a record of teaching progress from planning through evaluation. Updating the teaching plan by checking the description that currently applies to teaching in each subject area will alert other caregivers to

346 • DISCHARGE PLANNING GUIDE FOR NURSES

what has been done. They can then actively cooperate with the learning process by stimulating further patient interest in the subject and reinforcing learning. Following the completion of teaching, learning may be evaluated through tests, verbal questions, demonstrations, or other methods. Verifying that an objective has been successfully reached is positive feedback for both teacher and learner.

Motivation. Attention to a person's motivation to learn particular subjects is extremely important to effective and efficient teaching. If motivation is poor, the nurse will want to work on this before attempting to teach content in an area. Changes in motivation can be recorded with a check or an arrow. When several learners are involved, those with more motivation may be able to help the others understand the importance of the subject.

Prior Knowledge or Experience. A short phrase is usually enough to record the basis on which new learning can be built. Finding out what a learner already knows about a subject takes only moments, but it allows the teacher to start with relevant material, thereby improving both motivation and learning ability. It is best not to make any assumptions about what the learner knows; a person who has experienced the death of a number of close friends or relatives does not necessarily have a better understanding of the grief process, nor can he or she be expected to progress through it more quickly.

Learning Objective. The construction of learning objectives is a simple but often unfamiliar activity to those who are not full-time teachers. An objective or learning goal starts with the phrase *"The learner will be able to..."* This is followed by a verb indicating the **level of complexity** at which learning must take place. To "adapt" learning to different situations is, for example, much more complex than simply "remembering" it. We have suggested a number of possible words that may be used.

Next, a learning objective defines the **specific subject** of concern and states what kind of **behavior** is expected as a result of learning. Remember that the stated behavior must be observable in the time available, and therefore objectives for learning in acute care settings will necessarily be short-term and limited. The ultimate goal in teaching terminal patients about pain management, for example, might be that they experience a pain-free death. A realistic learning objective while they are in the hospital, however, might be that they demonstrate their ability to manage pain medications and state how they plan to use medical and emotional support as pain increases. Finally, writing down a **time** for learning to be completed gives both learners and teachers a target toward which to work.

Notes. Noting what teaching approaches have been used, (for example, "videotape on management of subcutaneous pumps") and the response learners have had to them, the priority given certain subjects, and plans for learning evaluation are all important pieces of information to share with other caregivers. Current notes kept in a known location are essential when several teachers are involved or learning needs are complex.

FORM 21. *DISCHARGE TEACHING PLAN FOR:* _____

OTHER THAN PATIENT, THOSE TO BE INVOLVED AS LEARNERS
INCLUDE: *(Note name and relationship to patient.)*
  #1:   #2:   #3:

1. MEDICAL NEEDS:
   Teaching: ___not needed   Motivation: ___present   Prior knowledge/
   ___planned   ___developing   experience: _____
   ___in progress   ___poor
   ___learning   _____
   evaluated

   Learner will be able to: _____ By _____
                            (level)   (specific subject)   (behavior)   (date)
               (e.g., remember, understand, apply information, make decisions about)

2. TREATMENTS AND PROCEDURES:
   Teaching: ___not needed   Motivation: ___present   Prior knowledge/
   ___planned   ___developing   experience: _____
   ___in progress   ___poor
   ___learning   _____
   evaluated

   Learner will be able to: _____ By _____
                            (level)   (specific subject)   (behavior)   (date)
               (e.g., remember, understand, apply information, perform, adapt, evaluate)

3. NUTRITIONAL NEEDS:
   Teaching: ___not needed   Motivation: ___present   Prior knowledge/
   ___planned   ___developing   experience: _____
   ___in progress   ___poor
   ___learning   _____
   evaluated

   Learner will be able to: _____ By _____
                            (level)   (specific subject)   (behavior)   (date)
               (e.g., remember, understand, apply information, prepare, adapt)

4. PAIN MANAGEMENT:
   Teaching: ___not needed   Motivation: ___present   Prior knowledge/
   ___planned   ___developing   experience: _____
   ___in progress   ___poor
   ___learning   _____
   evaluated
   Learner will be able to: _____ By _____
                            (level)   (specific subject)   (behavior)   (date)
               (e.g., remember, recognize, understand, apply information,
                                                   make decisions about, adapt)

5. PROGNOSIS/CRISIS MANAGEMENT:
   Teaching: ___not needed   Motivation: ___present   Prior knowledge/
   ___planned   ___developing   experience: _____
   ___in progress   ___poor
   ___learning   _____
   evaluated

   Learner will be able to: _____ By _____
                            (level)   (specific subject)   (behavior)   (date)
               (e.g., remember, recognize, understand, apply information, evaluate,
                                                   make decisions about)

FORM 21 *Continued*

6. FINANCIAL/LEGAL PLANNING:
   Teaching: ___not needed   Motivation: ___present   Prior knowledge/
   ___planned   ___developing   experience: _____
   ___in progress   ___poor   _____
   ___learning
   evaluated

   Learner will be able to: _____ By _____
   (level)   (specific subject)   (behavior)   (date)
   (e.g., recognize, understand, evaluate, adapt, make decisions about)

7. EMOTIONAL/SOCIAL ASPECTS OF CARE:
   Teaching: ___not needed   Motivation: ___present   Prior knowledge/
   ___planned   ___developing   experience: _____
   ___in progress   ___poor   _____
   ___learning
   evaluated

   Learner will be able to: _____ By _____
   (level)   (specific subject)   (behavior)   (date)
   (e.g., remember, understand, evaluate, apply information, realistically plan)

8. COMMUNITY SERVICES AND RESOURCES:
   Teaching: ___not needed   Motivation: ___present   Prior knowledge/
   ___planned   ___developing   experience: _____
   ___in progress   ___poor   _____
   ___learning
   evaluated

   Learner will be able to: _____ By _____
   (level)   (specific subject)   (behavior)   (date)
   (e.g., remember, understand, apply information, plan, utilize)

9. OTHER LEARNING OBJECTIVES:
   Learner will be able to _____ by _____

   Learner will be able to _____ by _____

   Teaching Plan initiated by _____ on _____

NOTES ON TEACHING (what was taught, methods/materials used, response, etc.)

C

Confirming the Plan Before Discharge

This third step toward effective continuing care is to confirm that all aspects of the discharge plan have been covered. Taken just before the patient's discharge, it presents an opportunity for the nurse to review relevant knowledge and skills, giving encouragement, positive feedback, and reinforcement for the learning that has taken place. It also allows clarification of the entire discharge plan, promotes discussion of both short- and long-term goals and provides the opportunity to ask lingering questions.

Form 22 is presented as a guideline for Step C. It lists topics that are commonly part of a comprehensive discharge plan. It may be used with the patient, a family member, a community caregiver, or a small group of people involved in the patient's continuing care. In situations in which care is complex, such as chronic disease management or rehabilitation, going over the list with both patient and caregiver together will serve to clarify interpretations of instructions that might cause confusion once the patient is at home.

In asking questions about each topic, the nurse will want to use "open" rather than "closed" questions (see Section 2.2). For example, the nurse might say: "Tell me about the medication you will be taking at home and how you are to take it," rather than ask: "Are you clear about how you are to take your medication?"

In the first example, the person is invited to demonstrate his or her knowledge, giving the nurse the opportunity to reinforce what has been learned and correct any details. In the second, especially when the person is defensive about appearing intelligent and knowledgeable, he or she may answer: "Yes" and go home with dangerously incomplete information.

If it is necessary to correct any misinterpretations of information or supply new knowledge just before the patient is discharged, it is very important that the nurse write it down as well as verbally explain

350

it. Just before discharge, patients and family members are concerned about the impending transition in responsibility, care, and social roles. It must be assumed that they will not reliably remember details given to them at that point.

Step C is best completed at least several hours prior to actual discharge, for two reasons. The first is that this will avoid the inevitable rush and confusion of the last moment. Discussion of plans and review of knowledge should be unhurried and presented non-threateningly rather than as a last-minute unexpected quiz. The second reason for doing the review well before discharge is that it allows a period of time in which to think of any additional questions. The review of information will encourage patients to imagine just what it will be like to be away from acute caregivers and to work through the kinds of decisions they will have to make on their own. They may be harboring some fantasies about the worst possible thing that could happen. Given time and opportunity, they can pose those questions and receive reassurance before departure.

FORM 22. *STEP C: CHECKLIST FOR REVIEW OF DISCHARGE PLAN FOR* _____

Instructions: Complete this checklist with the patient and/or family members prior to the patient's discharge.

REVIEW OF KNOWLEDGE AND SKILLS

1. Nutrition
—General diet instructions
—Foods to be included
—Foods to avoid
—Recommended eating pattern
—Desired fluid intake
—How diet/fluid to be monitored
—Reasons for diet/fluid orders
—Goals related to nutrition
—Other: _____

2. Medications
—Name of medications to be taken
—Identification of pills or capsules
—Proper dosage and instructions
—Time to be taken
—Reason for each medication
—What to do if forgotton
—Side effects or complications to watch for
—Who to contact if side effects occur and how
—When and how prescriptions are to be filled
—Other: _____

3. Treatments and Procedures
—Schedule of procedures or treatments
—Goals of procedures or treatments
—Supplies and equipment to be used
—Options available for equipment/ supplies
—When and how to refill supplies
—When and how to service/return equipment
—Step-by-step procedure protocol
—Procedure or treatment demonstration
—Monitoring and reporting response to treatment
—How to adapt procedures
—Who to contact with questions or problems
—Other: _____

4. Activities
—Activity limitations
—Reasons for limitatiaons
—Sequence of increasing activity
—Demonstrate safe ambulation
—Schedule of prescribed exercise(s)
—Demonstrate exercise(s)
—Adaptation of activities
—Other: _____

5. Management of Complications
—Danger signals to watch for
—Immediate procedures in event of complication
—Demonstration of emergency procedures
—How to report complications and to whom
—Who to contact for assistance
—How to minimize risk of complications
—Other: _____

6. Community Services and Resources
—Referrals made to services or resources
—Expected services to be offered
—Schedule of contact with community agencies
—Other services available in community
—When and how to contact other services
—Payment plan
—Other: _____

7. Health Promotion
—Plan to stop smoking
—Plan to alter eating habits
—Plan to alter other habits
—Plan for use of community support
—Goals for life-style changes
—Other: _____

FORM 22 *Continued*

REVIEW OF IMMEDIATE DISCHARGE PLANS

8. **Medical Follow-up**
___Schedule of medical appointments
___Reasons for follow-up
___Appointments with other health care
   workers
___Telephone numbers
___Written instructions
___Criteria for contacting doctor/nurse/
   others
___Payment plan for follow-up care
___Other:_____

9. **Leaving the Hospital**
___Immediate attendance of someone at
   destination
___Length of their stay
___Transportation to be used
___Arrangements for transport
___Appropriate clothing available
___Discharge orders written
___Doctor visit before discharge
___Billing office clearance
___Insurance forms in order
___Next medication to be taken
___Equipment and supplies ready
___Written instructions in hand

Checklist completed by: _____on: _____

A Sample Discharge Plan

The following pages contain an actual sample of the use of the discharge planning forms (Forms 1, 10, 11, and 13) described in Part II of this book. In this case, the patient was admitted for diarrhea and dehydration but was found to have hepatitis secondary to alcohol abuse. The surprise finding was that he was H.I.V. positive, although he had no active AIDs symptoms. Complicating his care was his wife's reaction to this finding, which exacerbated some long-standing feelings of anger and rejection related to the patient's alcohol abuse. At the same time the patient denied his alcohol problem.

The discharge plan shown here reflects the uncertainty of the patient's discharge destination, the nature of his continuing care, and the emotional issues involved. In spite of these difficulties, the nurse was able to initiate a useful discharge summary. She reported that the Detailed Needs Identification was especially useful as caregivers tried to give this patient and his family well-coordinated and comprehensive care.

FORM 1. *STEP A: INITIAL ASSESSMENT OF DISCHARGE NEEDS*

PATIENT IDENTIFICATION No.: *0000*   DATE: *2-23-90*
NAME: *Jerry M.*   UNIT or ROOM No.:
1. AGE: *32*   SEX: *m.*
2. MEDICAL DIAGNOSIS (at admission): Admitted on (date):_*2-22-90*_
     Diarrhea with dehydration, mental state changes
3. SELF-CARE RISK—Note abilities BEFORE admission.

Activities of Daily Living	Toileting	Mobility
__ independent for ADLs	✓ able to use toilet	__ able to walk unaided
✓ unable to feed self	__ continent	__ able to transfer
✓ unable to dress self	✓ variable continence	unaided
✓ unable to bathe self	__ incontinent bladder	✓ able to walk with aid
✓ unable to prepare own	__ incontinent bowels	✓ transfers with help
meals		__ confined to bed

4. MENTAL STATE

Memory	Orientation
__ not assessed	__ not assessed
__ good/normal	__ alert/aware
__ variable	✓ variable
✓ poor	__ disoriented

5. SOCIAL RISKS

Living situation (before admission)	Community involvement
✓ with spouse	__ not assessed
	__ resident for less than 1 year
__ alone	✓ relatives live in area
__ in residential care facility	__ no relatives in area
__ homeless	__ family not aware of admission
__ cares for dependent	

6. ECONOMIC RISKS

Finances	Insurance coverage
__ not assessed	✓ insurance for acute care
✓ employed or fully supported	__ belongs to HMO
__ unemployed or retired	__ Medicare/Medicaid
__ Social Security recipient	__ no insurance
__ receiving aid or welfare	

7. RISK IDENTIFICATION
Areas of special risk identified above or special risk factors that apply to this patient: *ADL/mobility/mental state*   *? Alcoholic hepatitis*
         ? HIV +

8. GOALS OF DISCHARGE PLANNING/CONTINUING CARE

	Patient will probably need	Person who will lead discharge planning:
__ Uncertain at this time	✓ high-intensity discharge planning	*J. Biggs*
__ Recuperation		
__ Rehabilitation	__ social work assistance	
✓ Chronic disease management	__ counseling assistance	
__ Residential care	__ special teaching	
__ Terminal care	✓ more extensive needs identification	

SIGNED *P. Rhodes R.N.* DATE *2-23-90*

FORM 10. *DISCHARGE PLAN SUMMARY FOR:* ___Jerry M.___

PATIENT IDENTIFICATION NO.: ___0000___ UNIT/ROOM: _____

GENERAL GOAL: Management of chronic disease while maintaining/improving other aspects of patient's health.

A. SPECIAL SERVICES DURING ACUTE CARE:
Note with + those that will/may need to be continued AFTER discharge.

___None
___Intensive care
✓ Isolation
___Surgery
✓ Blood transfusion
___Other: _____

___Radiation therapy
+✓ Respiratory therapy
+✓ Physical therapy
___Occupational therapy
___Speech therapy

+✓ Patient/family
   counseling
+✓ Social services
___Mental health/
   psychiatric
___Discharge planning
   team
___Rehabilitation team

B. IDENTIFICATION OF RISKS/DEFICITS   Patient's age is ___32___
*Note with * those risks present BEFORE admission.*
Note limitations expected to continue AFTER discharge.

___No special risks
   identified
✓ Activities of daily
   living
___Senses
✓ Communication
✓ Mobility

✓ Toileting
*✓ Mental state
___Motivation
*✓ Social situation
___Economic situation

Pt. wants to go home — wife uncertain

Pos. HIV not prev. known

C. TEACHING NEEDED FOR PATIENT OR FAMILY IN SUBJECTS OF:
___No separate teaching plan
Note names and phone numbers of family or others involved in teaching.

✓ Medical follow-up
  ✓ in progress
  ___completed
✓ Medications
  ✓ in progress
  ___completed
✓ Treatments/procedures
  ___in progress
  ___completed

✓ Activities
  ✓ in progress
  ___completed
✓ Nutrition/diet
  ___in progress
  ___completed
✓ Complication manag.
  ___in progress
  ___completed

✓ Health Promotion
  ✓ in progress
  ___completed
✓ Community services
  ___in progress
  ___completed
✓ Other: *HIV precautions*
  ___in progress
  ___completed

Form continued on following page

FORM 10 *Continued*

D. POST-HOSPITAL SERVICES: ___None needed.
Medical follow-up by: _____

Home Care: ✓Needed   ___Decision in progress

Referral made to ___J. Biggs___ on _2-27_ by __P. R._____

Extended Care: ___Needed   ✓Decision in progress

Referral made to _Dr. F. Andrews_ on _2-27_ by __P. R._____

Social Services: ✓Needed   ___Decision in progress

Referral made to ___B. Kelly___ on _2-27_ by __P. R._____

Mental Health: ___Needed   ✓Decision in progress

Referral made to _Dr. Andrews_ on _2-27_ by __P. R._____

Special Equip: ___Needed   ✓Decision in progress

Referral made to _Dr. Andrews_ on _2-27_ by __P. R._____

Note details of services needed, options considered, and agencies/caregivers involved. Continue on back of sheet if needed.

Home care vs SNF placement

E. SPECIFIC OBJECTIVES OF CONTINUING CARE: *Detail plans and goals for up to three months after discharge.*
   1. Pt. receive safe care & close monitoring
   2. Pt. start alcohol recovery prog.
   3. Pt. & wife cope with anxieties i.e. HIV+
ANTICIPATED DISCHARGE TO _____
ON OR ABOUT _____UNDER CARE OF DOCTOR_____

F. COORDINATION OF INFORMATION: *Note exactly where information can be located (e.g., "Nursing Care Plan" or "Form 111")*
   ✓Initial **assessment** of discharge risks can be found: behind face-sheet
   ✓Further details of continuing care **needs and plans** can be found: Nrsg. Care Plan
   ✓Details of **teaching** planned and/or completed can be found: Teaching plan
   ✓Copies of **referrals** or detailed plans can be found: following DPS

PLAN INITIATED BY: P. Rhodes RN ON: 2-28-90. UPDATED: _____

FORM 11. *DETAILED NEEDS IDENTIFICATION FOR* _Jerry M._
I.D. _____

INSTRUCTIONS: *Check all appropriate options for each item. Note individual aspects of need and how care will be affected.*

1. ACTIVITIES OF DAILY LIVING:

A. EATING	B. DRESSING	C. BATHING	D. ORAL CARE
__Indep.	__Indep.	__Indep.	__Indep.
✓Super.	__Super.	__Super.	__Super.
__Help	✓Help	✓Help	✓Help
__Total care	__Total care	__Total care	__Total care

Generalized weakness. ↓ ROM both arms. Tremors

2. SENSES:

A. VISION	B. HEARING	C. TOUCH	D. TASTE/SMELL
✓Full dist.	✓Normal	✓Normal	✓Normal
__Full close	__Aided	__Deficit	__Deficit
__Deficit	__Deficit		
__Under Rx	__Under Rx		

Glasses for distance

3. COMMUNICATION:

A. SPEECH	B. READING	C. WRITING
✓Normal	✓Normal	__Normal
__Deficit	__Deficit	✓Deficit
__Lang. dif.	__Non-Eng.	

Too weak

4. MOBILITY:

A. TRANSFER	B. AMBULATION	C. GROOMING	D. INSTRU. ADLs
__Indep.	__Indep.	__Indep.	*(meal prep., care of clothes)*
__Equip.	✓Equip.	__Super.	__Indep.
✓Help	__Help	✓Help	__Help
__Confined to bed	__Non-amb.	__Total care	✓Depen.

One person assist to commode. Walk 10' BID with walker,
but unsteady

5. HABITS AND PATTERNS:

A. APPETITE	B. SLEEP	C. BLADDER	D. BOWELS
✓Good	__Good	✓Continent	✓Continent
__Limited	__Poor	__Help	__Regular
__Spec. diet	✓Interrupted	✓Incont. *noc.*	__Help
	__Pre-bed rit.	__Frequen.	__Lax./Soft.
	__Naps	__Fluid def.	✓Incont. *noc.*

E. SMOKING/ALCOHOL/DRUG USE

__Tobacco	__Stop alco.	_Becomes confused, esp. at_
✓Stop tobac.	__Drugs	_night → incontinence_
__Alcohol	__Stop drugs	_Recently stopped smoking_
✓Alco. prob.		

Alcohol prob. long-standing → hepatitis

Form continued on following page

FORM 11 *Continued*

6. MENTAL STATE:

A. COGNITION	B. AWARENESS	C. RESP. TO CARE	D. MEMORY
—Normal	—Alert	✓Pos.	—Good
—Diminished	✓Aware of Dx.	—Neg.	✓Short
✓Variable	—Realistic	—Guard.	—Variable
—Poor concen.	✓Unreal.	—Upset	—Poor
—Disorient.	—Unaware		

Due to illness. Denies wife's reluctance to have him home.

7. MOTIVATION:

A. FOR SELF-CARE	B. LEARNING	C. PERSONAL-ITY	D. DECISION MAKING
—Active	—Interested	✓Present orien.	—Involved
—Self-respon.	✓Disabled	—Future orien.	—Near ready
✓Unreal.	—Uninterest.	—Time consc.	✓Unready
—Demoralized		✓Easygoing	✓Optimistic
			—Pessimistic

Imagines illness will disappear when home. Attn. span / memory short

8. SOCIAL SITUATION:

A. FAMILY IN-VOLVEMENT	B. COMMUNITY PARTICIP.	C. LIVING SITU-ATION	D. SPECIAL GROUP
—Active	—Soc. groups	—Ret. to former	—Minority
—Realistic	—Rel. groups	?Changing	—Handicap
—Supportive	✓Support	—Shared	✓Adjust. prob.
✓Limited	—Involved friends	—Alone	
—Not avail.	✓Few friends	—Resid. care	
—No support	—No support	—Needs modifi.	

Wife in emot. crisis. Pt. good rapport c̄ brother-in-law. Denies alcohol prob.

9. ECONOMIC SITUATION:

A. FINANCES	B. CONT. INS. BENEFITS	
—Ret. to employ.	—Medicare/-aid	*Some SNF care also covered*
✓Leave avail.	—H.M.O.	
—Supported	✓Pvt. insur. *Blue cross*	
—S.S./retir.	—Dr. visit	
—Receive aid	✓Home care	
—Uncertain	—No insur.	

10. CONTINUING CARE:

A. MEDICAL FOLLOW-UP	B. NURSING CARE	C. COMM. SERV.	D. EQUIPMENT
✓Reg. MD	—None	—Social work	✓Indoor mobil.
—Spec. MD	—Family	✓Counseling	—Outdoor mobil.
—Clinic	—Skilled	—Mental Hlth.	—Ventilation
—Other: _____	—Home care	✓Supp. group	—Communication
		—Therapies	—Other: _____

Walker

Needs Identification completed by *P. Rhodes* on *3-1-90*. Updated: _____

FORM 13. *DISCHARGE TEACHING PLAN FOR:* ___Jerry M.___

OTHER THAN PATIENT, THOSE TO BE INVOLVED AS LEARNERS
INCLUDE: *(Note name and relationship to patient.)*
#1: *Becky - wife*   #2: *Bill - Becky's bro.*   #3:

1. DIAGNOSIS/MEDICAL FOLLOW-UP:

Teaching: __not needed   Motivation: __present   Prior knowledge/
    ✓planned   ✓developing   experience: *use of gowns*
    ✓in progress   __poor   *+ gloves in hospital*
    __learning
    evaluated

Learner will be able to: *basic HIV precautions by describing* By *3-4-90*
    (level) (specific subject) (behavior)   (date)
    (e.g., remember, understand, apply information, make decisions about)

2. MEDICATIONS:

Teaching: __not needed   Motivation: __present   Prior knowledge/
    ✓planned   __developing   experience: *has taken*
    __in progress   ✓poor   *other meds in past*
    __learning
    evaluated

Learner will be able to: *by identifying meds & describing action* By *3-5-90*
    (level) (specific subject) (behavior)   (date)
    (e.g., remember, understand, apply information, respond, evaluate)

3. TREATMENTS/PROCEDURES:

Teaching: __not needed   Motivation: __present   Prior knowledge/
    ✓planned   __developing   experience: _____
    __in progress   ✓poor   _____
    __learning
    evaluated

Learner will be able to: _____ By _____
    (level) (specific subject) (behavior)   (date)
    (e.g., remember, understand, apply information, perform, adapt, evaluate)

4. ACTIVITIES:

Teaching: __not needed   Motivation: __present   Prior knowledge/
    ✓planned   ✓developing   experience: *has done*
    ✓in progress   __poor   *strengthening exercises*
    __learning
    evaluated

Learner will be able to: *safe ambulation c̄ walker* By *3-3-90*
    (level) (specific subject) (behavior)   (date)
    (e.g., remember, recognize, understand, apply information, perform, adapt)

5. NUTRITION/DIET:

Teaching: __not needed   Motivation: __present   Prior knowledge/
    ✓planned   __developing   experience: _____
    __in progress   __poor   _____
    __learning
    evaluated

Learner will be able to: _____ By _____
    (level) (specific subject) (behavior)   (date)
    (e.g., remember, recognize, understand, apply information, prepare, adapt)

Form continued on following page

FORM 13 *Continued*

6. COMPLICATION MANAGEMENT:

Teaching: ___not needed   Motivation: ___present   Prior knowledge/
     ✓planned   ___developing   experience: _____
     ___in progress   ✓poor   _____
     ___learning
     evaluated

Learner will be able to: _____ By _____
                    (level)   (specific subject)   (behavior)   (date)
(e.g., remember, recognize, understand, evaluate, perform, adapt)

7. HEALTH MAINTENANCE/PROMOTION:

Teaching: ___not needed   Motivation: ___present   Prior knowledge/
     ✓planned   ___developing   experience: *denies*
     ___in progress   ✓poor   *alcohol problem*
     ___learning
     evaluated

Learner will be able to: *need to seek help of AA by verbalizing* By *3-5-90*
                    (level)   (specific subject)   (behavior)   (date)
(e.g., remember, (understand) apply information, perform, realistically plan)

8. COMMUNITY SERVICES/RESOURCES:

Teaching: ___not needed   Motivation: ✓present   Prior knowledge/
     ✓planned   ___developing   experience: *aware of*
     ___in progress   ___poor   *resources*
     ___learning
     evaluated

Learner will be able to: *home care services by making detailed plan* By *3-5-90*
                    (level)   (specific subject)   (behavior)   (date)
(e.g., remember, understand, apply information, plan (utilize))

9. OTHER LEARNING OBJECTIVES:

Learner will be able to _____ by _____

Learner will be able to _____ by _____

Teaching Plan initiated by _____ *P. Rhodes R.N.* _____ on _*3-1-90*_

NOTES ON TEACHING (what was taught, methods/materials used, response, etc.)

B

Notes on Insurance for Senior Citizens

The provisions of both public and private insurance coverage are almost constantly in a state of change. Health care benefits for seniors, a growing and especially vulnerable group, is a national issue of such magnitude that some basic information should be included even though it may soon be out of date. We offer it as a basis of comparison as legislation and company policies bring about changes. We hope that this information will help readers become more aware of the issues as they are reported in public and professional press and that it helps them ask more insightful questions about current coverage.

There are three sections to this appendix. The first is a summary of the provisions of the Medicare "Catastrophic Care" law that was passed in 1988. Secondly, we have summarized some other possible sources of health care benefits. Finally, we have included a glossary of some terms (jargon) commonly used in discussing insurance benefits.

THE MEDICARE "CATASTROPHIC COVERAGE PLAN"

The Medicare Catastrophic Coverage Act of 1988 (Public Law 100–360) went into effect on January 1, 1989. Since that time the U.S. House of Representatives voted to rescind this Act; however, since the Senate did not follow suit, it remains law at this writing. The major provisions of the 1988 law are summarized in the following table. It limits the amount Medicare beneficiaries must pay for hospital care, physician services, medical supplies, and some medications. It increases home health care, skilled nursing care, and hospice care benefits (Department of Health and Human Services, 1988). These additional services are paid for by two new premiums: one an increase in the basic monthly Part B premiums and the other an annual income tax–related premium. (See Figure 1–2 in Chapter 1 for a description of Medicare Parts A and B.) It was a public outcry related to the income tax premium that led to the vote to reverse the entire Act by the House of Representatives. Hearings on compromise legislation are scheduled in 1990. It is most likely that the compromise will remove the objec-

	1988 LAW	**COMPARISONS**
HOSPITAL CARE	Starting in 1990, the patient pays a $592 hospital deductible once per year. ALL following days are covered by Medicare. The first day charges rise annually with medical inflation.	The provision of hospital care has been simplified. Copayments that were required after 60 days have been dropped and maximum days covered increased.
SKILLED NURSING-FACILITY (S.N.F.)	Patient pays $25.50 per day for first 8 days. Medicare pays 100% from 9th to 150th day. No Medicare coverage beyond 150 days.	Requirement that patient be hospitalized for acute care at least 3 days prior to admission to skilled nursing care has been dropped.
HOME CARE	Starting January 1, 1990, up to 6 days per week of home care for skilled nursing or home health aid is covered as long as it is ordered by a physician. If care is required 7 days per week, Medicare will pay for 38 consecutive days, with extensions under special circumstances.	Home care has been expanded.
DOCTOR AND OTHER OUT-PATIENT SERVICES	Starting in 1990, the patient pays a yearly deductible amount of $75 and 20% of additional approved charges until the patient's share reaches a cap of $1370. Medicare pays 100% of approved charges thereafter for the year. Doctors or suppliers may charge more than Medicare approves. These additional fees are paid by the patient and do not contribute to the "cap" amount.	The $75 deductible amount per year has been in effect for some time, as has the Medicare payment of 80% of approved charges. There was previously no "cap" amount, however.

	1988 LAW	**COMPARISONS**
PRESCRIPTION DRUGS	Starting in 1991, the patient pays the first $600 a year and 50% of additional charges for approved drugs. In 1992, the patient pays $642 and 40% of additional charges. After that, the deductible continues rising with medical inflation, but the patient copayment remains at 20%.	Coverage for prescription drugs was limited to hospital use.
RESPITE CARE	Starting in 1990, Medicare will pay for 80 hours of "personal care" providing that the patient is chronically dependent, needing help with at least two activities of daily living and has already paid either the cap amount of $1370 for outpatient services or the $600 deductible on drugs.	No previous coverage.
HOSPICE CARE	Beginning in 1989, unlimited hospice care is available for those certified as terminally ill.	Hospice care was previously limited to 210 days.
MAMMOGRAPHY	Beginning in 1990, Medicare will pay $50 toward cost of mammography every other year.	Previously covered only if cancer was suspected.

tionable income tax premium and limit some aspects of coverage—for example, on medications. The reader is encouraged to take note of public and legislative debate on this issue because it seriously affects access to care for a large segment of the population.

Starting in 1989, beneficiaries pay $31.90 a month for Medicare Part B coverage, plus a 15% surcharge on taxable federal income up to a maximum surcharge of $800 per person. Thus if an elderly person had a taxable income of $3000, he or she would pay a total of $832.80 in 1989 ($31.90 × 12 + 15% of $3000). The monthly premium rises with medical inflation.

Patients who need nursing home care but have no private insurance coverage or have exceeded the Medicare coverage for skilled nursing, may be eligible for state-regulated Medicaid. The rules for who is eligible are, at this writing, undergoing major change. Previously, states set income allowances for the spouse of someone in a nursing home.

In states that have community property laws, half the financial resources of a couple were protected, allowing one partner to become Medicaid eligible when their own resources became low enough. One of the provisions of the Medicare Catastrophic Coverage Act may override state community property laws, however. It would allow the spouse remaining at home to keep $786 a month of family income. A maximum of $60,000 plus the home itself would be considered protected assets, regardless of the source of those assets (e.g., inheritance or gift belonging to the unhospitalized spouse). While these rules were supposed to come into effect September 30, 1989, litigation may delay their implementation.

OTHER SOURCES OF HEALTH CARE BENEFITS FOR SENIORS

There are a number of sources of health care financing other than Medicare and Medicaid. They are summarized as follows:

Medigap Policies. These are policies written to supplement Medicare coverage. With changes in Medicare, these policies are either rewritten or amended. Policyholders should check with the company or their agent about current benefits.

Civilian Health and Medical Programs of the Uniformed Services (CHAMPUS). Families of active duty, retired, or deceased members of the Uniformed Services are eligible for basic in- and out-patient services. Skilled nursing in a facility or at home, equipment, and rehabilitative services may be covered.

Veteran Coverage. A veteran of the Uniformed Services may be eligible for care for both service and non-service connected illnesses and disabilities. The Veterans Administration determines eligibility. Coverage includes basic in- and out-patient services plus home care, residential care, equipment, and day care.

Health Maintenance Organizations. Health care is prepaid to an organization set up to provide or administer benefits. Eligibility and coverage vary according to plan.

Hill-Burton Funds. Any medical facility that has received Hill-Burton assistance must provide a reasonable amount of services to persons unable to pay for them and who are not eligible for other forms of assistance. Physicians' services are not covered.

A GLOSSARY OF INSURANCE TERMS

Approved Charge. The maximum fee that a third party (Medicare or an insurance company, for example) will allow in reimbursing a provider for a given service. A Medicare "approved" charge will be equal to the customary, prevailing, or actual charge, whichever is lowest.

Assignment. (1) Agreed transfer (usually written) of the benefits of the policy by an insured person to a provider, such as the hospital or doctor. (2) In Medicare, if a physician accepts assignment, he must agree to accept the Medicare **approved charge** as payment in full, except for the deductible or uncovered services, which must be paid by the patient.

Copayment. An amount paid by the insured person as a share of hospital or medical expenses (usually 20% or 30%).

Peer Review. Refers to the evaluation by physicians or other professionals of the effectiveness and efficiency of services ordered or performed by other practicing physicians or other members of the profession whose work is being reviewed. The term frequently refers to the activities of the Peer Review Organization (PRO) under contract with a state or locality to do their reviews.

Utilization Review. Evaluation of the necessity, appropriateness, and efficiency of the use of medical services, procedures, and facilities. In a hospital, this includes review of the appropriateness of admissions, services ordered and provided, length of stay, and discharge practices, both on a concurrent and retroactive basis.

REFERENCES AND BIBLIOGRAPHY

American Hospital Association *Discharge Planning Update.* 7(7), 1987.

Arnold, Elizabeth, and K. Boggs. *Interpersonal Relationships: Professional Communication Skills for Nurses.* Philadelphia: W. B. Saunders, 1989.

Baulch, Evelyn. *Home Care: A Practical Alternative to Extended Hospitalization.* Millbrae, Calif.: Celestial Arts, 1980.

Bauwens, Eleanor. *The Anthropology of Health.* St. Louis: C. V. Mosby Co., 1978.

Beatty, Sally R. (ed.). *Continuity of Care: The Hospital and the Community.* New York: Grune & Stratton, 1980.

Becker, M. H. "The Health Belief Model and Sick Role Behavior." *Health Education Monograph* 2:409–419, 1974.

Birmingham, J. J. *Home Care Planning Based on DRGs.* Philadelphia: J. B. Lippincott, 1986.

Bloom, Benjamin. *Taxonomy of Educational Objectives: The Classification of Educational Goals.* New York: David McKay Co., 1956.

Bradway, K. "Jung's Psychological Types." *Journal of Analytical Psychology* 9:129–135, 1964.

Bramson, Robert. *Coping With Difficult People.* New York: Ballantine Books, 1981.

Branch, L. G., and A. M. Jette. "A Prospective Study of Long-term Care Institutionalization Among the Aged." *American Journal of Public Health,* 72(12):1373–1379, 1982.

Bristow, O., C. Stickney, S. Thompson. *Discharge Planning for Continuity of Care.* Pub. No. 21–1604. New York: National League for Nursing, 1976.

Buckwalter, K. C. "Exploring the Process of Discharge Planning: Application to the Construct of Health." In McClelland, E., K. Kelly, and K. Buckwalter (eds.). *Continuity of Care: Advancing the Concept of Discharge Planning.* Orlando, Fl.: Grune & Stratton, 1985.

Burkey, Sylvia L. "An Audit Outcome: Home Going Instructions." *Supervisor Nurse,* May 1979.

Caplan, G. *Principles of Preventive Psychiatry.* New York: Basic Books, 1964.

Carkhuff, Robert. *The Art of Helping IV.* Amherst, Mass.: Human Resources Development Press, 1973.

Davis, J. W., M. Shapiro, and R. Kane. "Level of Care and Complications Among Geriatric Patients Discharged from the Medical Service of a Teaching Hospital." *Journal of the American Geriatrics Society* 32:427–430, 1984.

DeBellis, Robert, Austin Kutscher, M. R. Goldberg, *et al.* (eds.). *Continuing Care: For the Dying Patient, Family and Staff.* New York: Praeger, 1985.

Dempsey, Alice M. "Discharge-Referral Planning From the Viewpoint of the Community Health Nurse." In *Patient Discharge and Referral Planning—Whose Responsibility.* Pub. No. 20–1515, New York: National League for Nursing, 1974.

Egan, Gerard. *The Skilled Helper.* Monterey, Calif.: Brooks/Cole Publishing, 1975.

Elms, R. R., and R. C. Leonard. "Effects of Nursing Approaches During Admission." *Nursing Research* 15:39–48, Winter 1966.

Feather, J., and L. Nichols. "Hospital Discharge Planning for Continuity of Care: The National Perspective." In Hartigan, E., and D. J. Brown (eds.). *Discharge Planning for Continuity of Care.* Pub. No. 20–1977. New York: National League for Nursing, 1985.

Frank, T. "Trends in Health Care and Continuity of Care" (Ch. 2). In O'Hare, P. A., and M. A. Terry (eds.). *Discharge Planning: Strategies for Assuring Continuity of Care.* Rockville, Md.: Aspen Publ., 1988.

Freeman, Ruth. *Public Health Nursing Practice* (3rd ed.). Philadelphia: W. B. Saunders, 1963.

Gatchel, Robert, and Andrew Baum. *An Introduction to Health Psychology.* New York: Random House, 1983.

Gibson, R., and D. Waldo. "National Health Expenditures, 1980." *Health Care Financing Review* September 1981: 1–54.

Glaser, B., and H. Kirschenbaum. "Using Values Clarification in a Counseling Setting." *Personnel and Guidance Journal* 59:569–575, May 1980.

Glass, R. I., M. Mulvihill, H. Smith, R. Peto, D. Bucheister, and B. Stoll. "The 4 score: An Index for Predicting a Patient's Non-medical Hospital Days." *American Journal of Public Health* 67:751–755, 1977.

Glass, R. I., and M. Weiner. "Seeking a Social Disposition for the Medical Patient: CAAST, A Simple and Objective Clinical Index." *Medical Care* 14:637–641, 1976.

Goffman, E. *Presentation of Self in Everyday Life.* Harmondsworth, England: Penguin, 1971.

Halamandaris, Bill. "Federal Quality of Care Requirements: Intent and Impact on Health Care." In McClelland, E., K. Kelly, and K. Buckwalter (eds.). *Continuity of Care: Advancing the Concept of Discharge Planning.* Orlando, Fl.: Grune & Stratton, 1985.

Hall, Dale H. "Historical Perspective: Legislative and Regulatory Aspects of Discharge Planning." In McClelland, E., K. Kelly, and K. Buckwalter (eds.). *Continuity of Care: Advancing the Concept of Discharge Planning.* Orlando, Fl.: Grune & Stratton, 1985.

Hall, Lydia E. "Another View of Nursing Care and Quality." In Straub, K. M., and K.S. Parker (eds.). *Continuity of Patient Care: The Role of Nursing.* Washington D.C.: The Catholic University of America Press, 1966.

Hanser, J., E. Pross, and F. Oechsli. *Continuity of Nursing Care from Hospital to Home.* Code No. 11–1228. New York: National League for Nursing, 1966.

Hartigan, E. G., and D.J. Brown (eds.). *Discharge Planning for Continuity of Care.* Pub. No. 20–1977. New York: National League for Nursing, 1985

Henry, W. Lester. "The Changing Role of the Health Professions." In Straub, K. M., and K. S. Parker (eds.). *Continuity of Patient Care: The Role of Nursing.* Washington D.C.: The Catholic University of America Press, 1966.

Hobson, W. *The Theory and Practice of Public Health* (4th ed.). London: Oxford University Press, 1975.

Holmes, T., and R. Rahe. "Social Readjustment Rating Scale." *Journal of Psychosomatic Research* 11:213–218, 1967.

Houston, B. K. "Control Over Stress, Locus of Control and Response to Stress." *Journal of Personality and Social Psychology* 21:249–255, 1972.

Isler, Charlotte, "A Coordinated Home-Care Program." *RN,* Oct. 1967:42–51.

Ivey, A. E. *Microcounselling.* Springfield, Illinois: Charles C. Thomas, 1971.

Janis, I. L., and J. Rodin, "Attribution, Control and Decision-Making: Social Psychology and Health Care." In G. C. Stone, F. Cohen, and N. E. Adler, (eds.). *Health Psychology: A Handbook.* San Francisco: Jossey-Bass, 1979.

Jessee, W. F., and B. Doyle. "Discharge Planning: Using Audit to Identify Areas that Need Improvement." *Quality Review Bulletin,* May 1979.

Joint Commission for the Accreditation of Hospitals. *Accreditation Manual for Hospitals.* Chicago: The Commission, 1984.

Johnson, J. E., and H. Leventhal. "Effects of Accurate Expectations and Behavioral Instructions on Reactions During a Noxious Medical Examination." *Journal of Personality and Social Psychology* 29:710–718, May 1974.

Jung, Carl. *Personality Types.* New York: Harcourt Brace Jovanovich, 1923.

Katz, S., A. Ford, R. Moskowitz, B. Jackson, and M. Jaffe. "Studies of Illness in the Aged. The Index of ADL: A Standardized Measure of Biological and Psychosocial Function." *Journal of the American Medical Association* 185:914–919, 1963.

Kearney, P. and P. Gleason-Claydon. "Discharge Planning: A Clinical Dietician's Perspective" (Ch. 11). In McKeehan, Kathleen (ed.). *Continuing Care: A Multidisciplinary Approach to Discharge Planning.* St. Louis: C. V. Mosby, 1981.

Keirsey, D., and M. Bates. *Please Understand Me.* Del Mar, Calif.: Prometheus Nemesis Books, 1978.

Knowles, Malcolm. *The Modern Practice of Adult Education: From Pedagogy to Andragogy.* Chicago: Follett Pub. Co., 1984.

Kübler-Ross, E. *On Death and Dying.* London: Tavistock, 1970.

Kübler-Ross, E. *Death—The Final Stage of Growth.* Englewood Cliffs, N. J.: Prentice-Hall, 1975.

Lamont, C. T., S. Sampson, R. Matthias, and R. Kane. "The Outcome of Hospitalization for Acute Illness in the Elderly." *Journal of the American Geriatrics Society* 31:308–315, 1983.

Lau, R. "Origins of Health Locus of Control Beliefs." *Journal of Personality and Social Psychology* 42:322–334, 1982.

Leahy, K.M., M. Cobb, and M. Jones. *Community Health Nursing* (3rd *ed.*). New York: McGraw-Hill Book Co., 1977.

Lefcourt, H. *Locus of Control: Current Trends in Theory and Research.* Hillsdale, N. J.: Lawrence Erlbaum Assoc., 1982.

Lewin, Kurt. "Frontiers in Group Dynamics." *Human Relations* 1:5–41, 1947.

Mace, N. L., and P. Rabens. *The 36-hour Day: A Family Guide to Caring for Persons with Alzheimer's Disease, Related Dementing Illnesses and Memory Loss in Later Life.* Baltimore, Md.: Johns Hopkins University Press, 1981.

Mader, Joan P. "The Importance of Hope." *RN,* Dec. 1988:17–18.

Martinson, I. M., and A. Widmer (eds.). *Home Health Care Nursing.* Philadelphia: W. B. Saunders, 1989.

Maslow, A. H. "A Theory of Human Motivation." *Psychological Review* pp. 370–396, July 1943.

Maslow, A. H. *Toward a Psychology of Being.* Princeton, N. J.: D. Van Nostrand, 1962.

Maslow, A. H. *Motivation and Personality* (2nd ed.). New York: Harper & Row, 1970.

Master, R. J. "Discharge Planning: A Physician's Perspective" (Ch. 10). In McKeehan, Kathleen (ed.). *Continuing Care: A Multidisciplinary Approach to Discharge Planning.* St. Louis: C. V. Mosby, 1981.

McClelland, E. "National and International Comparisons of Continuity of Care." In McClelland, E., K. Kelly, and K. Buckwalter (eds.). *Continuity of Care: Advancing the Concept of Discharge Planning.* Orlando, Fl.: Grune & Stratton, 1985.

McClelland, E., K. Kelly, and K. Buckwalter (eds.) *Continuity of Care: Advancing the Concept of Discharge Planning.* Orlando, Fl.: Grune & Stratton, 1985.

McKeehan, Kathleen M. (ed.). *Continuing Care: A Multidisciplinary Approach to Discharge Planning.* St. Louis: C.V. Mosby, 1981.

Moore, L. G., P. Van Arsdale, J. Glittenberg, and R. Aldrich. *The Biocultural Basis of Health.* St. Louis: C. V. Mosby, 1980.

Muenchow, J. D., and B. Carlson. "Evaluating Programs of Discharge Planning." In McClelland, E., K. Kelly, and K. Buckwalter (eds.). *Continuity of Care: Advancing the Concept of Discharge Planning.* Orlando, Fl.: Grune & Stratton, Inc., 1985.

Muldary, T. W. *Interpersonal Relations for Health Professionals: A Social Skills Approach.* New York: Macmillan, 1983.

National League for Nursing. *Patient Discharge and Referral Planning: Whose Responsibility.* Pub. No. 201515 (Conference Report) New York: National League for Nursing, 1974.

O'Hare, P. A., and M. A. Terry (eds.). *Discharge Planning: Strategies for Assuring Continuity of Care.* Rockville, Md.: Aspen Publ., 1988.

Pender, Nola J. *Health Promotion in Nursing Practice.* Norwalk, Conn.: Appleton-Century-Crofts, 1982.

Phares, E. J. *Locus of Control in Personality.* Morristown, N. J.: General Learning Press, 1976.

Public Law 92–603, 92nd Congress, HR, 1, October 30, 1972, Washington D.C.

Rakich, J. S., B. Longest, and K. Darr. *Managing Health Services Organizations.* Philadelphia: W. B. Saunders, 1985.

Ridgeway, V., and A. Mathews. "Psychological Preparation for Surgery: A Comparison of Methods." *British Journal of Clinical Psychology* 21:271–280, 1982.

Roberts, Mary M. *American Nursing: History and Interpretation.* New York: The Macmillan Co., 1954.

Rogers, Carl. *On Becoming A Person.* Boston: Houghton Mifflin, 1961.

Rorden, J. W. *Nurses As Health Teachers: A Practical Guide.* Philadelphia: W. B. Saunders, 1987.

Rosenstock, I. M. "The Health Belief Model." *Milbank Memorial Fund Quarterly* 44:94, 1966.

Rosenstock, I. M. "The Health Belief Model and Preventative Health Behavior." *Health Education Monograph* 2:354–386, 1974.

Rosenstock, I. M., and J. Kirscht. "Why People Seek Health Care." In G. Stone, F. Cohen, and N. Adler (eds.). *Health Psychology: A Handbook.* San Francisco: Jossey-Bass, 1980.

Rotter, J. "Generalized Expectancies for Internal Versus External Control of Reinforcement." *Psychological Monographs: General and Applied.* 80, 1966.

Sandman, G. H. "Discharge Planning: A Social Worker's Perspective" (Ch. 9). In McKeehan, Kathleen (ed.). *Continuing Care: A Multidisciplinary Approach to Discharge Planning.* St Louis: C. V. Mosby, 1981.

Satir, Virginia. *Peoplemaking.* Palo Alto, Calif.: Science and Behavior Books, 1972.

Schultz, Duane. *Growth Psychology: Models of a Healthy Personality.* New York: D. Van Nostrand, 1977.

Schwartz, Doris. "Continuity of Patient Care Through an Interagency Referral System." *Hospitals and Public Health Nursing Services Plan Better Patient Care.* (Conference Report). New York: National League for Nursing, 1957.

Seligman, M. *Helplessness.* San Francisco: Freeman Press, 1975.

Selye, Hans. *Stress Without Distress.* New York: Lippincott & Crowell, 1974.

Shapiro, Evelyn, and Robert Tate. "Who is Really at Risk of Institutionalization?" *The Gerontologist,* 28(2):237–245, 1988.

Silver, George A. "Toward Better Patient Care." *Hospitals and Public Health Nursing Services Plan Better Patient Care.* (Conference Report). New York: National League for Nursing, 1957.

Sime, A. M. "Relationship of Preoperative Fear, Type of Coping, and Information Received About Surgery to Recovery from Surgery." *Journal of Personality and Social Psychology* 34:716–724, 1976.

Smith, Barbara. "When is 'Confusion' Translocation Syndrome?" *American Journal of Nursing,* 86(11):1280–81, 1986.

Smith, Judy Batson. "Home Care is More Than Medicare Regs." *American Journal of Nursing,* 87(3):305–6, 1987.

Smith, Louise C. *Factors Influencing Continuity of Nursing Service.* New York: National League for Nursing, 1962.

Social Security Act. Public Law No. 271, 74th Congress, H. R. 7260.

Sorensen, K. C., and J. Luckmann. *Basic Nursing: A Psychophysiologic Approach.* Philadelphia: W. B. Saunders, 1986.

Stoddard, Sandal. *The Hospice Movement: A Better Way of Caring for the Dying.* New York: Vintage Books, 1978.

Stone, G., F. Cohen, and N. Adler (eds.). *Health Psychology: A Handbook.* San Francisco: Jossey-Bass, 1980.

Straub, K. M., and K. S. Parker (eds.). *Continuity of Patient Care: The Role of Nursing.* Washington D.C.: The Catholic University of America Press, 1966.

Suther, Mary C. S., and Thomas Ricciardelli. "Impact of Discharge Planning and Home Care on Health Care Delivery in the United States." In McClelland, E., K. Kelly, and K. Buckwalter (eds.). *Continuity of Care: Advancing the Concept of Discharge Planning.* Orlando, Fl.: Grune & Stratton, Inc., 1985.

Task Force on Legal Issues in Discharge Planning. *Discharging Hospital Patients: Legal Implications for Institutional Providers and Health Care Professionals.* Legal Memorandum Number 9. Chicago: American Hospital Association, 1987.

Taylor, S. E. "Hospital Patient Behavior: Reactance, Helplessness, or Control." *Journal of Social Issues* 35:156–184, 1979.

Terry, Margaret A. "Essential Considerations in Setting Up a Discharge Planning Program." In O'Hare, P. A., and M. A. Terry (eds.). *Discharge Planning: Strategies for Assuring Continuity of Care.* Rockville, Md.: Aspen, 1988.

Terris, Milton. "The Future of Community Health Services." In *Community Nursing Services.* Code No. 21–1028. New York: National League for Nursing, 1962.

Wallston, B. S., K. A. Wallston, G. D. Kaplan, and S. A. Maides. "Development and Validation of the Health Locus of Control (HCL) Scale." *Journal of Consulting and Clinical Psychology* 44:580–585, 1976.

Wachtel, T. J., J. Fulton, and J. Goldfarb. "Early Prediction of Discharge Disposition After Hospitalization." *The Gerontologist* 27: (1):98–103, 1987.

Waring, J., and J. McLennan. *Community Health Nursing: Helping With Health*. Sydney: McGraw-Hill Book Co. (Int.), 1979.

Wensley, Edith. *Nursing Service Without Walls*. Code No. 11–1058. New York: National League for Nursing, 1963.

Wilson, C. R. M. *Hospital-wide Quality Assurance*. Toronto, Ont.: W. B. Saunders Co. Canada Ltd., 1987.

Young, Ernle. *Alpha and Omega: Ethics at the Frontiers of Life and Death*. Menlo Park, Calif.: Addison-Wesley, 1988.

Yura, H., and M. Walsh. *The Nursing Process* (4th ed.). Norwalk, Conn.: Appleton-Century-Crofts, 1983.

Index

Page numbers in *italics* indicate figures. Page numbers followed by (t) indicate tables, and those followed by (e) indicate case examples.

Body image, 85–86. See also *Self-perception.*

Transitions *(Continued)*
    stress during, 71, 211. See also *Stress.*
Trust. See *Communication; Relationships, trust.*
"Turf" battles, 29, 33, 126–127. See also *Relationships, professional.*

Utilization review, 19, 116–117, 214–215, 227

Videotape, use of, 36(e)
Visiting nursing association(s), 8, 103. See also *Community care; Resources, community.*

Warmth, quality of, 47. See also *Communication; Relationships.*
Who, when, where, what, how (4W-H), 209–210. See also *Discharge planning.*
Wickline vs. California, 226–227(e). See also *Issues.*

M.